Clinical Diagnosis and Management of Pregnancy Complications

Clinical Diagnosis and Management of Pregnancy Complications

Editor

Rinat Gabbay-Benziv

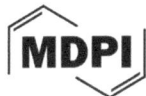

Basel • Beijing • Wuhan • Barcelona • Belgrade • Novi Sad • Cluj • Manchester

Editor
Rinat Gabbay-Benziv
Hillel Yaffe Medical Center
Hadera
Israel

Editorial Office
MDPI AG
Grosspeteranlage 5
4052 Basel, Switzerland

This is a reprint of articles from the Special Issue published online in the open access journal *Journal of Clinical Medicine* (ISSN 2077-0383) (available at: https://www.mdpi.com/si/jcm/Pregnancy_Complications_Diagnosis).

For citation purposes, cite each article independently as indicated on the article page online and as indicated below:

Lastname, A.A.; Lastname, B.B. Article Title. *Journal Name* **Year**, *Volume Number*, Page Range.

ISBN 978-3-7258-2457-1 (Hbk)
ISBN 978-3-7258-2458-8 (PDF)
doi.org/10.3390/books978-3-7258-2458-8

© 2024 by the authors. Articles in this book are Open Access and distributed under the Creative Commons Attribution (CC BY) license. The book as a whole is distributed by MDPI under the terms and conditions of the Creative Commons Attribution-NonCommercial-NoDerivs (CC BY-NC-ND) license.

Contents

Rinat Gabbay-Benziv
Special Issue: "Clinical Diagnosis and Management of Pregnancy Complications"
Reprinted from: *J. Clin. Med.* **2022**, *11*, 5644, doi:10.3390/jcm11195644 1

Yuval Atzmon, Efrat Ben Ishay, Mordechai Hallak, Romi Littman, Arik Eisenkraft and Rinat Gabbay-Benziv
Continuous Maternal Hemodynamics Monitoring at Delivery Using a Novel, Noninvasive, Wireless, PPG-Based Sensor
Reprinted from: *J. Clin. Med.* **2021**, *10*, 8, doi:10.3390/jcm10010008 5

Amir Naeh, Mordechai Hallak and Rinat Gabbay-Benziv
Parity and Interval from Previous Delivery—Influence on Perinatal Outcome in Advanced Maternal Age Parturients
Reprinted from: *J. Clin. Med.* **2021**, *10*, 460, doi:10.3390/jcm10030460 16

Fahimeh Ramezani Tehrani, Marzieh Saei Ghare Naz, Razieh Bidhendi Yarandi and Samira Behboudi-Gandevani
The Impact of Diagnostic Criteria for Gestational Diabetes Mellitus on Adverse Maternal Outcomes: A Systematic Review and Meta-Analysis
Reprinted from: *J. Clin. Med.* **2021**, *10*, 666, doi:10.3390/jcm10040666 24

Joon-Hyung Lee, Chan-Wook Park, Kyung-Chul Moon, Joong-Shin Park and Jong-Kwan Jun
Neutrophil to Lymphocyte Ratio in Maternal Blood: A Clue to Suspect Amnionitis
Reprinted from: *J. Clin. Med.* **2021**, *10*, 2673, doi:10.3390/jcm10122673 46

Yvan Gomez, Vincent Balaya, Karine Lepigeon, Patrice Mathevet and Martine Jacot-Guillarmod
Predictive Factors Involved in Postpartum Regressions of Cytological/Histological Cervical High-Grade Dysplasia Diagnosed during Pregnancy
Reprinted from: *J. Clin. Med.* **2021**, *10*, 5319, doi:10.3390/jcm10225319 59

Dana Anais Muin, Janina Sophie Erlacher, Stephanie Leutgeb and Anna Felnhofer
Facilitators and Strategies for Breaking the News of an Intrauterine Death—A Mixed Methods Study among Obstetricians
Reprinted from: *J. Clin. Med.* **2021**, *10*, 5347, doi:10.3390/jcm10225347 70

Patrocinio Rodríguez-Benitez, Irene Aracil Moreno, Cristina Oliver Barrecheguren, Yolanda Cuñarro López, Fátima Yllana, Pilar Pintado Recarte, et al.
Maternal-Perinatal Variables in Patients with Severe Preeclampsia Who Develop Acute Kidney Injury
Reprinted from: *J. Clin. Med.* **2021**, *10*, 5629, doi:10.3390/jcm10235629 83

Dana Anaïs Muin, Hanns Helmer, Hermann Leitner and Sabrina Neururer
Epidemiology of Antepartum Stillbirths in Austria—A Population-Based Study between 2008 and 2020
Reprinted from: *J. Clin. Med.* **2021**, *10*, 5828, doi:10.3390/jcm10245828 99

Josip Delmis and Marina Ivanisevic
Awakened Beta-Cell Function Decreases the Risk of Hypoglycemia in Pregnant Women with Type 1 Diabetes Mellitus
Reprinted from: *J. Clin. Med.* **2022**, *11*, 1050, doi:10.3390/jcm11041050 111

Héctor González-de la Torre, Adela Domínguez-Gil, Cintia Padrón-Brito, Carla Rosillo-Otero, Miriam Berenguer-Pérez and José Verdú-Soriano
Validation and Psychometric Properties of the Spanish Version of the Fear of Childbirth Questionnaire (CFQ-e)
Reprinted from: *J. Clin. Med.* **2022**, *11*, 1843, doi:10.3390/jcm11071843 119

Julja Burchard, George R. Saade, Kim A. Boggess, Glenn R. Markenson, Jay D. Iams, Dean V. Coonrod, et al.
Better Estimation of Spontaneous Preterm Birth Prediction Performance through Improved Gestational Age Dating
Reprinted from: *J. Clin. Med.* **2022**, *11*, 2885, doi:10.3390/jcm11102885 137

Agata Majewska, Paweł Jan Stanirowski, Mirosław Wielgoś and Dorota Bomba-Opoń
Efficacy of Continuous Glucose Monitoring on Glycaemic Control in Pregnant Women with Gestational Diabetes Mellitus—A Systematic Review
Reprinted from: *J. Clin. Med.* **2022**, *11*, 2932, doi:10.3390/jcm11102932 148

Hikari Yoshizawa, Haruki Nishizawa, Hidehito Inagaki, Keisuke Hitachi, Akiko Ohwaki, Yoshiko Sakabe, et al.
Characterization of the *MG828507* lncRNA Located Upstream of the *FLT1* Gene as an Etiology for Pre-Eclampsia
Reprinted from: *J. Clin. Med.* **2022**, *11*, 4603, doi:10.3390/jcm11154603 157

Ele Hanson, Inge Ringmets, Anne Kirss, Maris Laan and Kristiina Rull
Screening of Gestational Diabetes and Its Risk Factors: Pregnancy Outcome of Women with Gestational Diabetes Risk Factors According to Glycose Tolerance Test Results
Reprinted from: *J. Clin. Med.* **2022**, *11*, 4953, doi:10.3390/jcm11174953 168

Keita Hasegawa, Satoru Ikenoue, Yuya Tanaka, Maki Oishi, Toyohide Endo, Yu Sato, et al.
Ultrasonographic Prediction of Placental Invasion in Placenta Previa by Placenta Accreta Index
Reprinted from: *J. Clin. Med.* **2023**, *12*, 1090, doi:10.3390/jcm12031090 180

Dionysios Vrachnis, Nikolaos Antonakopoulos, Alexandros Fotiou, Vasilios Pergialiotis, Nikolaos Loukas, Georgios Valsamakis, et al.
Is There a Correlation between Apelin and Insulin Concentrations in Early Second Trimester Amniotic Fluid with Fetal Growth Disorders?
Reprinted from: *J. Clin. Med.* **2023**, *12*, 3166, doi:10.3390/jcm12093166 187

Moran Gawie-Rotman, Shoval Menashe, Noa Haggiag, Alon Shrim, Mordechai Hallak and Rinat Gabbay-Benziv
The Accuracy of Sonographically Estimated Fetal Weight and Prediction of Small for Gestational Age in Twin Pregnancy—Comparison of the First and Second Twins
Reprinted from: *J. Clin. Med.* **2023**, *12*, 3307, doi:10.3390/jcm12093307 197

Stefano Faiola, Maria Mandalari, Chiara Coco, Daniela Casati, Arianna Laoreti, Savina Mannarino, et al.
Long-Term Postnatal Follow-Up in Monochorionic TTTS Twin Pregnancies Treated with Fetoscopic Laser Surgery and Complicated by Right Ventricular Outflow Tract Anomalies
Reprinted from: *J. Clin. Med.* **2023**, *12*, 4734, doi:10.3390/jcm12144734 205

Esther Maor-Sagie, Mordechai Hallak, Yoel Toledano and Rinat Gabbay-Benziv
Oral Glucose Tolerance Test Performed after 28 Gestational Weeks and Risk for Future Diabetes—A 5-Year Cohort Study
Reprinted from: *J. Clin. Med.* **2023**, *12*, 6072, doi:10.3390/jcm12186072 216

Tiyasha Hosne Ayub, Brigitte Strizek, Bernd Poetzsch, Philipp Kosian, Ulrich Gembruch and Waltraut M. Merz
Placenta Accreta Spectrum Prophylactic Therapy for Hyperfibrinolysis with Tranexamic Acid
Reprinted from: *J. Clin. Med.* **2024**, *13*, 135, doi:10.3390/jcm13010135 227

Ohad Houri, Meytal Schwartz Yoskovitz, Asnat Walfisch, Anat Pardo, Yossi Geron, Eran Hadar and Ron Bardin
Neonatal Outcomes of Infants Diagnosed with Fetal Growth Restriction during Late Pregnancy versus after Birth
Reprinted from: *J. Clin. Med.* **2024**, *13*, 3753, doi:10.3390/jcm13133753 239

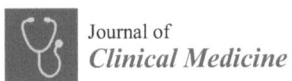

Editorial

Special Issue: "Clinical Diagnosis and Management of Pregnancy Complications"

Rinat Gabbay-Benziv [1,2]

1. Obstetrics and Gynecology Department, Hillel Yaffe Medical Center, Hashalom Street, PB 169, Hadera 38100, Israel; gabbayrinat@gmail.com; Tel.: +972-4-7748224
2. The Ruth and Bruce Rappaport Faculty of Medicine, Technion-Israel Institute of Technology, Haifa 32000, Israel

Citation: Gabbay-Benziv, R. Special Issue: "Clinical Diagnosis and Management of Pregnancy Complications". *J. Clin. Med.* 2022, 11, 5644. https://doi.org/10.3390/jcm11195644

Received: 15 September 2022
Accepted: 23 September 2022
Published: 25 September 2022

Publisher's Note: MDPI stays neutral with regard to jurisdictional claims in published maps and institutional affiliations.

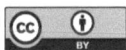

Copyright: © 2022 by the author. Licensee MDPI, Basel, Switzerland. This article is an open access article distributed under the terms and conditions of the Creative Commons Attribution (CC BY) license (https://creativecommons.org/licenses/by/4.0/).

Most pregnancies are uneventful and end with a healthy mother and a liveborn baby. Nevertheless, pregnancy poses a risk to the mother, the fetus, and the child. There is no single definition for high-risk pregnancy; however, broadly, any pregnancy in which a pre-pregnancy or new-onset condition poses an actual or potential risk to the wellbeing of the mother or fetus is considered a high-risk pregnancy [1].

In this Special Issue of "Clinical Diagnosis and Management of Pregnancy Complications", we will address some of the more common complications encountered during pregnancy.

Gestational diabetes mellitus (GDM) is one of the most common medical complication of pregnancy [2,3]. GDM prevalence is increasing and is currently estimated to be between 5 and 25% [3,4] in different populations with different criteria. GDM has serious implications for the mother, the fetus, and the child in the short- and long-term [5]; therefore, it is important to diagnose and treat it. In the short-term, GDM is associated with hypertensive disease during pregnancy, cesarean section, and traumatic deliveries. For the neonate, the main consequences are excessive growth and neonatal hypoglycemia. In the long-term, GDM is associated with increased incidence of type 2 diabetes, as well as metabolic syndrome, for both the mother and the child. Nevertheless, and despite numerous studies in the area, the appropriate diagnosis and management of GDM during pregnancy are still debated. Currently, a diagnosis can be made based on a 75 or 100 g glucose tolerance test, performed either as a diagnostic test for all parturients, according to risk factors (obesity, a family history of diabetes, previous GDM or macrosomia, etc.), or following a positive 50 g glucose challenge test. The accepted thresholds for 100 g OGTT were derived from mathematical extrapolation of values that correlated with the future development of type 2 diabetes in mothers [6]. The values for the 75 g test were determined via selected pregnancy outcomes [7]. Recent studies have shown that using the 75 g glucose tolerance test doubled the prevalence of GDM; however, without any proven clinical perinatal benefit [7,8], controversy remains, and both options are accepted as valid for GDM diagnosis. In this Special Issue, Hanson et al. [9] describe the pregnancy outcomes of a large cohort of un-selected parturients in Estonia over a 7-year period, according to GDM risk factors and diagnoses based on 75 g glucose tolerance test results. In their study, the authors found that the proportion of women with GDM risk factors increased from 43.5% in 2012 to 57.8% in 2018, and the diagnosis of GDM more than doubled (5.2% vs. 13.7%). More importantly, pregnancies in which the mother was predisposed to GDM but had normal 75 g glucose tolerance test results were accompanied by increased odds of delivering a large baby (AOR 2.3 (CI: 1.8–3.0)). As large babies are the hallmark of abnormal glucose exposure during pregnancy, and although 75 g glucose tolerance tests were used in this cohort for GDM diagnosis, this raises concern about the underdiagnosis of GDM using the accepted algorithms. In line with this paradigm, another study in this issue, published by Ramezani Tehrani et al. [10], examined the impact of different GDM diagnostic criteria on the risk of adverse maternal outcomes. In this meta-analysis—which included 49 population-based studies with a total of 1,409,018 pregnant women with GDM and 7,667,546 non-GDM counterparts—the authors found that GDM was associated with an increased risk of adverse maternal outcomes; these included primary cesarean, the induction of labor, maternal hemorrhage, and pregnancy-related-hypertension. Interestingly, this risk was increased regardless of the diagnostic criteria used to diagnose GDM. This finding further stresses the importance of conducting more studies to establish the correct algorithm and diagnostic criteria for GDM diagnosis that will have clinical benefit.

The debate does not end with GDM diagnosis, and controversies continue regarding management and treatment during pregnancy. Currently, establishing good glucose control during pregnancy relies mainly on maternal self-monitoring of blood glucose and fetal weight estimation. In recent years, continuous glucose monitoring (CGM) techniques have become widely available. CGM continuously measures maternal sugar levels, thus offering an alternative to the accepted periodic self-monitoring of blood glucose. Previous data have proven that CGM is safe during pregnancy, and it is now the method of choice for many parturients with pregestational diabetes, mainly with type 1 diabetes, to monitor their blood glucose values. To evaluate CGM's role and benefits in GDM, Majewska et al. [11] conducted a systematic review that aimed to assess the efficacy of CGM on glycemic control in GDM parturients. In addition, they evaluated the need for pharmacological treatment and perinatal outcomes in GDM parturients with CGM. Fourteen studies were included in their systematic review. The authors concluded that using CGM, when compared to the self-monitoring of blood glucose, improves glycemic control in parturients with GDM. Furthermore, CGM improved qualifications for insulin therapy. CGM demonstrated higher detection of hyperglycemia and hypoglycemia events, especially in insulin-treated parturients. A1c levels were better and gestational weight gain decreased in women using CGM. Nevertheless, neonatal outcomes remained similar without any robust improvement in the rates of macrosomia or neonatal hypoglycemia. Although using CGM to control sugar levels in GDM parturients seems intuitively logical and beneficial, there are still some concerns that should be considered. First, the majority of women with GDM will have good control under a proper diet and physical activity and will have favorable perinatal outcomes, with only mild interruptions to their daily routines. Twenty-four-hour knowledge of their sugar levels might shift their entire focus to their sugar levels, creating stress and anxiety in looking for "perfect" sugar status. This may become problematic, especially as the benefit of CGM has not yet been proven for short- and long-term maternal and child health. Second, as CGM is still considered new technology, there may be selection bias; parturients who are willing to join studies may be more aware and desire better control, thus skewing the results toward optimization of control with CGM. Lastly, the costs of using CGM should be carefully weighed against the yet-to-be-proven theoretical benefits.

Two other common complications of pregnancy are preterm delivery (PTD) and hypertensive disease of pregnancy (HDP). PTD refers to any delivery before 37 gestational weeks. PTD complicates about 5–13% of deliveries worldwide [12] and is the leading cause of neonatal mortality; moreover, it is the most common reason for antenatal hospitalization [13–17]. PTD may be spontaneous, or it may be indicated by a specific maternal or fetal complication. In this issue, a study by Burchard et al. [18] takes us back to the core of establishing PTD using the correct dating methodology. The authors compared the effect of using the last menstrual period (LMP) combined with first-trimester ultrasound-based dating vs. first-trimester ultrasound-based dating alone. The authors demonstrated an improvement in observed biomarker risk predictor performance in parturients who had more certain gestational age dating. In their simulation, a perfect PTD predictor showed a decrease in the AUC of 21% when gestational age was determined using LMP dating and confirmed via ultrasound, and a decrease of about half of that figure when gestational age was determined using ultrasound dating. While ultrasound dating is commonly accepted as a more certain dating method than LMP, its results demonstrate the novel suggestion that confirming LMP using ultrasound does not improve its certainty to the level achieved by using the actual ultrasound dates. This new concept may have wide application in obstetric practices based on accurate gestational age. Important decisions regarding fetal viability, antenatal steroids, the use of neuroprotective magnesium, and even everyday elective labor induction are determined and based on accurate gestation age. Regarding HDP, we present two important studies: The first, published by Yoshizawa et al. [19] explores the etiology and mechanistic base of preeclampsia using gene-expression profile analysis. The second evaluates the variables that are associated with kidney injury in pregnancies that are complicated by preeclampsia with severe features [20].

From a wider perspective on pregnancy complications, age, parity, and interpregnancy interval are crucial variables when predicting adverse outcomes of pregnancy. Over the years, maternal age has increased, particularly in high-income countries [21], and elderly gravida parturients are now relatively common. Numerous data support an increased rate of pregnancy complications with a short interval between pregnancies; however, there are fewer data on long pregnancy intervals, especially when combined with increased maternal age. The dual effect of parity and interpregnancy interval on the risk of pregnancy complications was elucidated in the study by Naeh et al. [22]. The authors performed a population-based retrospective cohort study utilizing all the birth certificate data in the United States in 2017. Parturients who were older than 40 years, and who had a singleton live birth after 24 weeks, were categorized into three groups based on parity and the interval from the last delivery: primiparas, multiparas with a pregnancy interval shorter than 5 years, and multiparas with a pregnancy interval of more than 5 years. The authors found that among multiparas with a pregnancy interval of more than 5 years, adverse outcomes (including PTD of <34 weeks, a birthweight of <2000 g, neonatal seizure, neonatal intensive care unit admission, an Apgar score of <7 at 5 min, or assisted ventilation >6 h) were higher and more like the nulliparity group. Moreover, among parturients older than 40 years, multiparity with a previous pregnancy within 5 years had a significant protective effect against adverse outcomes when compared to nulliparas. This finding has implications when consulting elderly multiparas who have had previous successful pregnancies

As the Guest Editor for this Special Issue, I would like to thank all of the contributing authors for sharing their valuable studies with us. Additionally, I appreciate and thank all the reviewers for their insightful remarks and the JCM team's support.

Funding: This research received no external funding.

Conflicts of Interest: The authors declare no conflict of interest.

References

1. Eunice Kennedy Shriver National Institute of Child Health and Human Development. What Are the Factors That Put a Pregnancy at Risk? Available online: https://www-nichd-nih-gov.yaffe.idm.oclc.org/health/topics/high-risk/conditioninfo/pages/factors.aspx (accessed on 29 April 2017).
2. Centers for Disease Control and Prevention. Diabetes during Pregnancy. Available online: https://www.cdc.gov/reproductivehealth/maternalinfanthealth/diabetes-during-pregnancy.htm (accessed on 17 September 2022).
3. Sacks, D.A.; Hadden, D.R.; Maresh, M.; Deerochanawong, C.; Dyer, A.R.; Metzger, B.E.; Lowe, L.P.; Coustan, D.R.; Hod, M.; Oats, J.J.; et al. Frequency of gestational diabetes mellitus at collaborating centers based on IADPSG consensus panel-recommended criteria: The Hyperglycemia and Adverse Pregnancy Outcome (HAPO) Study. *Diabetes Care* **2012**, *35*, 526–528. [CrossRef]
4. DeSisto, C.L.; Kim, S.Y.; Sharma, A.J. Prevalence estimates of gestational diabetes mellitus in the United States, Pregnancy Risk Assessment Monitoring System (PRAMS), 2007–2010. *Prev. Chronic. Dis.* **2014**, *11*, E104. [CrossRef]
5. American College of Obstetricians and Gynecologists. ACOG Practice Bulletin No. 190 Summary: Gestational Diabetes Mellitus. *Obstet. Gynecol.* **2018**, *131*, 406–408. [CrossRef]
6. Carpener, M.W.; coustan, D.R. Criteria for screening tests for gestational diabetes. *Am. J. Obstet. Gynecol.* **1982**, *144*, 768–773. [CrossRef]
7. HAPO Study Cooperative Research Group; Metzger, B.E.; Lowe, L.P.; Dyer, A.R.; Trimble, E.R.; Chaovarindr, U.; Coustan, D.R.; Hadden, D.R.; McCance, D.R.; Hod, M.; et al. Hyperglycemia and adverse pregnancy outcomes. *N. Engl. J. Med.* **2008**, *358*, 1991–2002.
8. Hillier, T.A.; Pedula, K.L.; Ogasawara, K.K.; Vesco, K.K.; Oshiro, C.E.S.; Lubarsky, S.L.; Van Marter, J. A Pragmatic, Randomized Clinical Trial of Gestational Diabetes Screening. *N. Engl. J. Med.* **2021**, *384*, 895–904. [CrossRef]

9. Hanson, E.; Ringmets, I.; Kirss, A.; Laan, M.; Rull, K. Screening of Gestational Diabetes and Its Risk Factors: Pregnancy Outcome of Women with Gestational Diabetes Risk Factors According to Glycose Tolerance Test Results. *J. Clin. Med.* **2022**, *11*, 4953. [CrossRef] [PubMed]
10. Ramezani Tehrani, F.; Naz, M.S.G.; Yarandi, R.B.; Behboudi-Gandevani, S. The Impact of Diagnostic Criteria for Gestational Diabetes Mellitus on Adverse Maternal Outcomes: A Systematic Review and Meta-Analysis. *J. Clin. Med.* **2021**, *10*, 666. [CrossRef] [PubMed]
11. Majewska, A.; Stanirowski, P.J.; Wielgoś, M.; Bomba-Opoń, D. Efficacy of Continuous Glucose Monitoring on Glycaemic Control in Pregnant Women with Gestational Diabetes Mellitus-A Systematic Review. *J. Clin. Med.* **2022**, *11*, 2932. [CrossRef]
12. WHO. Available online: http://www.who.int/topics/preterm_birth/en/ (accessed on 14 June 2022).
13. Tucker, J.M.; Goldenberg, R.L.; Davis, R.O.; Copper, R.L.; Winkler, C.L.; Hauth, J.C. Etiologies of preterm birth in an indigent population: Is prevention a logical expectation? *Obstet. Gynecol.* **1991**, *77*, 343–347.
14. Savitz, D.A.; Blackmore, C.A.; Thorp, J.M. Epidemiologic characteristics of preterm delivery: Etiologic heterogeneity. *Am. J. Obstet. Gynecol.* **1991**, *164*, 467–471. [CrossRef]
15. Kramer, M.S. Preventing preterm birth: Are we making any progress? *Yale J. Biol. Med.* **1997**, *70*, 227–232.
16. Coathup, V.; Boyle, E.; Carson, C.; Johnson, S.; Kurinzcuk, J.J.; Macfarlane, A.; Petrou, S.; Rivero-Arias, O.; Quigley, M.A. Gestational age and hospital admissions during childhood: Population based, record linkage study in England (TIGAR study). *BMJ* **2020**, *371*, m4075. [CrossRef] [PubMed]
17. American College of Obstetricians and Gynecologists' Committee on Practice Bulletins—Obstetrics. Prediction and Prevention of Spontaneous Preterm Birth: ACOG Practice Bulletin, Number 234. *Obstet. Gynecol.* **2021**, *138*, e65–e90. [CrossRef]
18. Burchard, J.; Saade, G.R.; Boggess, K.A.; Markenson, G.R.; Iams, J.D.; Coonrod, D.V.; Pereira, L.M.; Hoffman, M.K.; Polpitiya, A.D.; Treacy, R.; et al. Better Estimation of Spontaneous Preterm Birth Prediction Performance through Improved Gestational Age Dating. *J. Clin. Med.* **2022**, *11*, 2885. [CrossRef] [PubMed]
19. Yoshizawa, H.; Nishizawa, H.; Inagaki, H.; Hitachi, K.; Ohwaki, A.; Sakabe, Y.; Ito, M.; Tsuchida, K.; Sekiya, T.; Fujii, T.; et al. Characterization of the MG828507 lncRNA Located Upstream of the FLT1 Gene as an Etiology for Pre-Eclampsia. *J. Clin. Med.* **2022**, *11*, 4603. [CrossRef] [PubMed]
20. Rodríguez-Benitez, P.; Aracil Moreno, I.; Oliver Barrecheguren, C.; Cuñarro López, Y.; Yllana, F.; Pintado Recarte, P.; Arribas, C.B.; Álvarez-Mon, M.; Ortega, M.A.; De Leon-Luis, J.A. Maternal-Perinatal Variables in Patients with Severe Preeclampsia Who Develop Acute Kidney Injury. *J. Clin. Med.* **2021**, *10*, 5629. [CrossRef]
21. Royal College of Obstetricians & Gynaecologists. RCOG Statement on Later Maternal Age. 2009. Available online: http://www.rcog.org.uk/what-we-do/campaigningand-opinions/statement/rcogstatement-later-maternal-age (accessed on 17 September 2022).
22. Naeh, A.; Hallak, M.; Gabbay-Benziv, R. Parity and Interval from Previous Delivery-Influence on Perinatal Outcome in Advanced Maternal Age Parturients. *J. Clin. Med.* **2021**, *10*, 460. [CrossRef]

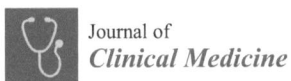

Article

Continuous Maternal Hemodynamics Monitoring at Delivery Using a Novel, Noninvasive, Wireless, PPG-Based Sensor

Yuval Atzmon [1,2], Efrat Ben Ishay [3], Mordechai Hallak [1,2], Romi Littman [3], Arik Eisenkraft [3,4] and Rinat Gabbay-Benziv [1,2,*]

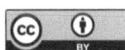

Citation: Atzmon, Y.; Ben Ishay, E.; Hallak, M.; Littman, R.; Eisenkraft, A.; Gabbay-Benziv, R. Continuous Maternal Hemodynamics Monitoring at Delivery Using a Novel, Noninvasive, Wireless, PPG-Based Sensor. *J. Clin. Med.* **2021**, *10*, 8. https://dx.doi.org/10.3390/jcm10010008

Received: 27 November 2020
Accepted: 21 December 2020
Published: 22 December 2020

Publisher's Note: MDPI stays neutral with regard to jurisdictional claims in published maps and institutional affiliations.

Copyright: © 2020 by the authors. Licensee MDPI, Basel, Switzerland. This article is an open access article distributed under the terms and conditions of the Creative Commons Attribution (CC BY) license (https://creativecommons.org/licenses/by/4.0/).

[1] Obstetrics and Gynecology Department, Hillel Yaffe Medical Center, Hadera 38100, Israel; atzmony@gmail.com (Y.A.); MottiH@hy.health.gov.il (M.H.)
[2] The Rappaport Faculty of Medicine, Technion, Haifa 32000, Israel
[3] Biobeat Technologies Ltd., POB 12272, Petah Tikva 44425, Israel; efratsand@gmail.com (E.B.I.); romi@bio-beat.com (R.L.); aizenkra@gmail.com (A.E.)
[4] Institute for Research in Military Medicine, Faculty of Medicine, The Hebrew University of Jerusalem, and The Israel Defense Force Medical Corps, Jerusalem 9112102, Israel
* Correspondence: gabbayrinat@gmail.com; Tel.: +972-4-6304313; Fax: +972-4-6314916

Abstract: Objective: To evaluate continuous monitoring of maternal hemodynamics during labor and delivery utilizing an innovative, noninvasive, reflective photoplethysmography-based device. Study design: The Biobeat Monitoring Platform includes a wearable wristwatch monitor that automatically samples cardiac output (CO), blood pressure (BP), stroke volume (SV), systemic vascular resistance (SVR), heart rate (HR) every 5 s and uploads all data to a smartphone-based app and to a data cloud, enabling remote patient monitoring and analysis of data. Low-risk parturients at term, carrying singletons pregnancies, were recruited at early delivery prior to the active phase. Big data analysis of the collected data was performed using the Power BI analysis tool (Microsoft). Next, data were normalized to visual presentation using Excel Data Analysis and the regression tool. Average measurements were compared before and after rupture of membranes, epidural anesthesia, fetal delivery, and placental expulsion. Results: Eighty-one parturients entered analysis. Epidural anesthesia was associated with a slight elevation in CO (5.5 vs. 5.6, L/min, 10 min before and after EA, $p < 0.05$) attributed to a non-significant increase in both HR and SV. BP remained stable as of counter decrease in SVR (1361 vs. 1319 mmHg·min·mL^{-1}, 10 min before and after EA, $p < 0.05$). Fetal delivery was associated with a peak in CO after which it rapidly declined (6.0 vs. 7.2 vs. 6.1 L/min, 30 min before vs. point of delivery vs. after delivery, $p < 0.05$). The mean BP remained stable throughout delivery with a slight increase at fetal delivery (92 vs. 95 vs. 92.1 mmHg, $p < 0.05$), reflecting the increase in CO and decrease in SVR (1284 vs. 1112 vs. 1280 mmHg·min·mL^{-1}, $p < 0.05$) with delivery. Placental expulsion was associated with a second peak in CO and decrease in SVR. Conclusions: We presented a novel application of noninvasive hemodynamic maternal monitoring throughout labor and delivery for both research and clinical use.

Keywords: remote patient monitoring; noninvasive monitoring; delivery; maternal hemodynamics

1. Introduction

Pregnancy, delivery, and the puerperium are characterized by ongoing major changes in maternal hemodynamics to adapt to the growing physiological demands [1–3]. Changes start as early as the first trimester and reach their peak during labor and delivery to adapt to the associated anxiety, exertion, pain, uterine contractions, uterine involution, and bleeding [4,5]. Understanding these changes is of paramount importance for allowing good clinical care in healthy parturients and especially in more challenging cases such as women with heart disease, preeclampsia, or peripartum hemorrhage. Despite advanced technology and numerous research contributions, data on maternal hemodynamics during labor are still inconsistent and lack validation. While some studies report rises in cardiac output (CO) beginning at the first stage of labor [2], others suggest that CO increment is mainly related to contractions at more advanced delivery [6]. In addition, the exact timing of CO decrease after labor is still uncertain [7,8]. Epidural anesthesia (EA) is known to influence maternal hemodynamics [1]; however, whether other events, such as rupture of membranes or placental separation, have any effect or reflection on maternal hemodynamics is not fully elucidated. Few methods for hemodynamic monitoring during labor and delivery exist. In the past, hemodynamic monitoring depended mainly on invasive techniques of pulmonary artery catheterization using the Fick method, dye dilution, or thermodilution [9–12]. However, the complexity of technique as well as the high risk for adverse events such as arrhythmias, pneumothorax, infection, thrombosis, and even death outweighed any presumed benefits except in very ill patients [13–15]. Echocardiography and tissue Doppler imaging are noninvasive alternatives for hemodynamic monitoring. Lung ultrasound can also serve as a helpful tool for detecting fluid intolerance. Although safe, these tools present logistical and cost issues and are operator dependent [16–18]. Over the recent years, technology has improved, allowing monitoring using whole-body bioimpedance and thoracic bioimpedance-based devices [19,20]. Both techniques are safe and easy to use; however, they still require maternal wiring, which is uncomfortable during labor. In addition, data on their correlation with invasive techniques are conflicting [21,22]. In this study, we assessed maternal hemodynamics during labor and delivery, by using continuous monitoring of cardiac output (CO), heart rate (HR), stroke volume (SV), systemic vascular resistance (SVR), and systolic-, diastolic-, and mean arterial blood pressure (SBP, DBP, and MAP) measured by a novel wearable, wireless, noninvasive reflective photoplethysmography (PPG) remote patient monitoring device

2. Materials and Methods

This was a prospective, observational, longitudinal data analysis study of continuous maternal hemodynamic monitoring using a novel PPG-based wearable device. The study was conducted at a single university-affiliated medical center between 1 April 2019 and 28 February 2020. The study was approved by the Hillel Yaffe Medical Center Institutional Review Board (HYMC-18-0101, NCT03838965) and each participant signed an informed consent form at enrollment.

2.1. Study Population

Women were eligible to participate if they were healthy, above 18 years old, and carrying term (37–42 gestational weeks), singleton pregnancy. Exclusion criteria included any major illness (e.g., heart disease, chronic hypertension, pregestational diabetes) or preeclampsia. Deliveries ending with cesarean section or subjects that removed the device prior to delivery were also excluded.

Women were enrolled in the delivery room prior to the onset of the active stage of labor. Following consent, women were given the device to be worn or their wrist. Initial calibration data including maternal age (years), height (cm), weight (Kg), and current heart rate and blood pressure were uploaded to the personal application provided with the device.

The wristwatch remained attached for at least two hours after delivery and was removed by study personnel prior to transferring the women to the maternity ward.

2.2. The PPG-Based Remote Patient Monitoring Device

The novel reflective PPG-based device (Biobeat Technologies Ltd., Petah Tikva, Israel) is a wearable, wireless, noninvasive medical-grade monitor that enables continuous remote patient monitoring, including the monitoring of maternal hemodynamics to assess cardiovascular changes during labor and delivery (Figure 1). Most commercially available PPG-based pulse oximeters transmit light in specific red and infrared wavelengths through the tissue. A detector measures the changing absorbance at each of the wavelengths, allowing it to determine the absorbance resulting from the pulsating arterial blood alone, excluding venous blood, skin, bone, muscle, and fat. Though PPG technology is commonly used for pulse oximetry, the device used in this study utilizes a unique reflective PPG technology in which the light source and sensor array are placed on the same side, and as the light is transmitted into the subject's skin, part of it is reflected from the tissue to a photodiode detector. The PPG signal is collected with a high temporal and quantitative resolution, and by employing pulse wave transit time and pulse wave analysis techniques' minute changes in tissue reflectance are captured, enabling measurement of numerous vital signs including HR, changes in blood pressure (BP), CO, SV, SVR, and more, every 5s. The PPG-based device has had both US Food and Drug Administration (FDA) clearance and a CE mark approval.

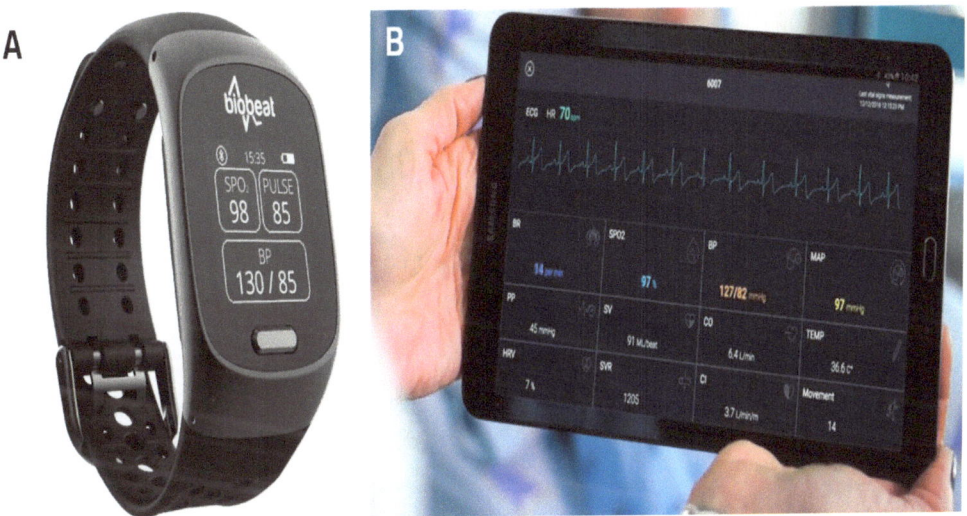

Figure 1. The Biobeat remote patient monitoring platform. (**A**)The wristwatch device. (**B**)Real-time measurement collected by the device.

2.3. Data Collection

Maternal and neonatal data were prospectively collected upon admission and during labor and delivery. Data included maternal characteristics and medical background such as age, pre-gestational weight and height, weight gain during pregnancy, known cardiovascular or metabolic illness, medications, smoking, etc. Obstetric characteristics included parity, previous obstetric history, and current pregnancy follow-up (first and second trimester genetic screening, anatomy scan, glucose status, any hypertensive disorders). Timing of all interventions during labor was documented at the time of event including rupture of membranes (spontaneous or artificial), epidural anesthesia (EA), exact time of fetal delivery, and placental expulsion. Delivery outcomes included gestational age at delivery, neonatal birth weight, and immediate neonatal outcome. Maternal outcome such as peripartum hemorrhage or puerperal fever were documented until discharge. The measurement rate of the monitoring devices was once every five seconds, and the data were uploaded through a smartphone application to a secured data cloud environment, from which it was remotely analyzed. Vital signs included in the analysis were CO, HR, SVR, SV, SBP, DBP, and MAP.

2.4. Data Analysis

Big data analysis of the collected physiological data was performed using the Power BI analysis tool (Microsoft). Next, the data were normalized to visual presentation using Excel Data Analysis and the regression tool. The data were presented as continuous time-series trend lines, identifying behavioral changes in the vital signs. In all, the X-axes represented the monitoring timeline, while the Y-axes represented changes in the values along the timeline. Average measurements calculated from all obtained measurements within the time interval that was defined were compared before and after rupture of membranes (representing the first stage of labor), EA, fetal delivery (representing the second stage of labor), and placental expulsion.

2.5. Statistical Analysis

Data were presented visually and numerically. Average measurements in 10-min time intervals were compared before and after each of the events. Statistical analysis was performed using SPSS version 21.0 software (SPSS, Inc., Chicago, IL, USA). A paired samples *t*-test was used to assess the change in vitals prior to and following each of the events. $p < 0.05$ was considered significant. Intervention studies involving animals or humans, as well as other studies requiring ethical approval must list the authority that provided approval and the corresponding ethical approval code.

3. Results

Of the 106 parturients that were enrolled to the study, only 81 remained eligible for the study. Five parturients were excluded due to hypertensive disorders (4 preeclampsia and 1 with gestational hypertension), fourteen deliveries ended with an emergency cesarean section, and the other 6 parturients were excluded due to technical issues (removing the device prior to delivery or incomplete data transmission). Study cohort characteristics are presented in Table 1. The median maternal age was 30 (21–42) years and 24/81(29.6%) were nullipara. The median body mass index (BMI) was 29.2, range 20.7–48.1, Kg/m^2. Continuous monitoring of all vitals was presented visually and numerically before and after EA, rupture of membranes, fetal delivery, and placental expulsion. Overall, 833,663 measurements were available for analysis. Video of ongoing continuous monitoring is available in the Supplementary File for selected women (Video S1–S5).

Table 1. Study cohort characteristics ($n = 81$).

Maternal age, years	30 (21–42)
Advanced maternal age (>35 years)	16 (19.7)
BMI, Kg/m^2	29.2 (20.7–48.1)
Class II–III BMI (>35 Kg/m^2)	36 (44.4)
Nulliparity	24 (29.6)
Gestational diabetes	14 (17.3)
Induction of labor	33 (40.7)
Epidural anesthesia	69 (85.2)
Artificial rupture of membranes	50 (61.7)
Gestational age at delivery in weeks	39.4 (37–41.9)
Birth weight in grams	3265 (2615–4494)

Data are presented as n (%) for categorical values and median (range), for continuous variables. BMI—body mass index.

3.1. Epidural Anesthesia

Sixty-nine (85.2%) parturients underwent EA. Visually, we noted a slight elevation in CO (5.5 vs. 5.6, L/min, 10 min before and after EA, $p < 0.05$) followed by decreased values. CO elevation seems attributed to a non-significant increase in both HR and SV. Overall, blood pressure values remained stable due to counter decrease in SVR (1361 vs. 1319, mmHg·min·mL^{-1}, 10 min before and after EA, $p < 0.05$) (Figure 2, Table 2).Continuous evaluation of measurements beyond 10 min after the epidural injection demonstrated a continuous decrease in SVR lasting only until 20 min after EA. The rest of the measurements were no longer statistically different (measured until 30 min after EA (Table 3).

3.1.1. Rupture of Membranes

Over half of the parturients (50/81, 61.7%) underwent artificial rupture of membranes. For the entire cohort, the median time (m) from the rupture of membranes to delivery was 3 h and 42 min, range (r) 0:05–23:49 h (artificial rupture: $m = 3:42$, $r = 0:15–23:49$; spontaneous rupture: $m = 3:20$, $r = 0:05–23:12$). Analysis was based on measurements taken 10 min prior and after rupture of membranes. For all variables measured, the rupture of membranes had no impact over maternal hemodynamics (Figure 3, Table 2).

3.1.2. Delivery

The greatest change in maternal hemodynamics appeared around fetal delivery. Cardiac output increased with labor, reaching a peak of 7.24 L/min at the point of fetal delivery, after which it rapidly declined (6.0 vs. 6.1 L/min, 30 min before and after delivery, $p < 0.05$) (Table 2, Figure 4). This was mainly due to marked changes in HR (88.8 vs. 104 vs. 90.5, bpm) and a slight change in SV (67 vs. 69 vs. 67.1, mL/beat), $p < 0.05$ for all. Mean BP remained clinically stable throughout delivery with a slight increase at fetal delivery (92 vs. 95 vs. 92.1, mmHg, $p < 0.05$), reflecting the increase in CO and decrease in SVR (1284 vs. 1112 vs. 1280, mmHg·min·mL^{-1}, $p < 0.05$) with delivery (Figure 4, Table 2).

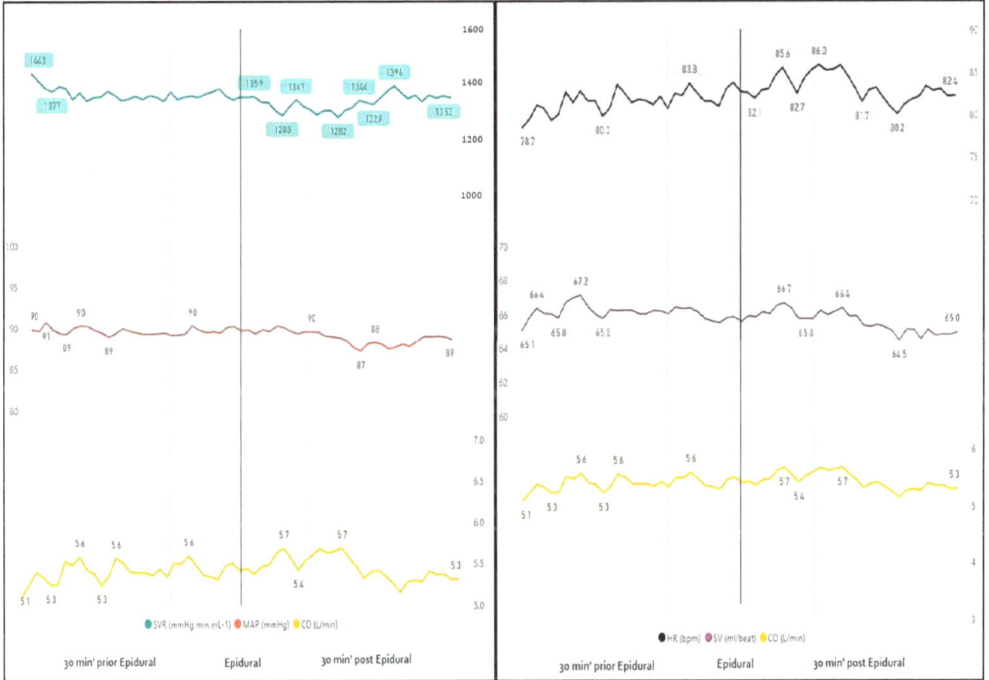

Figure 2. Continuous monitoring 30 min before and after epidural anesthesia. SVR—systemic vascular resistance; MAP—mean arterial blood pressure; $p < 0.05$ is marked in bold; CO—cardiac output.

3.1.3. Placental Expulsion

Evaluation of maternal hemodynamics around placental expulsion revealed increased CO (5.9 vs. peak value at delivery 7.1 vs. 6.6, L/min, $p < 0.05$) most probably due to increased HR (88.5 vs. 96, bpm) without any difference in SV, 10 min before and after the event. Similarly, blood pressure values remained stable with a decrease in SVR (1294 vs. 1130 vs. 1200 mmHg·min·mL^{-1}, $p < 0.05$), probably countering the CO increment. To note, the median time to placental expulsion was 8 min, consistent with peak values presented visually (a range of 0 to 57 min from delivery) (Figure 5, Table 2).

Table 2. Trends in vital signs during labor and delivery.

	Epidural Anesthesia		
	10 min prior	10 min after	*p*-Value
HR	81.9	84.0	0.0727
SVR	1361	1319	0.0177
CO	5.5	5.6	0.0079
SV	66.6	66.9	0.0733
MAP	89.4	89.8	0.2464
SBP	123.5	123.9	0.4724
DBP	72.2	72.7	0.1822
	Rupture of MEMBRANES		
	10 min prior	10 min after	*p*-Value
HR	88	85	0.3502
SVR	1233	1282	0.2601
CO	5.8	5.5	0.3113
SV	65.9	64.4	0.1309
MAP	87.9	86.6	0.0614
SBP	120	119.7	0.0832
DBP	71.6	70	0.0526
	Delivery		
	30 min prior	30 min after	*p*-Value
HR	88.8	90.5	0.0002
SVR	1284	1280	0.0000
CO	6.0	6.1	0.0003
SV	67.0	67.1	0.0001
MAP	92.0	92.1	0.0059
SBP	125.5	126.1	0.0071
DBP	75.2	75.1	0.0061
	Placental Expulsion		
	10 min prior	10 min after	*p*-Value
HR	88.5	96	0.0040
SVR	1294	1200	0.0464
CO	5.9	6.6	0.0049
SV	66.8	67.7	0.2182
MAP	92.2	93.4	0.6398
SBP	126	127	0.9658
DBP	75	76	0.6557

Numbers represent mean values of all obtained measurements within the time interval presented; CO—cardiac output; HR—heart rate; SV—stroke volume; SVR—systemic vascular resistance; SBP—systolic blood pressure; DBP—diastolic blood pressure; MAP—mean arterial blood pressure.

Table 3. Trends in vital signs 20 and 30 min before and after epidural anesthesia.

Epidural Anesthesia			
	10 min Prior	10–20 min after	*p*-Value
HR	81.9	83.5	0.1648
SVR	1361	1317.8	0.0240
CO	5.5	5.5	0.0854
SV	66.6	66.4	0.4080
MAP	89.4	88.3	0.5243
SBP	123.5	122.2	0.3459
DBP	72.2	71.3	0.7622
	10 min Prior	20–30 min after	*p*-Value
HR	81.9	81.6	0.1913
SVR	1361	1348.2	0.4167
CO	5.5	5.3	0.1128
SV	66.6	65.7	0.8424
MAP	89.4	87.9	0.0929
SBP	123.5	121.7	0.2257
DBP	72.2	70.9	0.0709

Numbers represent meanvalues of all obtained measurements within the time interval presented; CO—cardiac output; HR—heart rate; SV—stroke volume; SVR—systemic vascular resistance; SBP—systolic blood pressure; DBP—diastolic blood pressure; MAP—mean arterial blood pressure.

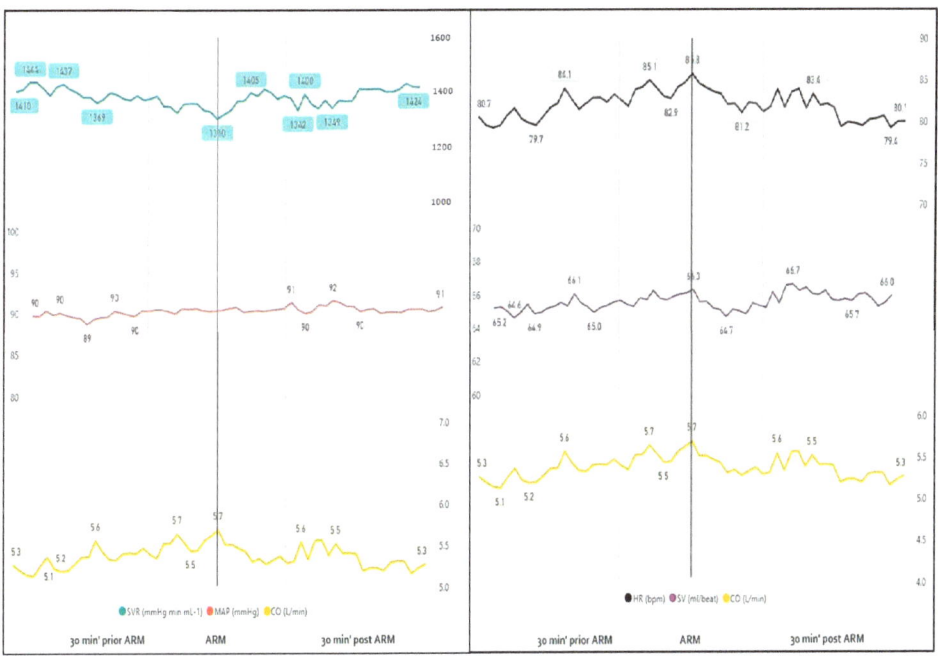

Figure 3. Continuous monitoring 30 min before and after rupture of membranes.

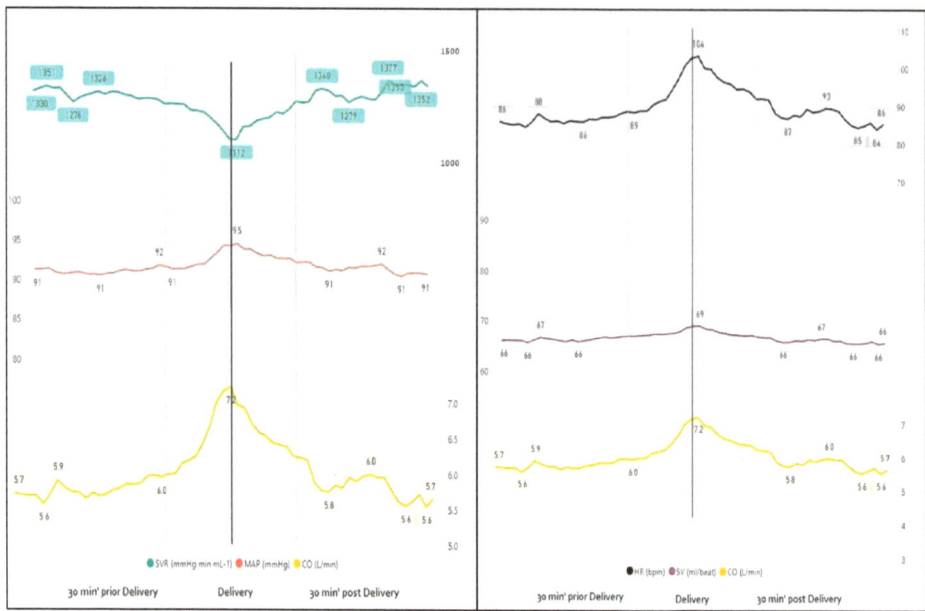

Figure 4. Continuous monitoring 30 min before and after delivery.

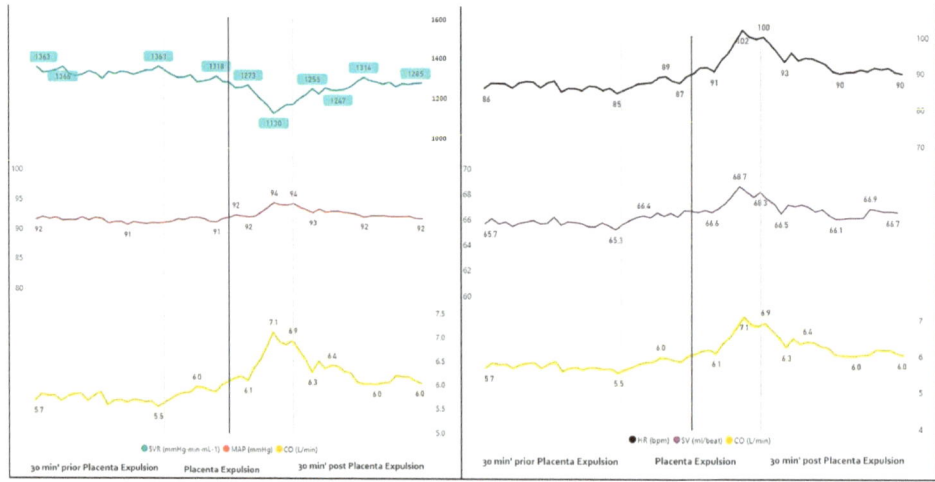

Figure 5. Continuous monitoring 30 min before and after placental expulsion.

4. Discussion

In this observational longitudinal study, we presented continuous maternal hemodynamic monitoring of low risk parturients undergoing vaginal deliveries using a novel PPG-based remote patient monitoring device. Our study presented the longitudinal adjustments of HR, SV, CO, SVR, SBP, DBP, and MAP sampled every 5 s throughout labor and delivery as well as their adaptation to "events" during labor and delivery: EA, rupture of membranes, fetal, delivery and placental expulsion. According to our results: (1) EA causes only minor changes in SVR and CO with stable blood pressure values up to 30 min after EA; (2) no maternal hemodynamics changes were documented following rupture of membranes; (3) fetal delivery was the point of maximal changes for all measured variables with a rapid onset significant reversal of changes after fetal delivery; and (4) placental expulsion was associated with a second peak in CO and HR, and a decrease in SVR, thus maintaining stable blood pressure values.

Thus far, studies investigating maternal hemodynamics during labor and delivery have yielded conflicting results, especially regarding magnitude and timing of hemodynamic adaptations. Previous studies suggested inconsistent results on the effect of EA on maternal hemodynamics during labor [19,23–26]. EA induces a sympathetic blockade that causes vasodilatation and a decrease in venous return to the heart, which can result in maternal hypotension. In addition, abrupt onset of pain relief may trigger a reduction in blood pressure. However, these effects are seen in only some of the studies and reported clinically in only 0–14% of laboring women receiving EA [23–27]. Recently, Ashwal et al. [19] compared maternal hemodynamics following vaginal and cesarean deliveries determined by a whole body bioimpedance-based device. They found a significant decrease in cardiac index and in MAP measured before and after EA. However, their sampling was continuous for only a 6-min interval before and after EA without standardization regarding the time interval before and after onset of anesthesia. In addition, data on fluid overload given prior to EA and its effect on measurements were not documented. In our study, we have documented the longitudinal changes in maternal hemodynamics following EA in a 5-s interval and found that blood pressure remained stable until 30 min after EA. This serves not only as a proof of concept for an easy, noninvasive, and accurate technique for longitudinal assessment of maternal hemodynamics, but also has clinical significance in terms of abandoning the fluid overload given prior to EA to allow real time adaptation of fluid management and fetal monitoring. The simplicity of this technology will enable us to further broaden our knowledge of maternal hemodynamics and individualize the management of high-risk parturients and complicated deliveries.

Rupture of membranes, although potentially relieving the tension within the uterus, did not impact any of the variable measured.

Like previous reports [1–6], the peak of changes was noted with fetal delivery. CO increased from early labor to the second stage, reaching 7.2 L/min with fetal delivery. This is most probably related to the strong contractions causing autotransfusion of uterine blood into the maternal systemic circulation, thus increasing the preload. Thirty minutes after fetal delivery, there was already a marked decrease in CO. Unlike the robust changes in CO, MAP remained relatively unchanged with only a mild increment found in the second stage and fetal delivery. To note, changes in blood pressure may differ between studies, as it is dependent upon many variables usually uncontrolled for between parturients such as: Duration and intensity of uterine contractions, maternal position, subjective maternal pain and anxiety, and timing of maternal pushing.

Placental expulsion was associated with a second peak in CO and HR that appeared minutes after delivery. Despite the rise in CO, MAP remained relatively unchanged due to a compensating decrease in SVR.

Our study benefitted from its longitudinal methodology with continuous monitoring of hemodynamic data every 5 s during labor and delivery. This was possible using the novel PPG-based technology that was previously validated as well as adjusted to specific maternal anthropometrics. In addition, as participants were derived from a single center, a standard approach was applied for all deliveries.

Our study was limited due to the small sample size. In addition, as our study was observational, we could not control measurements for variables such as maternal positioning, fluid management, maternal anxiety, timing of bearing down, etc. Lastly, we did not evaluate the change in hemodynamic parameters in different settings of maternal and obstetrical complications such as previous cardiovascular disease and acute bleeding.

5. Conclusions

In this study we utilized a novel PPG-based device to evaluate maternal hemodynamic adjustment during labor and delivery. Further studies should focus on hemodynamic monitoring in parturients with preexisting cardiovascular or obstetrical complications such as preeclampsia and use these data to define normal and abnormal values for creation of safety protocols during labor and delivery.

Supplementary Materials: The following are available online at https://www.mdpi.com/2077-0383/10/1/8/s1. Video S1: HR: In timeline and stage and events during labor and delivery; Video S2: SVR: In time line and stage and events during labor and delivery; Video S3: MAP: In time line and stage and events during labor and delivery. Video S4: CO: In timeline and stage and events during labor and delivery; Video S5: CO: In time line and stage and events during labor and delivery.

Author Contributions: Conceptualization, Y.A., R.G.-B.; methodology, Y.A., E.B.I., M.H., A.E., R.G.-B. software, E.B.I., R.L., A.E.; validation, E.B.I., M.H., R.L., A.E., R.G.-B.; formal analysis, E.B.I., M.H., R.L., A.E., R.G.-B.; investigation, Y.A., R.G.-B.; resources, Y.A., E.B.I., A.E.; data curation, Y.A., E.B.I., R.L.; writing—original draft preparation, Y.A., A.E., R.G.-B.; writing—Y.A., M.H., A.E., R.G.-B.; visualization, Y.A., E.B.I., R.G.-B.; supervision, M.H., R.G.-B. All authors have read and agreed to the published version of the manuscript.

Funding: This research received no external funding.

Conflicts of Interest: The authors declare no conflict of interest.

References

1. Ouzounian, J.G.; Elkayam, U. Physiologic changes during normal pregnancy and delivery. *Cardiol. Clin.* **2012**, *30*, 317–329. [CrossRef] [PubMed]
2. Hunter, S.; Robson, S.C. Adaptation of the maternal heart in pregnancy. *Br. Heart J.* **1992**, *68*, 540–543. [CrossRef] [PubMed]
3. Chapman, A.B.; Abraham, W.T.; Zamudio, S.; Coffin, C.; Merouani, A.; Young, D.; Johnson, A.; Osorio, F.; Goldberg, C.; Moore, L.G.; et al. Temporal relationships between hormonal and hemodynamic changes in early human pregnancy. *Kidney Int.* **1998**, *54*, 2056. [CrossRef]
4. Meah, V.L.; Cockcroft, J.R.; Backx, K.; Shave, R.; Stöhr, E.J. Cardiac output and related haemodynamics during pregnancy: A series of meta-analyses. *Heart* **2016**, *102*, 518. [CrossRef] [PubMed]
5. Duvekot, J.J.; Cheriex, E.C.; Pieters, F.A.; Menheere, P.P.; Peeters, L.H. Early pregnancy changes in hemodynamics and volume homeostasis are consecutive adjustments triggered by a primary fall in systemic vascular tone. *Am. J. Obstet. Gynecol.* **1993**, *169*, 1382. [CrossRef]
6. Maruta, S. The observation of thematernal hemodynamics during labor and cesarean section. *Nippon Sanka Fujinka Gakkai Zasshi* **1982**, *34*, 776–784.
7. Mahendru, A.A.; Everett, T.R.; Wilkinson, I.B.; Lees, C.C.; McEniery, C.M. A longitudinal study of maternal cardiovascular function from preconception to the postpartum period. *J. Hypertens.* **2014**, *32*, 849–856. [CrossRef]
8. Morris, E.A.; Hale, S.A.; Badger, G.J.; Magness, R.R.; Bernstein, I.M. Pregnancy induces persistent changes in vascular compliance in primiparous women. *Am. J. Obstet. Gynecol.* **2015**, *212*, 633.e1–633.e6. [CrossRef]
9. Sorensen, M.B.; Bille-Brahe, N.E.; Engell, H.C. Cardiac output measurement by thermal dilution: Reproducibility and comparison with the dye-dilution technique. *Ann. Surg.* **1976**, *183*, 67–72. [CrossRef]
10. Fegler, G. The reliability of the thermodilution method for determination of the cardiac output and the blood flow in central veins. *Q. J. Exp. Physiol. Cogn. Med. Sci.* **1957**, *42*, 254–266. [CrossRef]
11. Driul, L.; Meroi, F.; Sala, A.; Delrio, S.; Pavoni, D.; Barbariol, F.; Londero, A.; Dogareschi, T.; Spasiano, A.; Vetrugno, L.; et al. Vaginal delivery in a patient with severe aortic stenosis under epidural analgesia, a case report. *Cardiovasc. Ultrasound* **2020**, *18*, 43. [CrossRef] [PubMed]
12. Swan, H.J.; Ganz, W.; Forrester, J.; Marcus, H.; Diamond, G.; Chonette, D. Catheterization of the heart in man with use of a flow-directed balloontipped catheter. *N. Engl. J. Med.* **1970**, *283*, 447–451. [CrossRef] [PubMed]
13. Ventura, H.O.; Taler, S.J.; Strobeck, J.E. Hypertension as a hemodynamic disease: The role of impedance cardiography in diagnostic, prognostic, and therapeutic decision making. *Am. J. Hypertens.* **2005**, *18*, 26S–43S. [CrossRef] [PubMed]
14. Harvey, S.; Harrison, D.A.; Singer, M.; Ashcroft, J.; Jones, C.M.; Elbourne, D.; Brampton, W.; Williams, D.; Young, D.; Rowan, K. PAC-Man study collaboration. Assessment of the clinical effectiveness of pulmonary artery catheters in management of patients in intensive care (PAC-man): A randomized controlled trial. *Lancet* **2005**, *366*, 472–477. [CrossRef]
15. Peters, S.G.; Afessa, B.; Decker, P.A.; Schroeder, D.R.; Offord, K.P.; Scott, J.P. Increased risk associated with pulmonary artery catheterization in the medical intensive care unit. *J. Crit. Care* **2003**, *18*, 166–171. [CrossRef]
16. Vetrugno, L.; Dogareschi, T.; Sassanelli, R.; Orso, D.; Seremet, L.; Mattuzzi, L.; Scapol, S.; Spasiano, A.; Cagnacci, A.; Bove, T. Thoracic ultrasound evaluation and B-type natriuretic peptide value in elective cesarean section under spinal anesthesia. *Ultrasound J.* **2020**, *12*, 10. [CrossRef]
17. Arbeid, E.; Demi, A.; Brogi, E.; Gori, E.; Giusto, T.; Soldati, G.; Vetrugno, L.; Giunta, F.; Forfori, F. Lung Ultrasound Pattern Is Normal during the Last Gestational Weeks: An Observational Pilot Study. *Gynecol. Obstet. Investig.* **2017**, *82*, 398–403. [CrossRef]

18. Easterling, T.F.; Benedetti, T.J.; Schmucker, B.C.; Millard, S.P. Maternal hemodynamics in normal and preeclamptic pregnancies; a longitudinal study. *Obstet. Gynecol.* **1990**, *76*, 1061–1069.
19. Ashwal, E.; Shinar, S.; Orbach-Zinger, S.; Lev, S.; Gat, R.; Kedar, L.; Pauzner, Y.; Aviram, A.; Yogev, Y.; Hiersch, L. The Hemodynamics of Labor in Women Undergoing Vaginal and Cesarean Deliveries as Determined by Whole Body Bioimpedance. *Am. J. Perinatol.* **2018**, *35*, 177–183. [CrossRef]
20. Lavie, A.; Ram, M.; Lev, S.; Blecher, Y.; Amikam, U.; Shulman, Y.; Avnon, T.; Weiner, E.; Many, A. Maternal cardiovascular hemodynamics in normotensive versus preeclamptic pregnancies: A prospective longitudinal study using a noninvasive cardiac system (NICaS™). *BMC Pregnancy Childbirth* **2018**, *18*, 229. [CrossRef]
21. Young, J.D.; McQuillan, P. Comparison of thoracic electrical bioimpedance and thermodilution for the measurement of cardiac index in patients with severe sepsis. *Br. J. Anaesth.* **1993**, *70*, 58–62. [CrossRef] [PubMed]
22. Gotshall, R.W.; Wood, V.C.; Miles, D.S. Comparison of two impedance cardiographic techniques for measuring cardiac output in critically ill patients. *Crit. Care Med.* **1989**, *17*, 806–811. [CrossRef] [PubMed]
23. Nachman, D.; Gepner, Y.; Goldstein, N.; Kabakov, E.; Ishay, A.B.; Littman, R.; Azmon, Y.; Jaffe, E.; Eisenkraft, A. Comparing Blood Pressure Measurements Between a Photoplethysmography-Based and a Standard Cuff-Based Manometry Device. *Sci. Rep.* **2020**, *10*, 16116. [CrossRef] [PubMed]
24. Grant, G.J.; Susser, L.; Cascio, M.; Zakowski, M.I. Hemodynamic effects of intrathecal fentanyl in nonlaboring term parturients. *J. Clin. Anesth.* **1996**, *8*, 99. [CrossRef]
25. Palmer, C.M.; Van Maren, G.; Nogami, W.M.; Alves, D. Bupivacaine augments intrathecal fentanyl for labor analgesia. *Anesthesiology* **1999**, *91*, 84. [CrossRef] [PubMed]
26. Simmons, S.W.; Taghizadeh, N.; Dennis, A.T.; Hughes, D.; Cyna, A.M. Combined spinal-epidural versus epidural analgesia in labour. *Cochrane DatabaseSyst. Rev.* **2012**, *10*, CD003401. [CrossRef] [PubMed]
27. Grangier, L.; de Tejada, B.M.; Savoldelli, G.L.; Irion, O.; Haller, G. Adverse side effects and route of administration of opioids in combined spinal-epidural analgesia for labour: A meta-analysis of randomised trials. *Int. J. Obstet. Anesth.* **2020**, *41*, 83. [CrossRef]

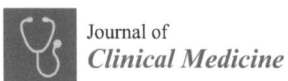

Journal of Clinical Medicine

Article

Parity and Interval from Previous Delivery—Influence on Perinatal Outcome in Advanced Maternal Age Parturients

Amir Naeh [1,2,*], Mordechai Hallak [1,2] and Rinat Gabbay-Benziv [1,2]

1. Obstetrics and Gynecology Department, Hillel Yaffe Medical Center, Hadera 38100, Israel; mottih@hy.health.gov.il (M.H.); gabbayrinat@gmail.com (R.G.-B.)
2. The Rappaport Faculty of Medicine, Technion, Haifa 32000, Israel
* Correspondence: amir_naeh@outlook.com; Tel.: +972-4-7748224

Abstract: Objective: To investigate the effect of parity and interpregnancy interval (IPI) on perinatal outcomes in advanced maternal age (AMA) parturients. Methods: A population-based retrospective cohort study of all women older than 40 years, who had a singleton live birth after 24 weeks in the United States in 2017 Women were categorized to three groups by parity and interval from last delivery: primiparas, multiparas with IPI $\leq$ 5 years, and multiparas with IPI > 5 years. Primary outcome was composite adverse neonatal outcome (preterm delivery <34 weeks, birthweight <2000 g, neonatal seizure, neonatal intensive care unit admission, Apgar score <7 at 5 min, or assisted ventilation >6 h). Secondary outcome was composite adverse maternal outcome and other adverse perinatal outcomes. Univariate and multivariate analysis were used to compare between groups. Results: During 2017, 3,864,754 deliveries were recorded into the database. Following exclusion, 109,564 AMA gravidas entered analysis. Of them, 24,769 (22.6%) were nulliparas, 39,933 (36.4%) were multiparas with IPI $\leq$ 5 years, and 44,862 (40.9%) were multiparas with IPI > 5 years. Composite neonatal outcome was higher in nulliparas and in multiparas with IPI > 5 years, in comparison to multiparas with IPI $\leq$ 5 years (16% vs. 13% vs. 10%, respectively, $p < 0.05$). Maternal composite outcome was similar between groups. In the multivariable analysis, relative to nulliparas, only multiparity with IPI $\leq$ 5 years had a protective effect against the composite neonatal outcome (aOR 0.97, 95% CI 0.95–0.99, $p < 0.001$). Conclusion: Among AMA gravidas, multiparity with IPI $\leq$ 5 years has a significant protective effect against adverse neonatal outcomes when compared to nulliparas. Multiparity with IPI > 5 years is no longer protective.

Keywords: advanced maternal age; adverse pregnancy outcome; elderly gravida; interpregnancy interval; nulliparity; pregnancy complications

Citation: Naeh, A.; Hallak, M.; Gabbay-Benziv, R. Parity and Interval from Previous Delivery—Influence on Perinatal Outcome in Advanced Maternal Age Parturients. *J. Clin. Med.* **2021**, *10*, 460. https://doi.org/10.3390/jcm10030460

Academic Editor: Eyal Sheiner
Received: 29 December 2020
Accepted: 21 January 2021
Published: 26 January 2021

Publisher's Note: MDPI stays neutral with regard to jurisdictional claims in published maps and institutional affiliations.

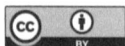

Copyright: © 2021 by the authors. Licensee MDPI, Basel, Switzerland. This article is an open access article distributed under the terms and conditions of the Creative Commons Attribution (CC BY) license (https://creativecommons.org/licenses/by/4.0/).

1. Introduction

During the last few decades, there has been an increasing trend for child bearing in the later reproductive years, particularly in high-income countries [1]. As age is a continuum rather than a categorical variable, the definition of advanced maternal age is not solid, and most studies refer to women over 35 to 40 years as such. Advanced maternal age gravidas have higher rates of adverse pregnancy outcomes including: pre-eclampsia, gestational diabetes mellitus, preterm birth, fetal growth restriction, cesarean delivery, stillbirth, and more [2–6].

Other than age, nulliparity is also associated with adverse pregnancy outcome [7,8], therefore, multiparity (assuming normal outcome) is considered protective. In multipara women, data suggests that interpregnancy interval (IPI), whether short (below 18 months) or long (above 60 month) has an impact on both maternal and neonatal outcome [9–15]. It is thought that following prolonged IPI, the maternal, physiologic, and anatomical pregnancy adaptations gradually decline and become comparable to those at their first pregnancy [9].

Therefore, the aim of this study was to investigate the combined effect of parity and IPI on perinatal outcomes in advanced maternal age parturients.

2. Materials and Methods

We performed a population-based cohort study of all parturients older than 40 years at time of delivery with singleton live birth at 2017 in the United States. We used de-identified natality data assembled by the National Vital Statistics System of the National Center for Health Statistics that provides demographic and health data for births occurring during the calendar year in the United States (available at: https://data.nber.org/data/vital-statistics-natality-data.html) [16]. The U.S. Standard Certificate of Live Birth, issued by the U.S. Department of Health and Human Services, has served for many years as the principal means for attaining uniformity in the content of the documents used to collect information on births in the United States. In 2003, birth certificates were revised to contains more detailed demographic, medical, and obstetric data compared to the previous 1989 version. The revised birth certificate was gradually adopted by the states and from 2016, represents 100% live births in the 50 states and Washington, DC.

Only livebirth deliveries at 24 or more gestational weeks with neonatal weights above 500 g were included. We excluded women if maternal age less than 40 years at time of delivery, carrying multifetal gestation, or had any known fetal anomalies or chromosomal abnormalities. Additionally, all births with unknown data on the time interval from previous delivery were excluded. This study was exempt from review by the institutional review board at our institution because the data we used do not meet the criteria for human subject research by federal standards. The STROBE (Strengthening the Reporting of Observational Studies in Epidemiology) guidelines for reporting observational studies were followed [17].

All parturients that entered analysis were categorized to three groups. Group 1 included nulliparas parturients. Group 2 included all multiparas with previous live birth delivery documented within 5 years from current delivery. Group 3 included multiparas with previous live birth delivery occurring at longer than 5 years interval from current delivery.

The primary outcome that was evaluated between groups was a composite of adverse neonatal outcome that included: preterm delivery <34 weeks, birthweight <2000 g, neonatal seizure, neonatal intensive care unit admission (NICU), Apgar score less than 7 at 5 min, or neonatal assisted ventilation for more than 6 h. Secondary outcomes included composite adverse maternal outcome (including uterine rupture, unplanned hysterectomy, maternal intensive care unit admission, and maternal blood transfusion) and other adverse perinatal outcomes including gestational diabetes, hypertensive disorders during pregnancy, induction of labor, mode of delivery, gestational age at delivery and birthweight, and any one of the variables included in the composite primary outcome separately. Newborns or women with more than one adverse outcome were counted once when formulating the composites.

Statistical Analysis

Statistical analysis was performed using R software (R version 3.6.2, R Foundation for Statistical Computing, Vienna, Austria). For univariate analyses of baseline differences, Student t-test and chi-square test were used for continuous data and categorical data, respectively. Multivariable logistic regression was performed to adjust the composite outcomes to potential confounders: maternal age, pregestational diabetes, chronic hypertension, smoking, race, body mass index, use of assisted reproductive technology, gestational diabetes, gestational hypertension, preeclampsia, and cesarean delivery. p-value was considered statistically significant of <0.05.

3. Results

During 2017, 3,864,754 live births were recorded into the database. In 124,574 (3.2%) of them, maternal age was older than 40 years at the time of delivery. Following exclusion, 109,564 cases met the inclusion criteria and entered analysis (Figure 1).

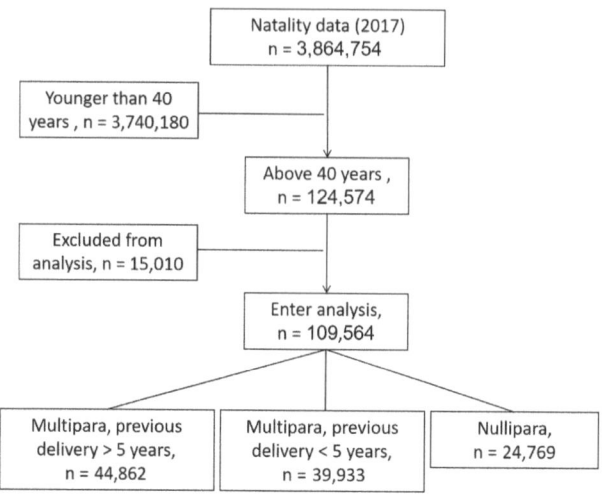

Figure 1. Flow chart of patients in each cohort after applying exclusion and inclusion criteria.

Almost quarter of the women delivering after 40 years of age were nulliparas (24,769/109,564, 22.6%). The rest were multiparas; 39,933 (36.4%) had their last previous delivery within 5 years from the current pregnancy and 44,862 (40.9%) had their last delivery at more than 5 years interval.

Maternal characteristics stratified by study group are presented in Table 1. For the entire cohort median maternal age was 41 years. For multipara women, median number of previous deliveries was four (range: 2–8). Group 2 had a mean IPI of 34 months and group 3 had mean IPI of 130 months. Maternal characteristics differed in race, smoking, BMI, presence of chronic hypertension or diabetes, and obstetrical history (previous preterm or cesarean deliveries). Surprisingly, there was no difference in assisted reproductive use between nulliparas and multiparas.

Table 1. Maternal characteristics stratified by parity and interval from previous delivery.

Maternal Characteristic	Group 1: Nulliparas $n = 24{,}769$	Group 2: Multiparas, Previous Delivery <5 Years $n = 39{,}933$	Group 3: Multiparas, Previous Delivery <5 Years $n = 44{,}862$	p-Value
Maternal age, years	41.65 ± 1.98	41.34 ± 1.67	41.54 ± 1.74	<0.001
		4.46 ± 2.08	4.14 ± 1.72	
Number of previous deliveries	-	Median 4 (range: 2–8)	Median 4 (range: 2–8)	<0.001
Previous delivery interval, months	-	34.16 ± 12.53	130 ± 57.12	<0.001
Race:				
White	17,661 (71%)	29,661 (74%)	31,042 (69%)	
Black	3193 (13%)	5315 (13%)	8152 (18%)	
American Indian or Alaskan Native	99 (0%)	384 (0%)	268 (0.7%)	
Asian or Pacific Islander	3816 (16%)	5284 (12%)	4689 (12%)	<0.001
Assisted reproduction *	3515 (82%)	1819 (82%)	1064 (80%)	0.14
Smoking	554 (2.2%)	1018 (2.6%)	2229 (5%)	<0.001
BMI (kg/m^2)	26.62 ± 6.45	27.11 ± 6.32	28.10 ± 6.53	<0.001
Pregestational diabetes	511 (2.1%)	648 (1.6%)	1172 (2.6%)	<0.001
Chronic hypertension	1217 (4.9%)	1361 (3.4%)	2533 (5.6%)	<0.001
Previous preterm delivery	-	2548 (6.4%)	2509 (5.6%)	<0.001
Number of previous cesarean deliveries	-	1.48 ± 0.87	1.53 ± 0.78	<0.001

Continuous variables are presented as mean ± SD or median (range); categorical values are n (%). Statistically significant p-values as marked in bold. * Data on ART was available for only part of the cohort; percentages are calculated from valid data.

Perinatal outcomes of the three study groups are shown in Table 2. Overall, for the entire cohort, 12.4% presented at least one adverse neonatal composite outcome (13,621/109,564). In the univariate analysis, neonatal composite outcome was statistically different between groups, i.e., nulliparas women had the highest rate of composite neonatal adverse outcome (16%), followed by multiparas with IPI longer than 60 months (13%).

Table 2. Perinatal outcome stratified by parity and interval from previous delivery.

Maternal Characteristic	Group 1: Nulliparas $n = 24{,}769$	Group 2: Multiparas, Previous Delivery <5 Years $n = 39{,}933$	Group 3: Multiparas, Previous Delivery <5 Years $n = 44{,}862$	p-Value
Pregnancy complications:				
Gestational diabetes	3108 (12.6)	4630 (11.6)	6790 (15.1)	<0.0001
Gestational hypertension	2675 (10.8)	1301 (5.8)	3707 (8.3)	<0.0001
Preeclampsia	143 (0.6)	98 (0.2)	173 (0.4)	<0.0001
Induction of labor	8712 (35.2)	8828 (22.1)	11,695 (26.1)	<0.0001
Cesarean delivery	14,344 (57.9)	16,269 (41.8)	19,994 (44.6)	<0.0001
Maternal blood transfusion	147 (0.6)	165 (0.4)	207 (0.5)	0.004
Uterine rupture	5 (0)	20 (0.1)	20 (0)	0.11
Maternal ICU admission	81 (0.3)	85 (0.2)	132 (0.3)	0.01
Unintended hysterectomy	27 (0.1)	72 (0.2)	60 (0.1)	0.05
Gestational age at delivery	38.3 ± 2.43	38.5 ± 2.07	38.1 ± 2.33	<0.0001
Birthweight	3169 ± 603	3379 ± 562	3324 ± 597	<0.0001
Birthweight by category:				
<1500 g	451 (1.8)	288 (0.7)	641 (1.4)	
1500–2499 g	2284 (9.2)	1935 (4.8)	3433 (7.7)	
>2500 g	22,034 (89)	37,710 (94.4)	40,788 (90.9)	<0.0001
Male gender	12,545 (50.6)	20,300 (50.8)	22,841 (50.9)	0.79
Apgar score:				
0–3	132 (0.5)	146 (0.4)	223 (0.5)	
4–6	472 (1.9)	426 (1.1)	641 (1.4)	
7–8	3433 (13.9)	4314 (10.9)	5249 (11.7)	
9–10	20,658 (83.7)	34,847 (87.7)	38,604 (86.3)	<0.0001
Neonatal ICU admission	3320 (13.4)	3218 (8.1)	4807 (10.7)	<0.0001
Neonatal seizures	8 (0)	9 (0)	14 (0)	0.69
Neonatal assisted ventilation >6 h	472 (1.9)	500 (1.3)	691 (1.5)	<0.0001
Neonatal composite	3869 (16)	3884 (10)	5868 (13)	<0.001
Maternal composite	104 (0.4)	145 (0.4)	178 (0.4)	0.5

Continuous variables are presented as mean ± SD; categorical values are n (%). Statistically significant p-values as marked in bold. Composite adverse neonatal outcome includes: preterm delivery <34 weeks, birthweight < 2000 g, neonatal seizure, neonatal intensive care unit admission, Apgar score less than 7 at 5 min or neonatal assisted ventilation for more than 6 h. Composite adverse maternal outcome includes uterine rupture, unplanned hysterectomy, maternal intensive care unit admission, and maternal blood transfusion.

Multiparas women with previous delivery at less than 5 years interval had the lowest rate of composite adverse neonatal outcome (10%, $p < 0.05$). For individual neonatal adverse outcomes, neonates of nulliparas had highest rates of low Apgar scores (<7 at 5 min), NICU admission, and required more assisted ventilation.

Only 0.4% (427/109,564) gravidas presented at least one of the composite adverse maternal outcomes with similar distribution between study groups. Nulliparas (Group 1) had highest rates of gestational hypertension (10.8% vs. 5.8% vs. 8.3%) and preeclampsia (0.6% vs. 0.2% vs. 0.4%) during pregnancy, with higher rates of induction of labor (35.2% vs. 22.1% vs. 26.1%) and cesarean deliveries (57.9% vs. 41.8% vs. 44.6%). Postpartum, they received more blood transfusions compared to other groups (0.6% vs. 0.4% vs. 0.5%), Group 1, 2, and 3 respectively.

Overall, Group 2 delivered later in pregnancy (38.3 vs. 38.5 vs. 38.1, gestational weeks) the largest babies (3169 vs. 3379 vs. 3324 g) Group 1, 2, and 3, respectively, $p < 0.05$ for all. For the majority of adverse outcomes, Group 3 was second to Group 1, leaving lowest rates of complications among multiparas with previous delivery within 5 years interval.

Results of multivariable analysis are shown in Table 3. Previous delivery within 5 years difference had a significant protective effect against the composite neonatal outcome (aOR 0.97, 95% confidence interval 0.95–0.99, $p < 0.001$) relative to nulliparas. Previous delivery at longer than 5 years was no longer protective from composite neonatal outcome.

Table 3. Adverse composite neonatal outcome evaluated by multivariable analysis to adjust for confounders.

	aOR B(EXP)	95% Confidence Interval	p-Value
Maternal group			
Group 1	Reference		
Group 2	0.97	0.95–0.99	<0.001
Group 3	0.99	0.97–1.02	0.651
Maternal age	1	0.99–1	0.154
Race:			
White	Reference		
Black	1.02	0.99–1.06	0.153
American Indian or Alaskan Native	0.94	0.79–1.11	0.471
Asian or Pacific Islander	0.99	0.97–1.02	0.804
Pregestational diabetes	1.16	1.08–1.24	<0.001
Chronic hypertension	1.13	1.08–1.17	<0.001
Smoking	1.27	1.1–1.46	0.001
BMI, kg/m^2			
<18.5	0.99	0.94–1.05	0.830
18.5–24.9	Reference		
25–29.9	1.02	1–1.04	0.045
30–34.9	1.03	1–1.06	0.022
35–39.9	1.03	0.99–1.06	0.151
>40	1.02	0.97–1.07	0.476
Assisted reproductive	1.01	0.99–1.03	0.524
Gestational diabetes	1.02	0.99–1.04	0.129
Gestational hypertension	1.12	1.09–1.15	<0.001
Preeclampsia	1.25	1.11–1.40	<0.001
Cesarean delivery	1.05	1.03–1.06	<0.001

4. Discussion

In this study, we aimed to evaluate the combined effect of parity and IPI on perinatal outcomes in advanced maternal age parturients. Our main findings were (1.) composite adverse neonatal outcome among advanced maternal age gravidas was overall high (12.4% of the cohort). Highest rate of adverse neonatal composite outcome was seen in nulliparas, followed by multiparas with IPI longer than 5 years and lastly, in multiparas with IPI within 5 years (16% vs. 13% vs. 10%, $p < 0.05$). Separate neonatal outcomes (low Apgar scores, NICU admission, assisted ventilation) were also more common among nulliparas. (2.) Nulliparas had higher rates of separate adverse maternal outcomes including hypertensive disorders of pregnancy, induction of labor, cesarean deliveries, and postpartum blood transfusions. However, parity had no influence on composite adverse maternal outcome. (3.) Utilizing a multivariable analysis and relative to nulliparas, a previous delivery within 5 years interval had a significant protective effect against the composite neonatal outcome. This effect did not persist when delivery interval was longer than 5 years.

Advanced maternal age is a well-established risk factor for adverse pregnancy outcomes [2–6]. Nulliparity adds further risk [7,8], putting the advanced maternal age nullipara gravida at the focus of research studies and pregnancy surveillance. Consistent with this assumption, multiparity is considered a protective factor among all maternal ages, including among advanced maternal age parturients. In this study, we aimed to evaluate this assumption stratified by the time interval from last delivery.

Reports differentiating older primiparas from multiparas are scarce. Shechter M.G. et al. [8] conducted a retrospective study that aimed to evaluate the impact of parity on adverse perinatal outcome among advanced maternal age parturients (over 35 years at time of delivery). The authors demonstrated higher rates of multifetal pregnancies, preterm deliveries, hypertensive disorders, diabetes, and fetal growth restriction among nulliparas compared to multiparas gravidas. Although their study demonstrated the protective effect of parity on risk for pregnancy complications, they did not take into account the time interval from last delivery for the multiparas women. Our study, not only refined the effect of age, including only parturients over 40 years, but also evaluated the protective effect of parity with regard to the time interval elapsed from last delivery.

Several studies have demonstrated an association between long IPI and pregnancy complications, including pre-eclampsia and eclampsia, preterm delivery, small for gestational age neonates, birth defects, higher rates of cesarean deliveries, and lower success rate for trial of labor after cesarean [9–14,18–22]. A recent study has also found that long IPI is associated with increased risk for long-term neurological morbidity of the offspring [15]. To note, there is no universal definition for long IPI, although most studies use the cutoff of 5 years. In our study, parity had a protective effect only when last delivery occurred within 5 years from the index pregnancy.

Various explanations were offered for the association between long IPI and pregnancy complications, including an age-related, physiological mechanisms, and other causes. Zhu et al. found that the optimal IPI for preventing adverse perinatal outcomes is 18–23 months [9]. They offered two hypotheses for the association between long IPI and pregnancy complications. The first was that vascular, physiological, and anatomical changes in pregnancy help parturients to gain growth-supporting capacities. If another fetus is not conceived for a long period of time, those capacities may gradually decline, and thus causing maternal physiologic characteristics to become more similar to those of the nullipara gravida. Second, with advanced time, metabolic or anatomical factors may cause both delayed fertility and adverse birth outcomes. Secondary infertility by itself is associated with an increased incidence of preterm birth [23]. Another possible explanation is that pregnancies conceived after a long IPI have higher probability of being unplanned, and they are more common in women with a low socioeconomic status, a significant risk factor for adverse pregnancy outcomes [24,25].

Our results demonstrate that IPI of less than 5 years had a significant protective effect against adverse neonatal outcomes. Since our study cohort included only women delivering after 40 years of age, this effect cannot be attributed to the parturients age. In addition, rates of assisted reproductive use were similar between the groups, excluding it as the cause for our results. BMI and rates of smoking, chronic hypertension, and pregestational diabetes were higher in the group with IPI > 5 years, and although adjusted in the multivariate analysis, they might also have contributed to the higher adverse outcomes in this group. The finding that this protective effect was lost in the group with IPI longer than 5 years is more compatible with a physiological mechanism, rather than an association with a categorical factor. We suggest that maternal physiological adaption to pregnancy, mainly vascular (e.g., increased uterine blood flow, reduced systemic resistance, and elevated cardiac output) is a fundamental process that is not everlasting and decreases over time. If this process is not regenerated, with time, the plasticity of these components declines, and therefore the protective effect is lost.

Our study also demonstrated the effect of parity and IPI on maternal adverse outcome. Similar to the neonatal outcomes, advanced maternal age nulliparas, as compared to multiparas, were at higher risk for hypertensive disorders of pregnancy, induction of labor, cesarean deliveries, and postpartum blood transfusions. Interestingly, multiparas with IPI > 5 years had significantly higher rate of gestational hypertension in comparison to multiparas with IPI < 5 years (8.3 vs. 5.3, $p < 0.001$). However, the overall impact of parity as well as of IPI for the mother, seems less significant compared to the impact on adverse neonatal outcome. One possible explanation for the diminished effect may be the association of maternal outcomes with age itself, unlike neonatal or pregnancy complications that may be more related to the maternal adaptation to pregnancy, other than to the absolute age-related risk [26].

Our study has several strengths. It is a population-based study that includes more than 100,000 parturients older than 40 years. The large sample size of our study enables evaluation of risk in subgroups within an overall high-risk cohort of parturients. In addition, the diverse population that derives from using a national data-base, with the use of multivariable logistic regression analysis allows us to control for risk factors that are already known to be associated with each adverse outcome. However, our study has also limitations, majority of them attributed to its retrospective design. The study is representative of all live birth in the United States in 2017 and, therefore, includes medical centers with heterogenicity in practice patterns that may have an effect on at least some of the measured outcomes. In addition, we excluded multiple gestations and pregnancies complicated by intrauterine fetal death, which is no doubt an important adverse outcome ignored in this study. Data on assisted reproductive therapy were available to only small part of the cohort and were possibly influenced by reporting bias. Lastly, this study is also prone to limitations of vital statistics data, which include likely underreporting of maternal comorbidities or other adverse outcomes.

5. Conclusions

In summary, our study demonstrates that among advanced maternal age gravidas, a previous delivery within 5 years interval has a significant protective effect against adverse neonatal outcomes when compared to nulliparas. In case of IPI of more than 5 years, this effect is lost, and the risk for adverse neonatal outcomes becomes comparable to that of advanced maternal age nullipara. We suggest that an IPI longer than 5 years should be considered as a significant risk factor for pregnancy complications and needs to be combined with other maternal characteristics when evaluating the individualized risk for adverse pregnancy complications. Early identification of parturient with an increased risk will enable to facilitate targeted surveillance and early intervention. Specifically, advanced maternal age gravidas with IPI > 5 years should be considered high-risk for pregnancy complications. Ideally, they should undergo prepregnancy consultation for possible lifestyle modifications to improve outcomes, and during pregnancy, they should be addressed with higher surveillance, including prophylactic aspirin treatment, close follow-up to detect fetal growth restriction, and serial monitoring for preterm labor and preeclampsia.

Author Contributions: A.N. contributed to the interpretation of data, wrote and revised the manuscript; M.H. contributed to interpretation of data and revision of the manuscript; R.G.-B. contributed to the design of the study, performed the statistical analysis, and wrote and revised the manuscript. All authors have read and agreed to the published version of the manuscript.

Funding: This research received no external funding.

Conflicts of Interest: The authors have no conflict to declare.

References

1. Royal College of Obstetricians & Gynaecologists. RCOG Statement on Later Maternal Age. 2009. Available online: http://www.rcog.org.uk/what-we-do/campaigningand-opinions/statement/rcogstatement-later-maternal-age (accessed on 2 July 2020).
2. Jacobsson, B.; Ladfors, L.; Milsom, I. Advanced Maternal Age and Adverse Perinatal Outcome. *Obstet. Gynecol.* **2004**, *104*, 727–733. [CrossRef] [PubMed]
3. Joseph, K.S.; Allen, A.C.; Dodds, L.; Turner, L.A.; Scott, H.; Liston, R. The Perinatal Effects of Delayed Childbearing. *Obstet. Gynecol.* **2005**, *105*, 1410–1418. [CrossRef] [PubMed]
4. Khalil, A.; Syngelaki, A.; Maiz, N.; Zinevich, Y.; Nicolaides, K.H. Maternal Age and Adverse Pregnancy Outcome: A Cohort Study. *Ultrasound Obstet. Gynecol. Off. J. Int. Soc. Ultrasound Obstet. Gynecol.* **2013**, *42*, 634–643. [CrossRef] [PubMed]
5. Lean, S.C.; Derricott, H.; Jones, R.L.; Heazell, A.E.P. Advanced Maternal Age and Adverse Pregnancy Outcomes: A Systematic Review and Meta-Analysis. *PLoS ONE* **2017**, *12*, e0186287. [CrossRef]

6. Frederiksen, L.E.; Ernst, A.; Brix, N.; Braskhøj Lauridsen, L.L.; Roos, L.; Ramlau-Hansen, C.H.; Ekelund, C.K. Risk of Adverse Pregnancy Outcomes at Advanced Maternal Age. *Obstet. Gynecol.* **2018**, *131*, 457–463. [CrossRef]
7. Bai, J.; Wong, F.W.S.; Bauman, A.; Mohsin, M. Parity and Pregnancy Outcomes. *Am. J. Obstet. Gynecol.* **2002**, *186*, 274–278. [CrossRef]
8. Shechter-Maor, G.; Sadeh-Mestechkin, D.; Ganor Paz, Y.; Sukenik Halevy, R.; Markovitch, O.; Biron-Shental, T. Does Parity Affect Pregnancy Outcomes in the Elderly Gravida? *Arch. Gynecol. Obstet.* **2020**, *301*, 85–91. [CrossRef]
9. Zhu, B.P.; Rolfs, R.T.; Nangle, B.E.; Horan, J.M. Effect of the Interval between Pregnancies on Perinatal Outcomes. *N. Engl. J. Med.* **1999**, *340*, 589–594. [CrossRef]
10. Ishaque, U.; Korb, D.; Poincare, A.; Schmitz, T.; Morin, C.; Sibony, O. Long Interpregnancy Interval and Mode of Delivery. *Arch. Gynecol. Obstet.* **2019**, *300*, 1621–1631. [CrossRef]
11. Rousso, D.; Panidis, D.; Gkoutzioulis, F.; Kourtis, A.; Mavromatidis, G.; Kalahanis, I. Effect of the Interval between Pregnancies on the Health of Mother and Child. *Eur. J. Obstet. Gynecol. Reprod. Biol.* **2002**, *105*, 4–6. [CrossRef]
12. Lin, J.; Liu, H.; Wu, D.-D.; Hu, H.-T.; Wang, H.-H.; Zhou, C.-L.; Liu, X.-M.; Chen, X.-J.; Sheng, J.-Z.; Huang, H.-F. Long Interpregnancy Interval and Adverse Perinatal Outcomes: A Retrospective Cohort Study. *Sci. China Life Sci.* **2020**, *63*, 898–904. [CrossRef] [PubMed]
13. Conde-Agudelo, A.; Belizán, J.M. Maternal Morbidity and Mortality Associated with Interpregnancy Interval: Cross Sectional Study. *BMJ* **2000**, *321*, 1255–1259. [CrossRef] [PubMed]
14. World Health Organization. *Report of a WHO Technical Consultation on Birth Spacing: Geneva, Switzerland 13–15 June 2005*; World Health Organization: Geneva, Switzerland, 2007.
15. Elhakham, D.; Wainstock, T.; Sheiner, E.; Sergienko, R.; Pariente, G. Inter-Pregnancy Interval and Long-Term Neurological Morbidity of the Offspring. *Arch. Gynecol. Obstet.* **2020**. [CrossRef] [PubMed]
16. NCHS' Vital Statistics Natality Birth Data. Available online: http://data.nber.org/data/vital-statistics-natality-data.html (accessed on 16 August 2020).
17. Von Elm, E.; Altman, D.G.; Egger, M.; Pocock, S.J.; Gøtzsche, P.C.; Vandenbroucke, J.P. The Strengthening the Reporting of Observational Studies in Epidemiology (STROBE) Statement: Guidelines for Reporting Observational Studies. *J. Clin. Epidemiol.* **2008**, *61*, 344–349. [CrossRef]
18. Rietveld, A.L.; Teunissen, P.W.; Kazemier, B.M.; De Groot, C.J.M. Effect of Interpregnancy Interval on the Success Rate of Trial of Labor after Cesarean. *J. Perinatol.* **2017**, *37*, 1192–1196. [CrossRef]
19. DaVanzo, J.; Hale, L.; Razzaque, A.; Rahman, M. Effects of Interpregnancy Interval and Outcome of the Preceding Pregnancy on Pregnancy Outcomes in Matlab, Bangladesh. *BJOG* **2007**, *114*, 1079–1087. [CrossRef]
20. Grisaru-Granovsky, S.; Gordon, E.-S.; Haklai, Z.; Samueloff, A.; Schimmel, M.M. Effect of Interpregnancy Interval on Adverse Perinatal Outcomes—A National Study. *Contraception* **2009**, *80*, 512–518. [CrossRef]
21. Chen, I.; Jhangri, G.S.; Chandra, S. Relationship between Interpregnancy Interval and Congenital Anomalies. *Am. J. Obstet. Gynecol.* **2014**, *210*, 564.e1–564.e8. [CrossRef]
22. Shachar, B.Z.; Mayo, J.A.; Lyell, D.J.; Baer, R.J.; Jeliffe-Pawlowski, L.L.; Stevenson, D.K.; Shaw, G.M. Interpregnancy Interval after Live Birth or Pregnancy Termination and Estimated Risk of Preterm Birth: A Retrospective Cohort Study. *BJOG Int. J. Obstet. Gynaecol.* **2016**, *123*, 2009–2017. [CrossRef]
23. Henriksen, T.B.; Baird, D.D.; Olsen, J.; Hedegaard, M.; Secher, N.J.; Wilcox, A.J. Time to Pregnancy and Preterm Delivery. *Obstet. Gynecol.* **1997**, *89*, 594–599. [CrossRef]
24. Silva, L.M.; Coolman, M.; Steegers, E.A.; Jaddoe, V.W.; Moll, H.A.; Hofman, A.; Mackenbach, J.P.; Raat, H. Low Socioeconomic Status Is a Risk Factor for Preeclampsia: The Generation R Study. *J. Hypertens.* **2008**, *26*, 1200–1208. [CrossRef] [PubMed]
25. Peacock, J.L.; Bland, J.M.; Anderson, H.R. Preterm Delivery: Effects of Socioeconomic Factors, Psychological Stress, Smoking, Alcohol, and Caffeine. *BMJ* **1995**, *311*, 531–535. [CrossRef] [PubMed]
26. Ling, H.Z.; Guy, G.P.; Bisquera, A.; Poon, L.C.; Nicolaides, K.H.; Kametas, N.A. Maternal Hemodynamics in Screen-Positive and Screen-Negative Women of the ASPRE Trial. *Ultrasound Obstet. Gynecol. Off. J. Int. Soc. Ultrasound Obstet. Gynecol.* **2019**, *54*, 51–57. [CrossRef] [PubMed]

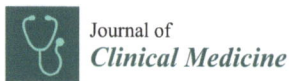

Review

The Impact of Diagnostic Criteria for Gestational Diabetes Mellitus on Adverse Maternal Outcomes: A Systematic Review and Meta-Analysis

Fahimeh Ramezani Tehrani [1], Marzieh Saei Ghare Naz [1], Razieh Bidhendi Yarandi [1] and Samira Behboudi-Gandevani [2,*]

1. Reproductive Endocrinology Research Center, Research Institute for Endocrine Sciences, Shahid Beheshti University of Medical Sciences, Tehran 1985717413, Iran; ramezani@endocrine.ac.ir (F.R.T.); saeigarenaz@gmail.com (M.S.G.N.); razi_bidhendi@yahoo.com (R.B.Y.)
2. Faculty of Nursing and Health Sciences, Nord University, 8049 Bodø, Norway
* Correspondence: samira.behboudi-gandevani@nord.no; Tel.: +47-75517670

Abstract: This systematic review and meta-analysis aimed to examine the impact of different gestational-diabetes (GDM) diagnostic-criteria on the risk of adverse-maternal-outcomes. The search process encompassed PubMed (Medline), Scopus, and Web of Science databases to retrieve original, population-based studies with the universal GDM screening approach, published in English language and with a focus on adverse-maternal-outcomes up to January 2020. According to GDM diagnostic criteria, the studies were classified into seven groups. A total of 49 population-based studies consisting of 1,409,018 pregnant women with GDM and 7,667,546 non-GDM counterparts were selected for data analysis and knowledge synthesis. Accordingly, the risk of adverse-maternal-outcomes including primary-cesarean, induction of labor, maternal-hemorrhage, and pregnancy-related-hypertension, overall, regardless of GDM diagnostic-criteria and in all diagnostic-criteria subgroups were significantly higher than non-GDM counterparts. However, in meta-regression, the increased risk was not influenced by the GDM diagnostic-classification and the magnitude of the risks among patients, using the IADPSG criteria-classification as the most strict-criteria, was similar to other criteria. In conclusion, a reduction in the diagnostic-threshold increased the prevalence of GDM, but the risk of adverse-maternal-outcome was not different among those women who were diagnosed through more or less intensive strategies. Our review findings can empower health-care-providers to select the most cost-effective approach for the screening of GDM among pregnant women.

Keywords: adverse maternal outcomes; diagnostic criteria; gestational diabetes; meta-analysis

Citation: Ramezani Tehrani, F.; Naz, M.S.G.; Yarandi, R.B.; Behboudi-Gandevani, S. The Impact of Diagnostic Criteria for Gestational Diabetes Mellitus on Adverse Maternal Outcomes: A Systematic Review and Meta-Analysis. *J. Clin. Med.* **2021**, *10*, 666. https://doi.org/10.3390/jcm10040666

Academic Editor: Rinat Gabbay-Benziv
Received: 12 January 2021
Accepted: 3 February 2021
Published: 9 February 2021

Publisher's Note: MDPI stays neutral with regard to jurisdictional claims in published maps and institutional affiliations.

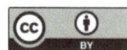

Copyright: © 2021 by the authors. Licensee MDPI, Basel, Switzerland. This article is an open access article distributed under the terms and conditions of the Creative Commons Attribution (CC BY) license (https://creativecommons.org/licenses/by/4.0/).

1. Introduction

Gestational diabetes mellitus (GDM) is one of the most prevalent endocrinopathies during pregnancy and affects 4–12% of all pregnancies depending on the type of diagnostic criteria as well as the prevalence of associated risk factors such as type 2 diabetes (T2DM), body mass index (BMI), advanced maternal age, and ethnicity [1–4]. Chronic disturbances in maternal β-cell, release of diabetogenic peptides from the placenta, and hormones may play a key role in the pathophysiology of GDM [5]. However, GDM is strongly associated with a higher risk of adverse pregnancy outcomes [6,7], lifelong risk of abnormal glucose tolerance, and diabetes later in life [8,9]. However, appropriate treatment strategies for GDM including lifestyle modifications and pharmacotherapy such as insulin or metformin can significantly decrease related adverse outcomes. In addition, inositol as a nutritional supplementation has been shown to improve glycemic homeostasis during pregnancy and prevent GDM [9,10].

There are ongoing debates regarding the optimum GDM screening strategy. In this respect, the risk of developing postpartum T2DM among women with a history of GDN has been used as the first criteria for the definition of GDM; subsequently, GDM has been defined based on adverse pregnancy outcomes [11] after the Hyperglycemia and Adverse Pregnancy Outcomes' (HAPO) study, which has shown a linear continuous association between the increasing values of maternal blood glucose and adverse pregnancy outcomes [12]. The International Association of Diabetes in Pregnancy Study Group (IADPSG) [13] and the World Health Organization (WHO) [14] have recommended 75-g oral glucose tolerance test (75 g-OGTT), as the diagnostic criteria for GDM. Although this definition is one of the lowest thresholds for GDM definition, the evidence supporting this endorsement is consensus-based.

Previous reviews have shown associations between GDM and adverse perinatal outcomes just based on the WHO and IADPSG criteria [6] or the IADPSG and Carpenter and Coustan definition [15].

Lack of an evidence-based international definition of GDM may potentially influence the accurate estimation of the risk of adverse maternal outcomes. Therefore, this systematic review and meta-analysis examined the impact of various GDM criteria on the risk of adverse maternal outcomes.

2. Materials and Methods

The standard guideline for conducting and reporting meta-analysis [16] was used in this review. The review objectives were as follows:

- To study the pooled risk of adverse maternal outcomes among pregnant women with GDM compared to non-GDM counterparts, regardless of diagnostic criteria;
- To study the pooled risk of adverse maternal outcomes among pregnant women with GDM compared to non-GDM women, according to the various diagnostic criteria;
- To study the association between adverse maternal outcomes and GDM criteria.

2.1. Eligibility Criteria

Satisfaction with fulfilling the following criteria was considered for selecting studies: universal screening of GDM; having a population-based design; full description of the GDM screening method and glucose cutoff point in the screening test; reporting the prevalence or risk of short-term maternal outcomes in both GDM and non-GDM groups. Non-original studies and also those with unclear data or insufficient information about the review topic were excluded.

2.2. Search Strategy

The authors systematically searched on online databases such as PubMed [including Medline], Scopus, and Web of Science to retrieve original studies published in English on the prevalence, incidence, and risk of adverse maternal outcomes among women with GDM up to January 2020, using the following keywords: (adverse pregnancy outcomes OR pregnancy outcomes OR pregnancy complications OR preeclampsia OR pregnancy-induced hypertension OR gestational hypertension OR PIH OR hemorrhage OR postpartum hemorrhage OR PPH OR placenta abruption OR decolman OR placenta previa OR antepartum hemorrhage OR maternal weight gain OR pregnancy weight gain OR induction of labor OR labor induction OR induced labor OR cesarean sections OR c-section OR abdominal deliveries) AND (pregnancy-induced diabetes OR diabetes in pregnancy OR gestational diabetes mellitus OR gestational diabetes OR GDM).

In addition, the reference lists of the included articles and relevant reviews were manually searched to enhance the possibility of identifying eligible studies.

2.3. Study Selection and Data Extraction

Two investigators (M.S.G.N, S.B.G) independently selected manuscripts by the title, abstract, and full text. Next, the following information from each study were extracted: the first author's name, publication year, study location, sample size, research design, GDM screening characteristics including the screening strategy, details of GDM definition, quality assessment, and outcome measurements in terms of number and prevalence, incidence, or risk of adverse events.

2.4. Study Subgroups and Outcomes of Study

The studies were classified into seven sub-groups according to the GDM definition as follows:

(i) IADPSG criteria, one step screening with oral glucose tolerance test (2 h, 75 g GTT); GDM diagnosis: any of the given values are met or exceeded (fasting: 92 mg/dL, BS-1 h: 180 mg/dL, BS-2 h: 153 mg/dL);
(ii) One step screening with 2 h, 75 g OGTT. GDM diagnosis: any of the given valued are met or exceeded (fasting 100 mg/dL, 2 h: 144 mg/dL);
(iii) One step screening with 2 h, 75 g OGTT. GDM diagnosis: any of the given valued are met or exceeded (fasting: 110 mg/dL, 2 h: 140 mg/dL);
(iv) Group 4, one step screening with 2 h, 75 g OGTT. GDM diagnosis: any of the given values are met or exceeded (fasting 100 mg/dL, BS 2 h: 162 mg/dL);
(v) Two step screening with 1 h-50 g Glucose challenge test (1 h-50 g-GCT), values > 140 mg/dL following 100 g OGTT. GDM diagnosis: two values are met or exceeded (fasting: 95 mg/dL, BS-1 h: 180 mg/dL, BS-2 h: 155 mg/dL, BS-3 h: 140 mg/dL or two step screening with 1 h-50 g-GCT, values > 140 mg/dL following 75 g OGTT. GDM diagnosis: two values are met or exceeded (fasting: 95 mg/dL, BS-1 h: 180 mg/dL, BS-2 h: 155 mg/dL, BS-3 h: 140 mg/dL);
(vi) Two step screening with 1 h-50 g-GCT, values > 140 mg/dL following 100 g OGTT. GDM diagnosis: two values are met or exceeded (fasting: 105 mg/dL, BS-1 h: 155 mg/dL, BS-2 h: 165 mg/dL, BS-1 h: 145 mg/dL);
(vii) One step screening with 75 g OGTT. GDM diagnosis: any of the given valued are met or exceeded (fasting: 128 mg/dL, BS2 h: 140 mg/dL).

The adverse maternal outcomes in this review were primary cesarean; gestational weight gain; induction of labor; maternal hemorrhage including antepartum or postpartum hemorrhage, placenta previa, placenta abruption; hypertension-related pregnancy including pregnancy-induced hypertension, preeclampsia, eclampsia.

For quality appraisal, the modified Newcastle-Ottawa Quality Assessment Scale was used [17]. As a validated and standard scale, it assessed nonrandomized studies for inclusion to meta-analyses in terms of the selection of participants, comparability of the study, and assessment of outcomes. Scores above 6, 3–5, and below 3 were interpreted as high, moderate, and low quality, respectively.

The (ROBINS) tool in non-randomized studies of interventions and observational studies was used for assessing the risk of bias [18], which has been recommended by the Cochrane [19]. Five domains of (i) assessment of exposure, (ii) development of outcome of interest in case and controls, (iii) selection of cases, (iv) selection of cases, and (v) control of prognostic variable in cross-sectional studies and 7 domains of (i) selection of exposed and nonexposed cohort, (ii) assessment of exposure, (iii) presence of outcome of interest at the start of the study, (iv) control of prognostic variables, (v) assessment of the presence or absence of prognostic factors, (vi) assessment of outcome, (vii) adequacy of follow up for cohort studies were used for appraisal. The authors classified their judgment on the quality of each study into high risk, unclear risk, or low risk of bias [19].

2.5. Statistical Analysis

The Stata version 12 was used for data analysis. Heterogeneity was estimated by I^2 statistic. The pooled effect size including pooled odds ratio and pooled standardized mean differences of events was calculated using the fixed or random-effects models with Mantel–Haenszel method. Publication bias was evaluated using Begg's test. The association between the risk of adverse outcome of GDM and its diagnostic criteria as a potential source of heterogeneity was assessed using meta-regression. IADPSG definition criteria were used as the reference group for the comparison. All tests were two-sided and $p < 0.05$ was considered statistically significant.

3. Results

3.1. Literature Search Results and Quality assessment

Figure 1 illustrates the flow diagram of the search strategy and study selection.

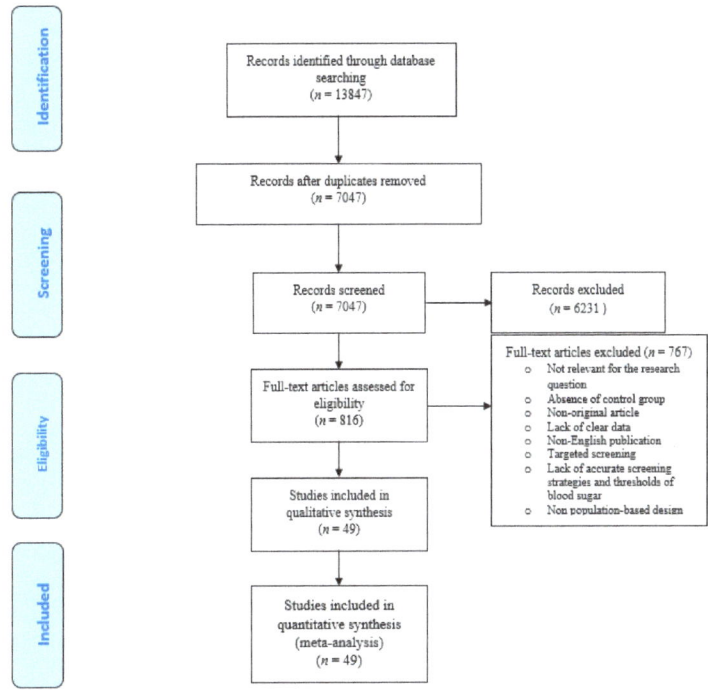

Figure 1. Flow diagram of literature search.

The search led to 13,847 studies of which 49 studies had the required inclusion criteria and were included in the meta-analysis. The studies' populations were 1,409,018 pregnant women with GDM and 7,667,546 non-GDM counterparts. Table 1 shows the summary of the studies evaluating the risk of adverse maternal outcomes among GDM and non-GDM populations.

Table 1. Characteristics of studies assessing the adverse pregnancy outcome in gestational diabetes mellitus (GDM) and non-GDM population.

Author, Year	Country	GDM Diagnostic Criteria	GDM Characteristics *	Non-GDM Characteristics *	Adverse Maternal Outcome in Women with vs. without GDM, % or Mean (SD)
Capula et al., 2013	Italy	IADPSG	n = 171, Age: 30.8 (3.2), BMI: 22.8 (1.9)	n = 367, Age: 29.3 (3.5), BMI: 21.4 (2.0)	Hypertension: 4.1 vs. 1.6; Preeclampsia: 2.9 vs. 1.4; Labor induction: 1.2 vs. 0.3; gestational weight gain: 10.3 (3.4) vs. 8 (2.8); Primary cesarean section: 29.8 vs. 15.3
Karmon et al., 2009	Israel	CC	n = 10,227	n = 174,029	Hypertensive disorders: 11.6 vs. 5.5 Abruption: 0.8 vs. 0.7; Labor induction: 42.1 vs. 27.0.
Moses et al., 1995	Australia	ADIPS	n = 138, Age: 29.5 (5.3)	n = 144, Age: 28.2 (5.4)	PIH:13.8 vs. 13.2; Labor induction: 26.8 vs. 26.4
Waters et al., 2016	North American	(1) IADPSG (2) CC	(1) n = 878, Age: 31.0 (5.6), BMI: 31.5 (6.4) (2) n = 261, Age: 32.3 (5.3), BMI: 31.6 (5.8)	n = 5020, Age: 30.1 (5.8), BMI: 28.2 (4.9)	(1) Preeclampsia: 14.9 vs. 6.4; Primary cesarean section: 23.9 vs. 17.2 (2) Preeclampsia: 14 vs. 6.4; Primary cesarean section: 30.4 vs. 17.2
Gu et al., 2019	China	WHO-1999	GDM with hypertensive disorders of pregnancy: n = 91, Age: 33.8 (3.59), Pre-pregnancy BMI: 25.1 (3.64) GDM without hypertensive disorders of pregnancy: n = 1172, Age: 33.3 (3.49), Pre-pregnancy BMI: 22.9 (3.24)	Non-GDM with hypertensive disorders of pregnancy: n = 261, Age: 32.9 (2.68), Pre-pregnancy BMI: 22.2 (3.04) Non-GDM without hypertensive disorders of pregnancy: n= 261, Age: 32.9 (2.84), Pre-pregnancy BMI: 21.4 (2.96)	Non hypertensive disorder: Gestational weight gain, kg: 16.6 (5.87) vs. 18.2 (6.67) Hypertensive disorder: Gestational weight gain, kg: 19.0 (7.01) vs. 21.3 (6.14)
Shand et al., 2008	Australia	ADIPS	n = 16,727	n = 349,933	Pre-eclampsia: 6.7 vs. 4.4; Gestational hypertension: 6.9 vs. 4.2; Placenta Previa or abruption: 1.6 vs. 1.1; APH: 1.5 vs. 1.1; PPH: 6.3 vs. 6; Severe PPH: 0.9 vs. 0.7; Labor induction: 32.7 vs. 23.9
Anderberg et al., 2010	Sweden	WHO-1999	n = 306, Age: 32 (18–46)	n = 329, Age: 31 (20–42)	Labor induction: 18.6 vs. 6.4
Avalos et al., 2013	Ireland	IADPSG	n = 622, Age: 32.8	n = 4225, Age: 31 (4.9)	GDM without risk factor vs. GDM with risk factor vs. Non-GDM Hypertension: 13 vs. 15 vs. 7
Wahabi et al., 2017	Saudi Arabia	WHO-2013	n = 2354, Age: 31.5 (5.9)	n = 6951, Age: 29.5 (5.7)	Gestational hypertension: 1.8 vs. 1.3; Preeclampsia/superimposed: 1 vs. 1.1; Labor induction: 17.9 vs. 16
Meek et al., 2015	UK	(1) IADPSG (2) NICE	(1) n = 387, Age: 32.6, BMI: 27.4 (2) n = 261, Age: 32.1, BMI: 25.5	n = 2406, Age: 31.4, BMI: 26	(1) Pre-eclampsia: 10.1 vs. 7.2; PPH:1 vs. 2; APH: 1.6 vs. 2.4 (2) Pre-eclampsia: 9.2 vs. 7.2; PPH:0.4 vs. 2; APH: 2.7 vs. 2.4
Boghossian et al., 2014	USA	ICD-9	n = 1279, Age: 30.3 (4.9); Prepregnancy BMI: 28.9 (7.2)	n = 58,224, Age: 28.1 (4.5), Prepregnancy BMI: 24.9 (5.6)	Gestational hypertension: 4.7 vs. 2.2; Preeclampsia: 3 vs. 1.6; Labor induction: 40.2 vs. 39.4
Kawakita et al., 2017	USA	ICD-9	n = 11,327, Age: 30.8 (6.0), BMI: 34.1 (7.5)	n= 208,355, Age: 27.4 (6.1), BMI: 30.6 (6.1)	Pregnancy-associated hypertension: 11.7 vs. 7.2

Table 1. Cont.

Author, Year	Country	GDM Diagnostic Criteria	GDM Characteristics *	Non-GDM Characteristics *	Adverse Maternal Outcome in Women with vs. without GDM, % or Mean (SD)
Brand et al. 2018	UK	Modified WHO-1999	White European: n = 210, Age: 30.2 (5.4), BMI: 28.6 (6.3) South Asian: n = 622, Age: 30.7 (5.3), BMI: 28.2 (5.8)	White European: n = 4537, Age: 26.6 (6.0), BMI: 26.5 (5.9) South Asian: n = 5336, Age: 27.7 (5.0), BMI: 25.2 (5.3)	White European Hypertensive disorders of pregnancy: 6.7 vs. 6.7 South Asian Hypertensive disorders of pregnancy: 5.6 vs. 5.2
Kaul et al., 2014	Canada	CDA-2013	GDM only: n = 7332, Age: 31.9 (5.5) GDM and overweight: n = 1399, Age: 31 (5.2)	n = 213,765, Age: 28.6 (5.6)	GDM only vs. GDM and overweight vs. No GDM, not overweight Pre-eclampsia or eclampsia: 1.9 vs. 5.5 vs. 1.2; Labor induction: 42.1 vs. 58.4 vs. 28.5
Kgosidialwa et al., 2015	Ireland	IADPSG	n = 567, Age: 33.4 (4.9), BMI: 30.5 (6.1)	n = 2499, Age: 31.5 (5.2), BMI: 26.7 (4.8)	Pre-eclampsia: 4.2 vs. 3.8; Hypertensive pregnancy disorders: 11.6 vs. 8.3 PIH: 11.6 vs. 7.7
Donovan et al., 2017	Canada	CDA IADPSG	HAPO 1.75: n = 4308, Age: 31.2 (5.1) HAPO 2-1: n = 5528, Age: 31.6 (5.2) HAPO 2-2: n = 3252, Age: 32.1 (5.2)	Normal 50 g screen: n = 144,191, Age: 28.8 (5.3) Normal 75 g OGTT: n = 21,248, Age: 30.3 (5.3)	Normal 50 g screen: Hypertensive disorders of pregnancy: 5.6; Labor induction: 27.5 Normal 75 g OGTT: Hypertensive disorders of pregnancy: 7.3; Labor induction: 27.7 HAPO 1.75: Hypertensive disorders of pregnancy: 9.1; Labor induction: 29.6 HAPO 2-1: Hypertensive disorders of pregnancy: 9.6; Labor induction: 38.2 HAPO 2-2: Hypertensive disorders of pregnancy: 11.7; Labor induction: 42.3
Kieffer et al., 1999	Michigan	NDDG	n = 19, Age: 29.4 (6.2), BMI: 28.7 (5.7)	n = 353, Age: 24.79 (4.85), BMI: 25.1 (4.21)	Hypertensive disorder: 21.1 vs. 7.16
Ekeroma et al., 2014	New Zealand	(1) NZSSD (2) IADPSG (3) ADIPS	(1) n = 381, Age: 31.7 (5.5), BMI: 31.8 (10.8) (2) n = 238, Age: 31.4 (5.8), BMI: 32.9 (11.7) (3) n = 608, Age: 31.5 (5.4), BMI: 30.5 (9.8)	n = 1672, Age: 30.0 (5.7), BMI: 30.7 (9.1)	(1) Pre-eclampsia: 8 vs. 6 (2) Pre-eclampsia: 7 vs. 6 (3) Pre-eclampsia: 7 vs. 6
Aung et al., 2015	Cook Islands	Modified IADPSG	n = 94, Age: 36 (28–40), BMI: 34 (30–39)	n = 28 (23–34), Age: 24.79 (4.85), BMI: 31 (26–36)	Pregnancy weight gain (kg): 6 (3–11) vs. 10 (6–14)
Erjavec et al., 2016	Croatia	(1) WHO-1999 (2) IADPSG	(1) n = 953, Age: 30.88 (5.23), BMI: 25.84 (5.28) (2) n = 1829, Age: 31.34 (5.19), BMI: 26.03 (5.64)	(1) n = 41,703, Age: 28.77 (5.23), BMI: 23.38 (3.99) (2) n = 37,263, Age: 29.49 (5.33), BMI: 23.38 (4.11)	(1) Weight gain: 12.57 (5.62) vs. 14.51 (5.29) (2) Weight gain: 12.50 (5.76) vs. 14.19 (5.71)
Gortazar et al., 2018	Spain	NDDG	n = 35,729, Age: 33.42	n = 704,148, Age: 31.27	Pre-eclampsia: 2.56 vs. 1.44
Zamstein et al., 2018	Israel	ACOG	GDM A1: n = 9460, Age: 32.1 (5.8) GDM A2: n = 724, Age: 33.7 (5.6)	n = 206,013, Age: 28 (5.7)	GDM A1 vs. GDM A2 vs. Non-GDM Hypertensive disorders of pregnancy: 11.2 vs. 18.1 vs. 4.8

Table 1. Cont.

Author, Year	Country	GDM Diagnostic Criteria	GDM Characteristics *	Non-GDM Characteristics *	Adverse Maternal Outcome in Women with vs. without GDM, % or Mean (SD)
Hedderson et al., 2003	California	(1) NDDG (2) CC	(1) n = 1523 (2) n = 840	n = 38,515	(1) Pregnancy-induced hypertension: 3.4 vs. 1.9; Preeclampsia or eclampsia:5.8 vs. 2.9; Placenta previa: 0.6 vs. 0.1; Abruptio placentae: 1 vs. 0.8; Labor induction: 18.4 vs. 14.5 (2) Pregnancy-induced hypertension: 3.6 vs. 1.9; Preeclampsia or eclampsia: 5.6 vs. 2.9; Placenta previa: 0.8 vs. 0.1; Abruptio placentae: 0.5 vs. 0.8; Labor induction: 13.5 vs. 14.5
Hosseini et al., 2018	Iran	IADPSG	Early-onset GDM: n = 93, Age: 30.7 (4.6), Pre-pregnancy BMI: 26.5 (4.2) Late-onset GDM: n = 78, Age: 31.1 (4.9), Pre-pregnancy BMI: 26.2 (4.7)	n = 758, Age: 28.8 (4.6), Pre-pregnancy BMI: 24.2 (4.1)	Early-onset GDM vs. Late-onset GDM vs. Normal Preeclampsia: 6.5 vs. 6.4 vs. 3.6 Gestational hypertension: 8.6 vs. 12.8 vs. 6.1
Hosseini et al., 2018	Iran	(1) IADPSG (2) CC	(1) n = 78, Age: 18–45 (2) n = 35, Age: 18–45	(1) n = 35, Age: 18–45 (2) n = 801, Age: 18–45	(1) Preeclampsia (OR): 1.5; Gestational hypertension (OR): 1.9 (2) Preeclampsia (OR): 2.8; Gestational hypertension (OR): 2.4
Jain et al., 2016	India	DIPSI	N = 8000	n = 7641	PIH: 9 vs. 6; APH/PPH: 0.84 vs. 0.32
Kun et al., 2010	Tolna	WHO-1999	n = 139, Age: 29.6 (5.2), Pregnancy BMI: 25.4 (5.3)	n = 2583, Age: 27.1 (4.9), Pregnancy BMI: 23.1 (4.5)	Weight gain, kg: 9.1 (4.8) vs. 12.9 (5.0)
Leybovitz-Haleluya et al., 2018	Israel	ACOG	GDM A1: n = 9460, Age: 32.1 (5.8) GDM A2: n = 724, Age: 33.7 (5.6)	n = 206,013, Age: 28 (5.7)	GDM A1 vs. GDM A2 vs. No GDM Preeclampsia: 7 vs. 6.4 vs. 3.9
Jacobson et al., 1989	California	NDDG	n = 97, Age: 28.8 (0.5), BMI: 27.6 (0.8)	n = 2107, Age: 26.3 (0.1), BMI: 22.8 (0.1)	Pregnancy-induced hypertension: 3.8 vs. 3.7; Weight gain: 30.2 (1.8) (pounds) vs. 33.0 (0.3)
Pan et al., 2015	China	(1) WHO-1999 (2) IADPSG	(1) n = 257, Age: 29 (2.6), Prepregnancy BMI: 22.9 (3.5) (2) n = 429, Age: 28.8 (2.9), Prepregnancy BMI: 23.9 (4)	(1) n = 16 173, Age: 28.4 (2.8), Prepregnancy BMI: 22.1 (3.3)	(1) PIH: 15.8 vs. 4.8 (2) PIH: 7.5 vs. 4.8
Son et al., 2014	Korea	ICD-10	n = 78,716, Age: 15–49	n = 11171575, Age: 15–49	Pregnancy-induced hypertension without significant proteinuria: 1.71 vs. 1; Pregnancy-induced hypertension with significant proteinuria: 1.66 vs. 1.13; Eclampsia: 0.08 vs. 0.05; Placenta previa: 1.41 vs. 1.16; Premature separation of placenta: 0.42 vs. 0.42; Postpartum hemorrhage: 7.03 vs. 7.30; Antepartum hemorrhage: 2.29 vs. 2.39
Katterfeld et al., 2011	Australia	ADIPS	Australian born n = 4765 CALD n = 1686 Non-CALD n = 1273	Australian born n = 142,537 CALD n = 23,541 Non-CALD n = 31,814	Australian born Pre-eclampsia: 8.4 vs. 5; Labor induction: 54.3 vs. 37.3 CALD Pre-eclampsia: 5.6 vs. 3.6; Labor induction: 37.6 vs. 25.7 Non-CALD Pre-eclampsia: 7.2 vs. 4.6; Labor induction: 51.9 vs. 35

Table 1. Cont.

Author, Year	Country	GDM Diagnostic Criteria	GDM Characteristics *	Non-GDM Characteristics *	Adverse Maternal Outcome in Women with vs. without GDM, % or Mean (SD)
Sacks et al., 2015	California	IADPSG	(1) GDM-1: n = 771, Age: 30.9 (5.6) (2) GDM-2: n = 1121, Age: 31 (5.7)	n = 7943, Age: 26.3 (0.1)	GDM-1 vs. GDM-2 vs. normal Preeclampsia–eclampsia: 4.3 vs. 7.7 vs. 4.4; Primary cesarean delivery: 20.6 vs. 22.3 vs. 16.6
Soliman et al., 2018	Qatar	IADPSG	n = 3027	n = 8995	Hypertensive disorders: 5.5 vs. 3.5; Labor induction: 26.5 vs. 12.4
Xiong et al., 2001	Canada	CDA	n = 2755	n = 8995	Gestational hypertension: 11.4 vs. 4.8; Pre-eclampsia: 1.1 vs. 1.1
Oster et al., 2014	Canada	CDA	n = 1224, Age: 28.8 (6.27)	n = 26,793, Age: 24.7 (5.8)	Pregnancy induced hypertension: 11.3 vs. 4.4; Labor induction: 43.6 vs. 23.8
Sugaya et al., 2000	Japan	(1) JSOG (2) WHO-1998	(1) n = 55, Age: 29.7 (4.3), BMI: 26.2 (3.4) (2) n = 51, Age: 32.8 (4.3), BMI: 26.5 (4.3)	(1) n = 55, Age: 30 (4.7), BMI: 25.5 (3.3)	(1) preeclampsia: 18 vs. 17 (2) preeclampsia: 28 vs. 17
Nerenberg et al., 2013	Canada	CDA	n = 15,404, Age: 31.5 (5.4)	n = 407,268, Age: 28.4 (5.6)	Preeclampsia/eclampsia: 2.6 vs. 1.2; Labor induction: 41.9 vs. 27.1
Edith Kieffer et al., 2006	Mexico	ADA-2003	n = 68, Age: 28.6 (0.6), BMI: 25.7 (0.2)	n = 933, Age: 24.8 (0.2), BMI: 28.4 (0.8)	Weight gain (kg): 10.0 (0.6) vs. 13 (0.2)
Goswami Mahanta et al., 2014	India	DIPSI	N = 28	n = 749	Gestational hypertension: 53.6 vs. 28.1
Ellerbe et al., 2013	USA	ICD-9	Non-Hispanic White: n = 8567, Age: 29.6 (5.9), BMI: 29.3(7.3) Non-Hispanic Black n = 4724, Age: 27.5 (6.2), BMI: 31.7 (7.5)	Non-Hispanic White: n = 126,524, Age: 27.0 (5.9), BMI: 25.7 (6.1) Non-Hispanic Black n = 71,939, Age: 24.3 (5.6), BMI: 28.1(7.0)	Non-Hispanic White Gestational weight gain (kg): 11.7 (7.7) vs. 13.7 (7.6). Non-Hispanic Black Gestational weight gain (kg): 11.5 (8.3) vs. 11.1 (8.0)
Sletner et al., 2017	Norway	WHO-1999	Europe Mild: n = 30, Age: 31.2 (29.5), BMI: 25.5 (23.8, 27.2) Moderate/severe: n = 9, Age: 30.6 (27.6, 33.5); BMI: 30.5 (27.4, 33.6) South Asia Mild: n = 9, Age: 30.7 (28.3, 33.0), BMI: 25.3 (23.2, 27.5) Moderate/severe: n = 4724, Age: 30.4 (28.0, 32.7), BMI: 22.7 (20.6, 24.9)	Europe n = 310, Age: 30.6 (30.1, 31.1), BMI: 24.3 (23.8, 24.8) South Asia n = 156, Age: 28.4 (27.7, 29.1), BMI: 23.7 (23.0, 24.3)	Europe Mild vs. Moderate/Severe vs. Non-GDM Mild hypertension/preeclampsia: 10 vs. 0 vs. 7; Severe hypertension/preeclampsia: 2 vs. 0 vs. 2; inclusion to week 28 GWG: 6.2 (5.2, 7.2) vs. 5.2 (3.4, 7.1) vs. 7.1 (6.8, 7.4), week 28 to birth: 4.0 (2.6, 5.5) vs. 2.0 (-0.4, 4.4) vs. 5.9 (5.5, 6.4) South Asia Mild hypertension/preeclampsia: 7 vs. 14 vs. 3; Severe hypertension/preeclampsia: 0 vs. 7 vs. 2; inclusion to week 28, GWG: 5.6 (3.9, 7.4) vs. 6.5 (4.7, 8.2) vs. 6.6 (6.0, 7.1), week 28 to birth, GWG: 5.1 (2.9, 7.4) vs. 4.8 (2.5, 7.0) vs. 5.2 (4.5, 5.9)
Zeki et al., 2018	Australia	ADIPS	n = 51135, Age: 32.2 (5.3)	n = 950 678, Age: 29.9 (5.6)	Primary Cesarean: Relative % 13.8 vs. 13.5
Hoorn et al., 2002	Australia	ADIPS	n = 51, Age: 30.9 (5.7), BMI:31.5 (.1)	n = 258, Age: 24.9 (6.3), BMI: 25.5 (5.9)	Gestational hypertension: 45.1 vs. 29.1; Preeclampsia: 19.6 vs. 17.1

Table 1. Cont.

Author, Year	Country	GDM Diagnostic Criteria	GDM Characteristics *	Non-GDM Characteristics *	Adverse Maternal Outcome in Women with vs. without GDM, % or Mean (SD)
Su et al., 2019	China	China National criteria	Underweight n = 1466, BMI: 17.55 (0.79) Normal weight n = 6905, BMI: 20.80 (1.21) Overweight n = 2220, BMI: 23.86 (0.57) Obese n = 2252, BMI: 27.21 (2.15)	Underweight n = 12,336, BMI: 17.54 (0.79) Normal weight n = 36,935, BMI: 20.54 (1.2) Overweight n = 6654, BMI: 23.82 (0.56) Obese n = 4730, BMI: 26.97 (1.97)	Normal weight weight gain, kg: 11.45 (3.98) vs. 13.15 (0.25) Underweight weight gain, kg: 12.53 (3.94) vs. 13.76 (3.93) Overweight weight gain, kg: 10.92 (4.49) vs. 12.29 (4.48) Obese weight gain, kg: 8.87 (4.38) vs. 10.50 (4.35)
Metcalfe et al., 2017	Canada	ICD-10	n = 149,780	n = 2,688,231	Gestational hypertension: 7.93 vs. 4; Mild/unspecified Preeclampsia: 0.32 vs. 0.1; Severe preeclampsia: 2.05 vs. 1.18; Placenta previa: 0.9 vs. 0.58; Labor induction: 35.33 (Rate per 100 deliveries) vs. 22.04
Carr et al., 2011	USA	ICD-9&10	n = 1314, Age: 32.7 (5.7)	One abnormal: n= 1242, Age: 32.3 (5.3) Non abnormal: n= 3620, Age: 32 (5.7)	Preeclampsia (n): 111 vs. 102 vs. 226
Lamminpää et al., 2014	Finland	ICD-10	<35 y: n = 19,422 >35 y: n = 7732	<35 y: n = 210,581 >35 y: n = 45,589.00	<35 y: Normal glucose tol. vs. Diet-treated vs. Insulin-treated Preeclampsia: 4.2 vs. 6.7 vs. 7.7; Placenta previa: 0.2 vs. 0.2 vs. 0.2 Late pregnancy bleeding: 1 vs. 1.2 vs. 1.8 >35 y: Normal glucose tol. vs. Diet-treated vs. Insulin-treated Preeclampsia: 5.1 vs. 8.2 vs. 8.6; Placenta previa: 0.4 vs. 0.5 vs. 0.1; Late pregnancy bleeding: 1.3 vs. 1.3 vs. 1.4
Black et al., 2010	California	IADPSG	single isolated impaired glucose tolerance (i-IGT1) n =391, Age: 32.1 (5.4), BMI: 28.1 (5.6) isolated impaired fasting glucose (i-IFG) n = 886, Age: 30.4 (5.6), BMI: 30.8 (7.1) double-isolated impaired glucose tolerance (i-IGT2) n = 83, Age: 32.3 (5.2), BMI: 27.5 (4.7) IFG + IGT n = 331, Age: 32 (5.1), BMI: 31.8 (7)	n = 7020, Age: 28.6 (5.9), BMI: 26.9 (5.8)	i-IGT1 vs. i-IFG vs. i-IGT2 vs. IFG + IGT vs. No GDM Gestational hypertension: 9.8 vs. 10.8 vs. 13.6 vs. 15.4 vs. 7.2; Primary cesarean section: 12.8 vs. 9.1 vs. 18.1 vs. 8.2 vs. 6.6; gestational weight gain: 119 (30.4) (lb) vs. 427 (48.2) vs. 23 (27.7) vs. 175 (52.9) vs. 1737 (24.7)

IADPSG: International Association of Diabetes and Pregnancy Study Groups; CC: Carpenter and Coustan; ADIPS: The Australasian Diabetes in Pregnancy Society; WHO: World Health Organization; NICE: The National Institute for Health and Care Excellence; ICD: International Classification of Diseases; CDA: Canadian Diabetes Association; NZSSD: New Zealand Society for the Study of Diabetes; NDDG: National Diabetes Data Group; ACOG: American College of Obstetricians and Gynecologists; DIPSI: Diabetes In Pregnancy Study group India; JSOG: Japan Society of Obstetrics and Gynecology; BMI: Body mass index; CALD: culturally and linguistically diverse. * age and BMI are reported as mean (standard deviation).

The Supplementary Tables S1 and S2 contain the results of quality assessment. All studies were categorized as high quality [20–68]. A total of 95.9% studies were prospective or retrospective cohorts [22–68] and 4% were cross-sectional studies [20,21]. In addition, 17 (34.6%) studies used the GDM classification of group 1 [21,22,26,35,38,40,47,48,50,51,53,54, 59–61,64,67] and IADPSG; 7 (14.2%) group 2 [20,27,28,51,59,65,68], 3 (6.1%) group 3 [32,46, 56], 1 (2%) group 4 [51], 19 (38.7%) group 5 [23–25,29,31,33,34,36,39,40,42,44,47,53,55,57,58, 64,66], 6 (12.2%) group 6 [37,41,43,44,49,52] and 6 (12.2%) group 7 [21,29,30,45,62,63].

It should be noted that 9 studies used more than one GDM classification [21,29,40,44, 47,51,53,59,64] as follows: 4 studies used classifications 1 and 5 [40,47,52,63], one used 1 and 2 classifications [59], one used classifications 1, 2 and 4 [51], one used classifications 1 and 7 [21], one used classifications 5 and 6 [44], and finally one used classifications 5 and 7 [29].

In addition, 34.69% of the studies were conducted in the U.S. [22,24,25,31,33,34,36–38,41,44,52,53,55,57,58,64], 14.2% in Australia [20,27,28,50,51,65,68], 28.5% in Asia [26,29, 32,35,39,40,42,46–49,60,63,66], and 22.4% in Europe [21,23,30,43,45,54,56,59,61,62,67].

3.2. Meta-Analysis and Meta-Regression Results

The overall pooled OR/mean difference (95% CI) of adverse maternal outcomes, its heterogeneity, and the estimation of publication bias among various subgroups of GDM diagnosis criteria, compared to non-GDM counterparts have been presented in Table 2.

Table 2. Results of meta-analyses for risk/standardized mean difference adverse maternal outcome among women with gestational diabetes according to different GDM screening strategy group.

Outcomes [£]	GDM Classification	Sample Size		Heterogeneity		Publication Bias Begg's Test	Effect Size * (95% CI)	p-Value from Meta-Regression
		GDM Group	Non-GDM Group	I^2 (%)	p-Value			
Primary Cesarean	1	4632	49,353	21.1	0.262	0.621	1.3 (1.2, 1.5)	Ref
	Overall	4990	56,480	41	0.084	0.655	1.4 (1.2, 1.5)	–
Induction of labor	1	10,098	183,424	95.2	0.001	0.327	1.3 (0.9, 1.8)	Ref
	2	25,197	549,639	94.7	0.001	0.851	1.8 (1.5, 2.1)	0.144
	5	196,263	4,151,466	97.4	0.001	0.371	1.8 (1.6, 2.0)	0.112
	Overall	233,767	4,925,044	97.5	0.001	0.766	1.7 (1.6, 1.9)	–
Maternal Hemorrhage	2	67,430	1,404,544	79.9	0.001	0.348	1.2 (1.0, 1.4)	[£] Ref
	5	609,575	9,821,846	95	0.001	0.680	1.1 (1.0, 1.3)	0.867
	6	3046	77,031	91.9	0.001	0.317	2.6 (0.5, 12.6)	0.126
	Overall	688,825	11,315,874	93	0.001	0.523	1.2 (1.0, 1.3)	–
Pregnancy related Hypertension	1	20,021	269,637	38.2	0.031	0.766	1.5 (1.4, 1.7)	Ref
	2	42,287	902,497	1.6	0.424	0.325	1.6 (1.5, 1.6)	0.784
	3	8860	18,263	74.2	0.009	0.497	1.3 (0.9, 1.9)	0.535
	5	771,027	14,009,374	98.7	0.001	0.207	2.0 (1.8, 2.4)	0.38
	6	42,762	959,991	76.4	0.005	0.051	2.1 (1.7, 2.6)	0.160
	7	751	18,674	0	0.471	0.484	1.8 (1.3, 2.5)	0.248
	Overall	886,089	1,618,008	96.3	0.001	0.541	1.7 (1.6, 1.9)	–
Gestational weight gain	1	18,518	142,679	99.5	0.001	0.337	−0.307 (−0.560, −0.054)	Ref
	5	14,689	257,901	90	0.001	0.624	−0.353 (−0.569, −0.137)	0.911
	7	2410	45,271	84.7	0.001	1.000	−0.400 (−0.567, −0.233)	0.988
	Overall	35,714	447,958	99.4	0.001	0.564	−0.333 (−0.492, −0.174)	–

* Effect size represents the odds ratio for all variables, except for weight gain that is the standardized mean difference. [£] Analysis was not performed in all subgroups of GDM classifications due to insufficient data. [€] As there were not enough studies in the first classification, the second one as a reference group for comparison was used.

The odds ratio of primary cesarean among women with GDM, regardless of GDM classification, was 1.4 folds greater than in healthy controls (Pooled overall OR = 1.4, 95% CI: 1.2, 1.5) (Figure 2).

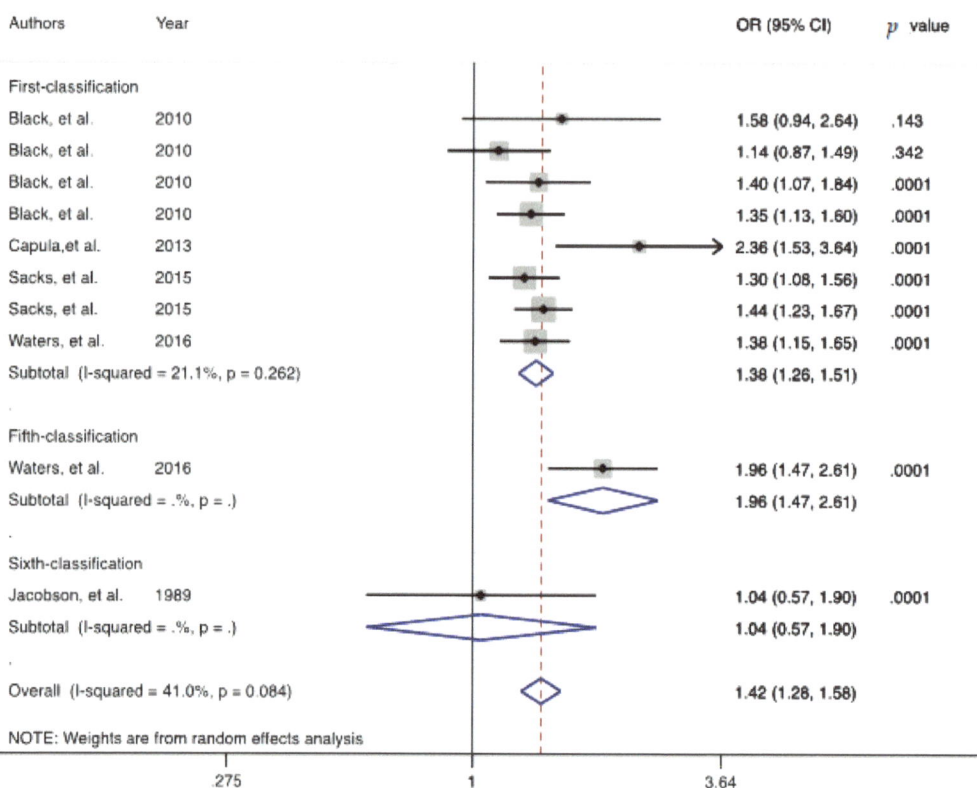

Figure 2. Meta-analysis forest plot of odds ratio (OR) OR for primary cesarean in women with and without Gestational Diabetes Mellitus (GDM) based on different diagnostic criteria.

In addition, risk of other adverse maternal outcomes, including induction of labor (Pooled overall OR = 1.7, 95% CI: 1.6, 1.9), maternal hemorrhage (Pooled overall OR = 1.2, 95% CI: 1.0, 1.3), and pregnancy-related hypertension (Pooled overall OR = 1.7, 95% CI: 1.6, 1.9) among women with GDM, regardless of GDM diagnostic classification, were significantly higher than non-GDM counterparts (Table 2, Figures 3–5).

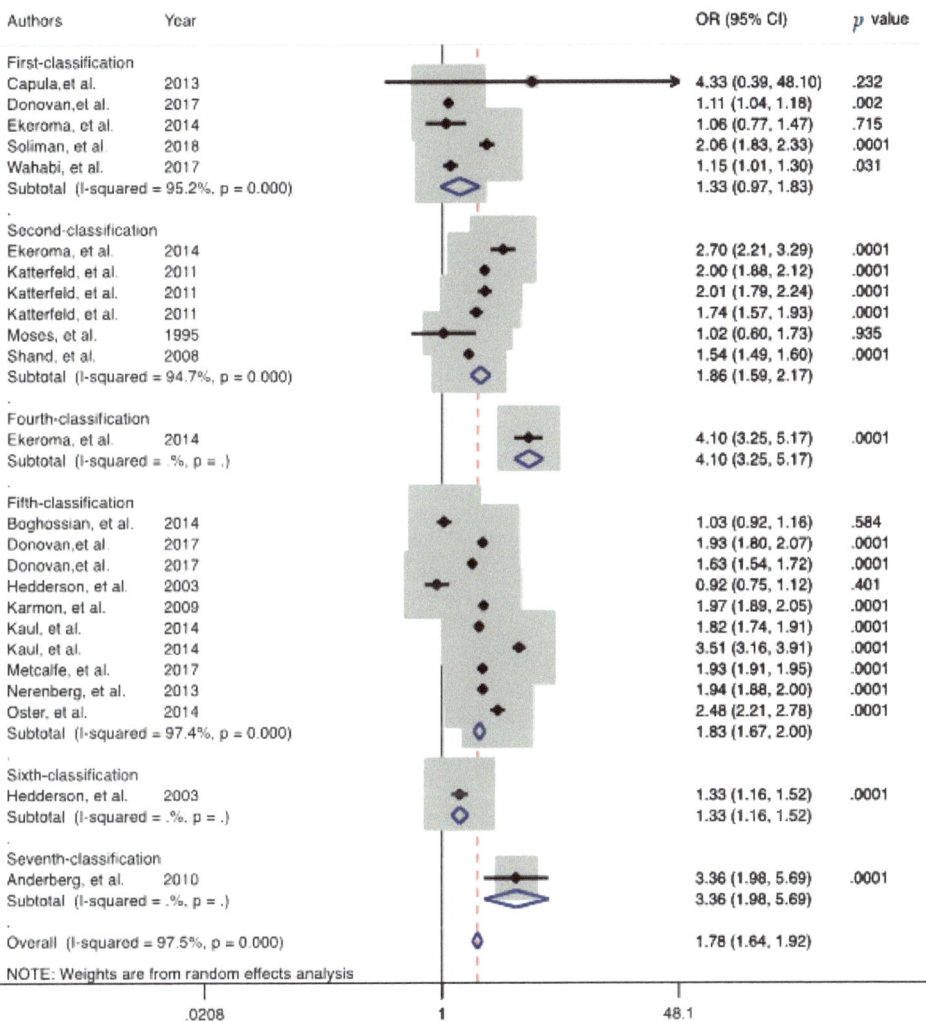

Figure 3. Meta-analysis forest plot of OR for the induction of labor among women with and without GDM based on different diagnostic criteria.

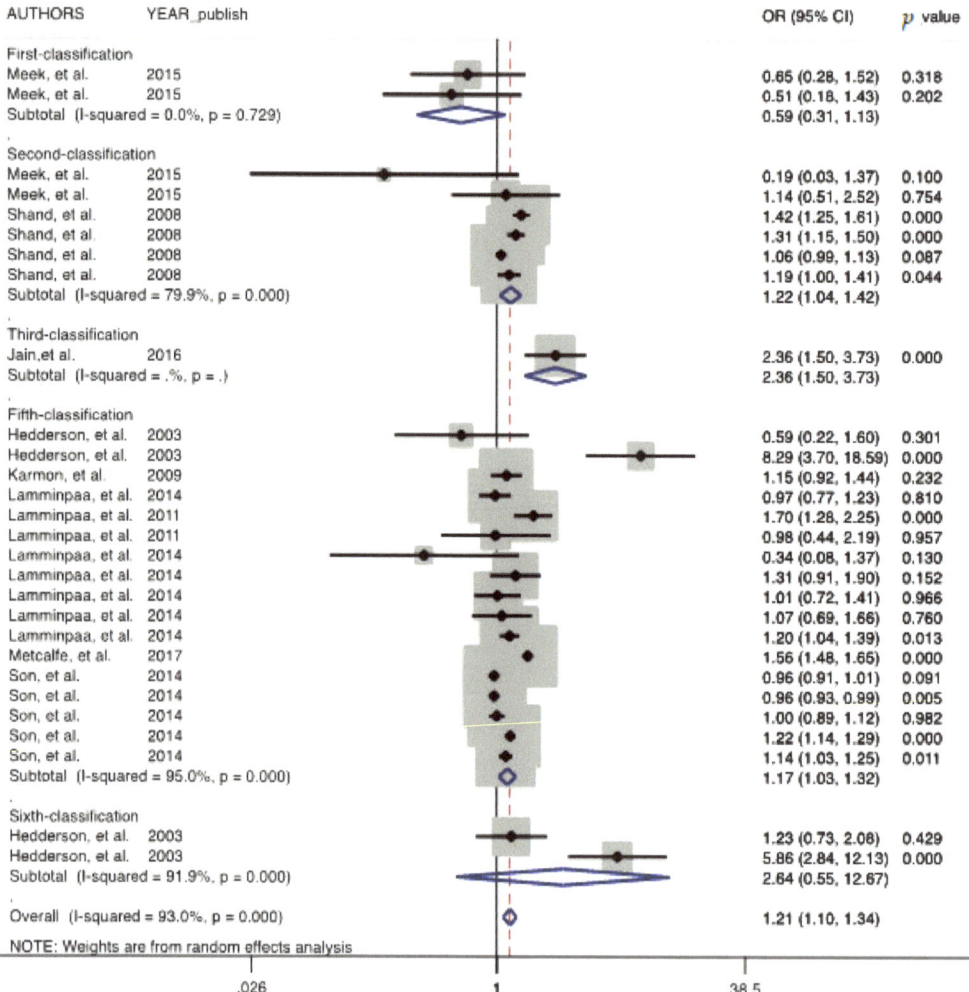

Figure 4. Meta-analysis forest plot of OR for maternal hemorrhage among women with and without GDM based on different diagnostic criteria.

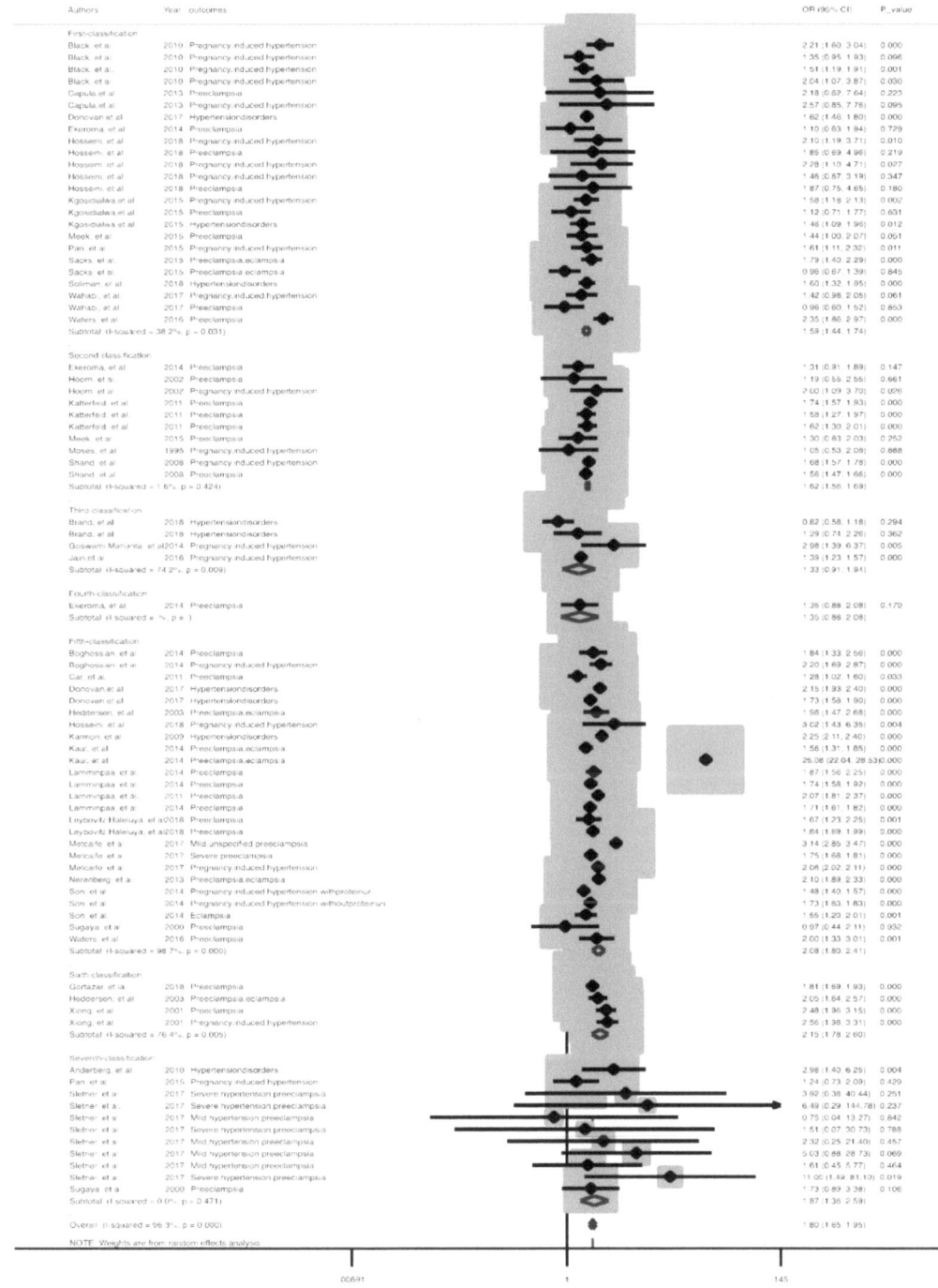

Figure 5. Meta-analysis forest plot of OR for pregnancy-related hypertension among women with and without GDM based on different diagnostic criteria.

The gestational weight gain among women with GDM was significantly lower than the non-GDM population, (Pooled overall mean difference = −0.333, 95% CI (−0.492, −0.174) (Figure 6).

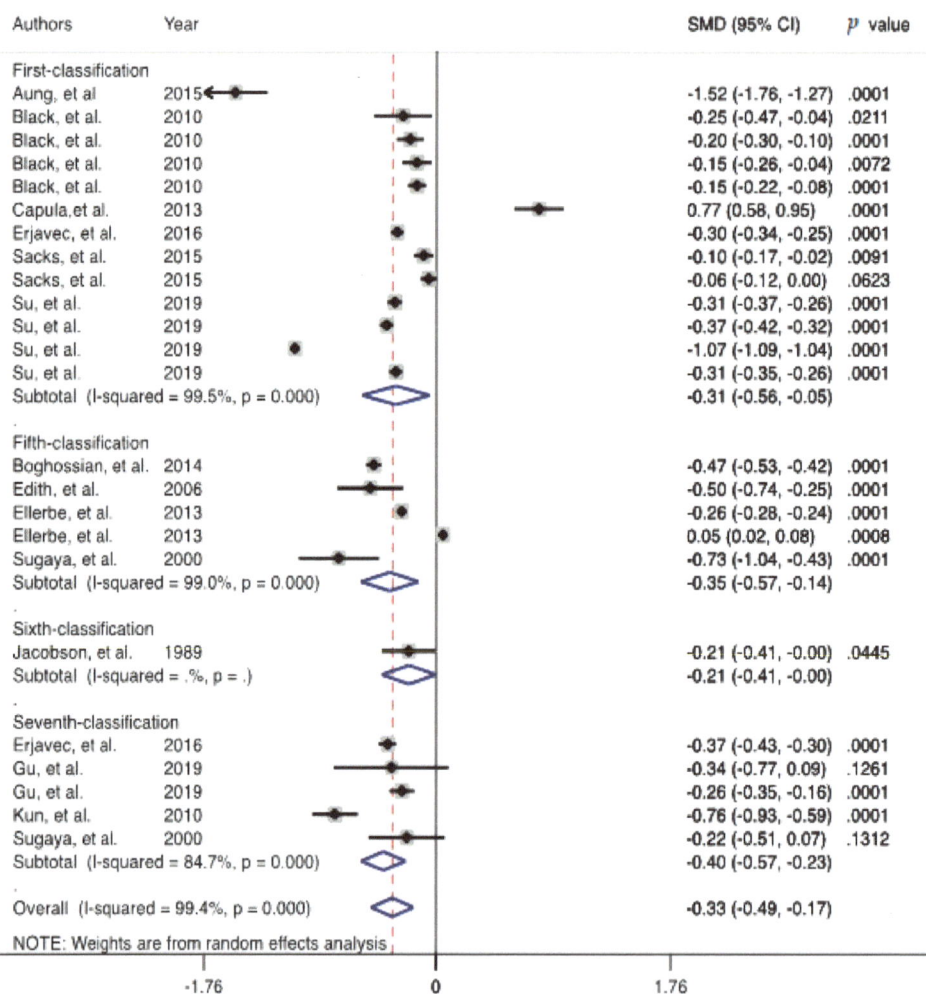

Figure 6. Meta-analysis forest plot of the mean difference of gestational weight gain among women with and without GDM based on different diagnostic criteria.

Subgroup analysis revealed that the risk of adverse maternal outcomes in women with GDM in all GDM diagnostic classifications were significantly higher than the non-GDM population (Table 2).

The results of meta-regression showed that the odds ratio/mean difference were not influenced by GDM diagnostic classification. The risk of adverse maternal outcomes in the IADPSG criteria classification, as the strictest criteria, was similar to others (Figure 7).

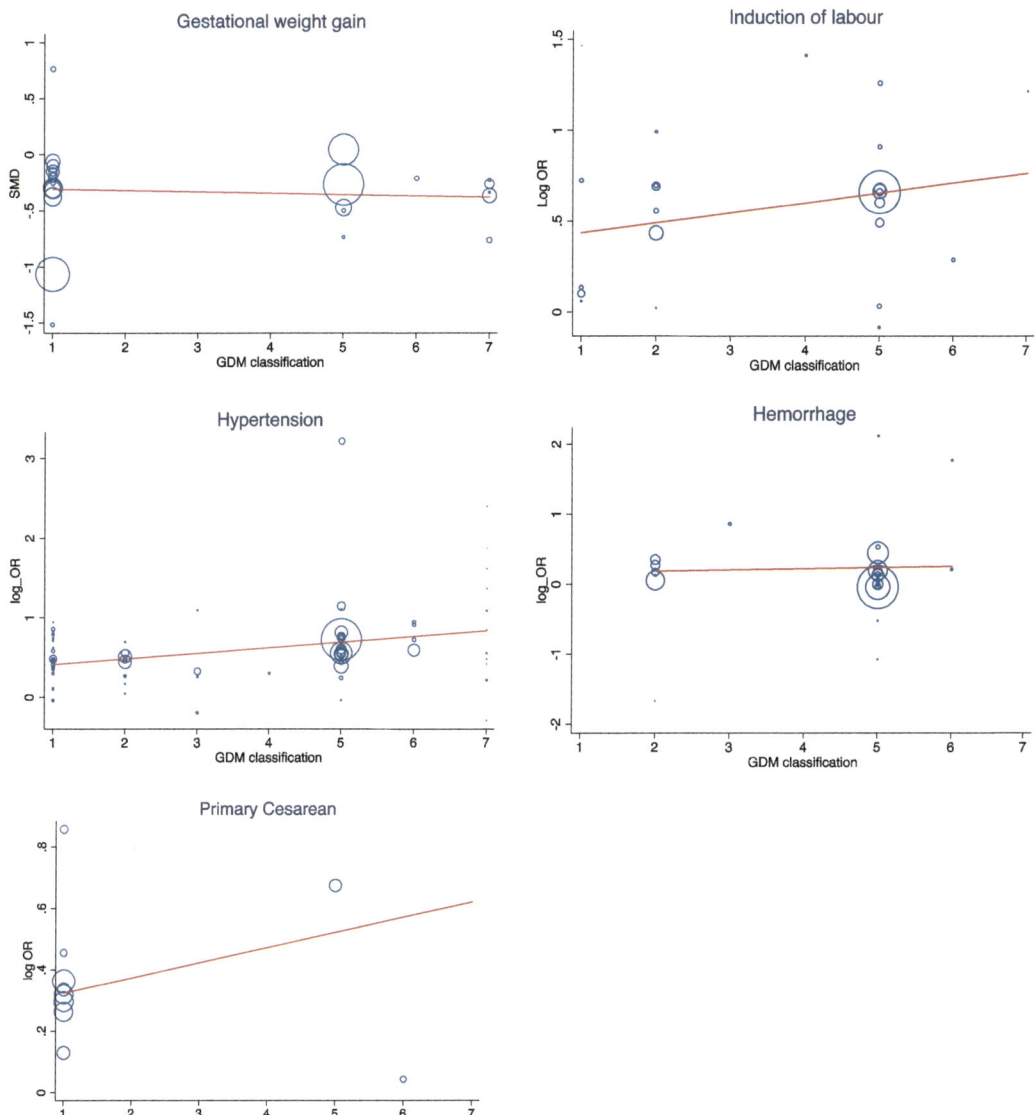

Figure 7. Bubble plot of the meta-regression relationships adverse outcomes and GDM classification.

3.3. Results of Publication Bias and Risk of Bias evaluation

According to Begg's test, no considerable publication bias for various meta-analyses was observed (Table 2). Results of the Risk of Bias evaluation are presented in Supplementary Figures S1A,B and S2A,B. Given that all included studies were observational, the overall risk of bias was low or probably low. However, half of the cross-sectional studies had a probably high risk of bias in the control of prognostic variables. 10% of cohort studies had a probable or high risk of bias in the assessment of exposure and bias in controlling prognostic variables.

4. Discussion

Results of this systematic review and meta-analysis demonstrated that GDM, regardless of its diagnostic classification, could increase the risk of adverse maternal outcomes; however, the key finding is that, despite variations in screening approaches, screening methods, and diagnostic threshold values, the increased risk was not influenced by the GDM diagnostic classification.

Despite the wide range of endorsements and guidelines for the diagnosis of GDM in pregnant women recommended by international societies [1,13,69–74], there is a strong controversy over the definition of GDM including advice on selective approaches such as universal or risk-based screening, the optimal time for screening in the first and second trimesters, appropriate screening method or criteria for diagnosis, and proper threshold values. Furthermore, there are ongoing debates concerning the risk of adverse pregnancy outcomes and the cost-effectiveness of different screening or diagnostic strategies. However, the aim of almost six decades of research and tremendous efforts has been to reach a global consensus and uniformly accepted guideline with regard to the optimum and cost-effective approach for screening by which the risk of adverse pregnancy outcome is reduced.

The risk of adverse perinatal events using two main GDM diagnostic criteria has been studied by previous reviews. Given that our systematic review and meta-analysis compared all available criteria, it can have a complementary role to the findings of other reviews. For instance, Wendland et al. (2012) [6] in a systematically review and meta-analysis of the relationship between GDM based on the WHO and IADPSG criteria, and adverse events of preeclampsia and cesarean delivery, reported that these criteria could identify women with an elevated risk of adverse perinatal events. The same magnitude for both criteria was reported in our review. Another meta-analysis by Hosseini et al. (2018) [15] assessed the magnitude of the association between GDM using the IADPSG or Carpenter and Coustan criteria and selected adverse perinatal events. They demonstrated that the risk of adverse pregnancy events including preeclampsia, cesarean section, and gestational hypertension increased in both GDM criteria. Although associations with the Carpenter and Coustan criteria were slightly greater, it was not confirmed by the statistical test.

The results of our review demonstrated that despite an increased risk of adverse maternal outcomes among women with GDM, this risk had a similar magnitude for all GDM diagnostic classification. Considering that the use of the strict IADPSG criteria has a significant impact on health care costs and infrastructure capacity with a similar magnitude on short term adverse maternal outcomes, the cost-effectiveness of their use should be defined. Until now, there are not sufficient data to demonstrate the cost-effectiveness superiority of one screening and diagnostic approach over the other [75,76]. In addition, most available cost-effectiveness studies [75,77–80] were performed in developed societies with higher health economic resources and a lower rate of annual birth than developing and transitional countries [81].

Moreover, the label of GDM, its exhausting treatment, concerns about pregnant women, and unborn health status are some sources of stress, which may lead to a serious psychological problem for some pregnant women and families and could diminish the quality of life [82–84]. However, using the optimum cost-effective GDM diagnosis approach with an improved adverse outcome such problems can be prevented.

It is believed that GDM is associated with adverse perinatal events and our meta-analysis confirmed the findings of available literature. Diagnosis of GDM is associated with more pregnancy-related hypertension, and higher rates of induction of labor and primary cesarean section, irrespective of the diagnostic criteria used for GDM. However, insulin resistance has also been hypothesized to contribute to the pathophysiology of adverse outcomes [85]. In our review despite the lower gestational weight gain, an increase in the rate of primary cesarean was seen, which was associated with GDM and an increase in the frequency of induction of labor. It is assumed that gestational weight gain may not be the important factor responsible for the higher odds of cesarean section or induction of labor among women with GDM compared to non-GDM counterparts [7]. Fetal size and macrosomia given fetal insulin response to the elevated glucose level in the body of pregnant women or overtreatment may be associated with an elevated prevalence of cesarean section [7,86]. Moreover, the label of GDM can lead to a tendency toward cesarean section.

Ass the limitations of this review, studies that used the universal screening strategy were selected for inclusion in the meta-analysis. Therefore, studies from north Europe with a low prevalence of GDM that might use a targeted high-risk screening strategy were not included in our review. The short-term maternal outcomes of GDM were considered in our review indicating the need to evaluate the long-term adverse outcomes of GDM based on different diagnostic criteria. Also, given the lack of data on some GDM diagnostic criteria, subgroup analysis for classifications could not be carried out and the lack of a unique definition for each adverse pregnancy outcome may have affected our review findings and their generalizability. Additionally, the effect of diagnostic criteria on outcomes irrespective of GDM treatment strategies might have influenced the results.

5. Conclusions

The use of the straighten criteria of the IAPDSG definition can increase the prevalence of GDM among pregnant women. Also, the magnitude of the increased risk of adverse maternal outcomes in all diagnostic criteria was similar. The finding of our review can empower health care providers to select the cost-effective GDM screening approach for pregnant women.

Supplementary Materials: The following are available online at https://www.mdpi.com/2077-0383/10/4/666/s1, Table S1: Quality assessment of studies using the Newcastle–Ottawa Quality Assessment Scale for cohort studies., Table S2: Quality assessment of included studies using the Newcastle–Ottawa Quality Assessment Scale for cross-sectional study, Figure S1: Risk of bias in cross-sectional studies, Figure S2: Risk of bias in cohort studies.

Author Contributions: Conceptualization, F.R.T. and S.B.-G.; methodology, F.R.T. and S.B.-G.; software, M.S.G.N. and R.B.Y.; formal analysis, R.B.Y. and F.R.T.; investigation, M.S.G.N., S.B.-G. and F.R.T.; data curation, F.R.T., S.B.-G. and M.S.G.N.; writing—original draft preparation, F.R.T. and M.S.G.N.; writing—review and editing, S.B.-G. and R.B.Y.; supervision, F.R.T. and S.B.-G.; project administration, F.R.T.; funding acquisition, S.B.-G. All authors have read and agreed to the published version of the manuscript.

Funding: This research was funded by National Institutes for Medical Research Development (NIMAD), grant number 972438.

Institutional Review Board Statement: Not applicable.

Informed Consent Statement: Not applicable.

Data Availability Statement: The data presented in the study are available on request from the corresponding author.

Acknowledgments: The authors would like to thank Marzieh Atashkar, the library staff of the Research Institute for Endocrine Sciences, for assistance with the literature search. Also, Nord University, Bodø, Norway covered the article processing charges.

Conflicts of Interest: The authors declare no conflict of interest.

References

1. American Diabetes Association. Classification and Diagnosis of Diabetes: Standards of Medical Care in Diabetes—2020. *Diabetes Care* **2020**, *43*, S14–S31. [CrossRef]
2. Behboudi-Gandevani, S.; Amiri, M.; Yarandi, R.B.; Tehrani, F.R. The impact of diagnostic criteria for gestational diabetes on its prevalence: A systematic review and meta-analysis. *Diabetol. Metab. Syndr.* **2019**, *11*, 1–18. [CrossRef]
3. Gabbay-Benziv, R.; Doyle, L.E.; Blitzer, M.; Baschat, A.A. First trimester prediction of maternal glycemic status. *J. Périnat. Med.* **2015**, *43*, 283–289. [CrossRef]

4. Giannakou, K.; Evangelou, E.; Yiallouros, P.; Christophi, C.A.; Middleton, N.; Papatheodorou, E.; Papatheodorou, S.I. Risk factors for gestational diabetes: An umbrella review of meta-analyses of observational studies. *PLoS ONE* **2019**, *14*, e0215372. [CrossRef]
5. Plows, J.F.; Stanley, J.L.; Baker, P.; Reynolds, C.M.; Vickers, M.H. The Pathophysiology of Gestational Diabetes Mellitus. *Int. J. Mol. Sci.* **2018**, *19*, 3342. [CrossRef]
6. Morikawa, M.; Sugiyama, T.; Sagawa, N.; Hiramatsu, Y.; Ishikawa, H.; Hamada, H.; Kameda, T.; Hara, E.; Toda, S.; Minakami, H. Perinatal mortality in Japanese women diagnosed with gestational diabetes mellitus and diabetes mellitus. *J. Obstet. Gynaecol. Res.* **2017**, *43*, 1700–1707. [CrossRef] [PubMed]
7. Gorgal, R.; Gonçalves, E.; Barros, M.; Namora, G.; Magalhães, Â.; Rodrigues, T.; Montenegro, N. Gestational diabetes mellitus: A risk factor for non-elective cesarean section. *J. Obstet. Gynaecol. Res.* **2011**, *38*, 154–159. [CrossRef]
8. Corrado, F.; D'Anna, R.; Laganà, A.S.; Di Benedetto, A. Abnormal glucose tolerance later in life in women affected by glucose intolerance during pregnancy. *J. Obstet. Gynaecol.* **2014**, *34*, 123–126. [CrossRef] [PubMed]
9. Vitagliano, A.; Saccone, G.; Cosmi, E.; Visentin, S.; Dessole, F.; Ambrosini, G.; Berghella, V. Inositol for the prevention of gestational diabetes: A systematic review and meta-analysis of randomized controlled trials. *Arch. Gynecol. Obstet.* **2019**, *299*, 55–68. [CrossRef] [PubMed]
10. Facchinetti, F.; Appetecchia, M.; Aragona, C.; Bevilacqua, A.; Espinola, M.S.B.; Bizzarri, M.; D'Anna, R.; Dewailly, D.; Diamanti-Kandarakis, E.; Marín, I.H.; et al. Experts' opinion on inositols in treating polycystic ovary syndrome and non-insulin dependent diabetes mellitus: A further help for human reproduction and beyond. *Expert Opin. Drug Metab. Toxicol.* **2020**, *16*, 255–274. [CrossRef]
11. Jacklin, P.B.; Maresh, M.J.; Patterson, C.C.; Stanley, K.P.; Dornhorst, A.; Burman-Roy, S.; Bilous, R.W. A cost-effectiveness comparison of the NICE 2015 and WHO 2013 diagnostic criteria for women with gestational diabetes with and without risk factors. *BMJ Open* **2017**, *7*, e016621. [CrossRef] [PubMed]
12. Metzger, B.E.; Lowe, L.; Dyer, A.; Trimble, E.; Chaovarindr, U.; Coustan, D.; Hadden, D.; McCance, D.; Hod, M.; McIntyre, H.; et al. Hyperglycemia and Adverse Pregnancy Outcomes. *Obstet. Anesth. Dig.* **2009**, *29*, 39–40. [CrossRef]
13. International Association of Diabetes and Pregnancy Study Groups Consensus Panel. International association of diabetes and pregnancy study groups recommendations on the diagnosis and classification of hyperglycemia in pregnancy. *Diabetes Care* **2010**, *33*, 676–682. [CrossRef] [PubMed]
14. World Health Organization. *Diagnostic Criteria and Classification of Hyperglycaemia First Detected in Pregnancy*; World Health Organization: Geneva, Switzerland, 2013.
15. Hosseini, E.; Janghorbani, M. Systematic review and meta-analysis of diagnosing gestational diabetes mellitus with one-step or two-step approaches and associations with adverse pregnancy outcomes. *Int. J. Gynaecol. Obstet.* **2018**, *143*, 137–144. [CrossRef] [PubMed]
16. Moher, D.; Liberati, A.; Tetzlaff, J.; Wong, C.S. Preferred reporting items for systematic reviews and meta-analyses: The PRISMA statement. *Int. J. Sur.* **2010**, *8*, 336–341. [CrossRef]
17. Stang, A. Critical evaluation of the Newcastle-Ottawa scale for the assessment of the quality of nonrandomized studies in meta-analyses. *Eur. J. Epidemiol.* **2010**, *25*, 603–605. [CrossRef] [PubMed]
18. Sterne, J.A.; Hernán, M.A.; Reeves, B.C.; Savović, J.; Berkman, N.D.; Viswanathan, M.; Henry, D.; Altman, D.G.; Ansari, M.T.; Boutron, I.; et al. ROBINS-I: A tool for assessing risk of bias in non-randomised studies of interventions. *BMJ* **2016**, *355*, i4919. [CrossRef]
19. Higgins, J. *Analysing data and undertaking meta-analyses In Cochrane Handbook for Systematic Reviews of Interventions (Version 5.1. 0)*; Higgins, J., Green, S., Eds.; Wiley: New York, NY, USA, 2011.
20. Shand, A.W.; Bell, J.C.; McElduff, A.; Morris, J.; Roberts, C.L. Outcomes of pregnancies in women with pre-gestational diabetes mellitus and gestational diabetes mellitus; a population-based study in New South Wales, Australia, 19982002. *Diabet. Med.* **2008**, *25*, 708–715. [CrossRef] [PubMed]
21. Erjavec, K.; Poljičanin, T.; Matijević, R. Impact of the Implementation of New WHO Diagnostic Criteria for Gestational Diabetes Mellitus on Prevalence and Perinatal Outcomes: A Population-Based Study. *J. Pregnancy* **2016**, *2016*, 1–6. [CrossRef] [PubMed]
22. Black, M.H.; Sacks, D.A.; Xiang, A.H.; Lawrence, J.M. Clinical Outcomes of Pregnancies Complicated by Mild Gestational Diabetes Mellitus Differ by Combinations of Abnormal Oral Glucose Tolerance Test Values. *Diabetes Care* **2010**, *33*, 2524–2530. [CrossRef]
23. Lamminpää, R.; Vehviläinen-Julkunen, K.; Gissler, M.; Gissler, M.; Selander, T.; Heinonen, S. Pregnancy outcomes in women aged 35 years or older with gestational diabetes—A registry-based study in Finland. *J. Matern. Fetal Neonatal Med.* **2016**, *29*, 55–59. [CrossRef] [PubMed]
24. Carr, D.B.; Newton, K.M.; Utzschneider, K.M.; Faulenbach, M.V.; Kahn, S.E.; Easterling, T.R.; Heckbert, S.R. Gestational Diabetes or Lesser Degrees of Glucose Intolerance and Risk of Preeclampsia. *Hypertens. Pregnancy* **2010**, *30*, 153–163. [CrossRef]
25. Metcalfe, A.; Sabr, Y.; Hutcheon, J.A.; Donovan, L.; Lyons, J.; Burrows, J.; Joseph, K.S. Trends in Obstetric Intervention and Pregnancy Outcomes of Canadian Women with Diabetes in Pregnancy From 2004 to 2015. *J. Endocr. Soc.* **2017**, *1*, 1540–1549. [CrossRef] [PubMed]
26. Su, W.-J.; Chen, Y.-L.; Huang, P.-Y.; Shi, X.-L.; Yan, F.-F.; Chen, Z.; Yan, B.; Song, H.-Q.; Lin, M.-Z.; Li, X. Effects of Prepregnancy Body Mass Index, Weight Gain, and Gestational Diabetes Mellitus on Pregnancy Outcomes: A Population-Based Study in Xiamen, China, 2011–2018. *Ann. Nutr. Metab.* **2019**, *75*, 31–38. [CrossRef] [PubMed]

27. Van Hoorn, J.; Dekker, G.; Jeffries, B. Gestational diabetes versus obesity as risk factors for pregnancy-induced hypertensive disorders and fetal macrosomia. *Aust. N. Z. J. Obstet. Gynaecol.* **2002**, *42*, 35–40. [CrossRef] [PubMed]
28. Zeki, R.; Oats, J.J.; Wang, A.Y.; Li, Z.; Homer, C.S.E.; Sullivan, E.A. Cesarean section and diabetes during pregnancy: An NSW population study using the Robson classification. *J. Obstet. Gynaecol. Res.* **2018**, *44*, 890–898. [CrossRef]
29. Sugaya, A.; Sugiyama, T.; Nagata, M.; Toyoda, N. Comparison of the validity of the criteria for gestational diabetes mellitus by WHO and by the Japan Society of Obstetrics and Gynecology by the outcomes of pregnancy. *Diabetes Res. Clin. Pr.* **2000**, *50*, 57–63. [CrossRef]
30. Sletner, L.; Jenum, A.K.; Yajnik, C.S.; Mørkrid, K.; Nakstad, B.; Rognerud-Jensen, O.H.; Birkeland, K.I.; Vangen, S. Fetal growth trajectories in pregnancies of European and South Asian mothers with and without gestational diabetes, a population-based cohort study. *PLoS ONE* **2017**, *12*, e0172946. [CrossRef]
31. Ellerbe, C.N.; Gebregziabher, M.; Korte, J.E.; Mauldin, J.; Hunt, K.J. Quantifying the Impact of Gestational Diabetes Mellitus, Maternal Weight and Race on Birthweight via Quantile Regression. *PLoS ONE* **2013**, *8*, e65017. [CrossRef]
32. Mahanta, T.G.; Deuri, A.; Mahanta, B.N.; Bordoloi, P.; Rasaily, R.; Mahanta, J.; Baruah, S.; Gogoi, P. Maternal and foetal outcome of gestational diabetes mellitus in a rural block of Assam, India. *Clin. Epidemiol. Glob. Health* **2014**, *2*, 9–15. [CrossRef]
33. Kieffer, E.C.; Tabaei, B.P.; Carman, W.J.; Nolan, G.H.; Guzman, J.R.; Herman, W.H. The Influence of Maternal Weight and Glucose Tolerance on Infant Birthweight in Latino Mother–Infant Pairs. *Am. J. Public Health* **2006**, *96*, 2201–2208. [CrossRef] [PubMed]
34. Nerenberg, K.A.; Johnson, J.A.; Leung, B.; Savu, A.; Ryan, E.A.; Chik, C.L.; Kaul, P. Risks of Gestational Diabetes and Preeclampsia Over the Last Decade in a Cohort of Alberta Women. *J. Obstet. Gynaecol. Can.* **2013**, *35*, 986–994. [CrossRef]
35. Soliman, A.; Salama, H.; Al Rifai, H.; De Sanctis, V.; Al-Obaidly, S.; Al Qubasi, M.; Olukade, T. The effect of different forms of dysglycemia during pregnancy on maternal and fetal outcomes in treated women and comparison with large cohort studies. *Acta Biomed. Atenei Parm.* **2018**, *89*, 11–21.
36. Oster, R.T.; King, M.; Morrish, D.W.; Mayan, M.; Toth, E.L. Diabetes in pregnancy among First Nations women in Alberta, Canada: A retrospective analysis. *BMC Pregnancy Childbirth* **2014**, *14*, 136. [CrossRef]
37. Xiong, X.; Saunders, L.; Wang, F.; Demianczuk, N. Gestational diabetes mellitus: Prevalence, risk factors, maternal and infant outcomes. *Int. J. Gynecol. Obstet.* **2001**, *75*, 221–228. [CrossRef]
38. Sacks, D.A.; Black, M.H.; Li, X.; Montoro, M.N.; Lawrence, J.M. Adverse pregnancy outcomes using the International Association of the Diabetes and Pregnancy Study Groups criteria: Glycemic thresholds and associated risks. *Obstet. Gynecol.* **2015**, *126*, 67–73. [CrossRef]
39. Son, K.H.; Lim, N.K.; Lee, J.; Cho, M.; Park, H. Comparison of maternal morbidity and medical costs during pregnancy and delivery between patients with gestational diabetes and patients with pre-existing diabetes. *Diabet. Med.* **2015**, *32*, 477–486. [CrossRef]
40. Pan, L.; Leng, J.; Liu, G.; Zhang, C.; Liu, H.; Li, M.; Tan, L.; Tian, H.; Chan, J.C.; Hu, G.; et al. Pregnancy outcomes of Chinese women with gestational diabetes mellitus defined by the IADPSG's but not by the 1999 WHO's criteria. *Clin. Endocrinol.* **2015**, *83*, 684–693. [CrossRef]
41. Jacobson, J.D.; Cousins, L. A population-based study of maternal and perinatal outcome in patients with gestational diabetes. *Am. J. Obstet. Gynecol.* **1989**, *161*, 981–986. [CrossRef]
42. Leybovitz-Haleluya, N.; Wainstock, T.; Landau, D.; Sheiner, E. Maternal gestational diabetes mellitus and the risk of subsequent pediatric cardiovascular diseases of the offspring: A population-based cohort study with up to 18 years of follow up. *Acta Diabetol.* **2018**, *55*, 1037–1042. [CrossRef] [PubMed]
43. Gortazar, L.; Roux, J.A.F.-L.; Benaiges, D.; Sarsanedas, E.; Payà, A.; Mañé, L.; Pedro-Botet, J.; Goday, A. Trends in prevalence of gestational diabetes and perinatal outcomes in Catalonia, Spain, 2006 to 2015: The Diagestcat Study. *Diabetes Metabol. Res. Rev.* **2019**, *35*, e3151. [CrossRef] [PubMed]
44. Hedderson, M.M.; Ferrara, A.; Sacks, D.A. Gestational diabetes mellitus and lesser degrees of pregnancy hyperglycemia: Association with increased risk of spontaneous preterm birth. *Obstet. Gynecol.* **2003**, *102*, 850–856. [CrossRef]
45. Kun, A. Insulin Resistance Is Associated with Gestational Hypertension and Not with Preeclampsia: A Population-Based Screening Study. *Gynecol. Obstet. Investig.* **2011**, *71*, 256–261. [CrossRef]
46. Davey, S.; Jain, R.; Davey, A.; Raghav, S.K.; Singh, J.V. Can the management of blood sugar levels in gestational diabetes mellitus cases be an indicator of maternal and fetal outcomes? The results of a prospective cohort study from India. *J. Fam. Community Med.* **2016**, *23*, 94–99. [CrossRef]
47. Hosseini, E.; Janghorbani, M.; Aminorroaya, A. Incidence, risk factors, and pregnancy outcomes of gestational diabetes mellitus using one-step versus two-step diagnostic approaches: A population-based cohort study in Isfahan, Iran. *Diabetes Res. Clin. Pr.* **2018**, *140*, 288–294. [CrossRef] [PubMed]
48. Hosseini, E.; Janghorbani, M.; Shahshahan, Z. Comparison of risk factors and pregnancy outcomes of gestational diabetes mellitus diagnosed during early and late pregnancy. *Midwifery* **2018**, *66*, 64–69. [CrossRef]
49. Zamstein, O.; Sheiner, E.; Wainstock, T.; Landau, D.; Walfisch, A. Maternal gestational diabetes and long-term respiratory related hospitalizations of the offspring. *Diabetes Res. Clin. Pr.* **2018**, *140*, 200–207. [CrossRef]
50. Aung, Y.Y.M.; Sowter, M.; Kenealy, T.; Herman, J.; Ekeroma, A. Gestational diabetes mellitus screening, management and outcomes in the Cook Islands. *N. Z. Med. J.* **2015**, *128*.

51. Ekeroma, A.J.; Chandran, G.S.; McCowan, L.; Ansell, D.; Eagleton, C.; Kenealy, T. Impact of using the international association of diabetes and pregnancy study groups criteria in South Auckland: Prevalence, interventions and outcomes. *Aust. N. Z. J. Obstet. Gynaecol.* **2014**, *55*, 34–41. [CrossRef]
52. Kieffer, E.C.; Nolan, G.H.; Carman, W.J.; Sanborn, C.Z.; Guzman, R.; Ventura, A. Glucose Tolerance During Pregnancy and Birth Weight in a Hispanic Population. *Obstet. Gynecol.* **1999**, *94*, 741–746. [CrossRef] [PubMed]
53. Donovan, L.; Edwards, A.; Savu, A.; Butalia, S.; Ryan, E.A.; Johnson, J.A.; Kaul, P. Population-level outcomes with a 2-step approach for gestational diabetes screening and diagnosis. *Can. J. Diabetes* **2017**, *41*, 596–602. [CrossRef]
54. Kgosidialwa, O.; Egan, A.M.; Carmody, L.; Kirwan, B.; Gunning, P.; Dunne, F.P. Treatment with Diet and Exercise for Women With Gestational Diabetes Mellitus Diagnosed Using IADPSG Criteria. *J. Clin. Endocrinol. Metab.* **2015**, *100*, 4629–4636. [CrossRef] [PubMed]
55. Kaul, P.; Savu, A.; Nerenberg, K.A.; Donovan, L.; Donovan, E.; Chik, C.L.; Ryan, E.A.; Johnson, J.A. Impact of gestational diabetes mellitus and high maternal weight on the development of diabetes, hypertension and cardiovascular disease: A population-level analysis. *Diabet. Med.* **2015**, *32*, 164–173. [CrossRef]
56. Brand, J.S.; West, J.; Tuffnell, D.; Bird, P.K.; Wright, J.; Tilling, K.; Lawlor, D.A. Gestational diabetes and ultrasound-assessed fetal growth in South Asian and White European women: Findings from a prospective pregnancy cohort. *BMC Med.* **2018**, *16*, 203. [CrossRef]
57. Kawakita, T.; Bowers, K.; Hazrati, S.; Zhang, C.; Grewal, J.; Chen, Z.; Sun, L.; Grantz, K.L.; Gtantz, K. Increased Neonatal Respiratory Morbidity Associated with Gestational and Pregestational Diabetes: A Retrospective Study. *Am. J. Perinatol.* **2017**, *34*, 1160–1168. [CrossRef] [PubMed]
58. Boghossian, N.S.; Yeung, E.; Albert, P.S.; Mendola, P.; Laughon, S.K.; Hinkle, S.N.; Zhang, C. Changes in diabetes status between pregnancies and impact on subsequent newborn outcomes. *Am. J. Obstet. Gynecol.* **2014**, *210*, 431.e1. [CrossRef] [PubMed]
59. Meek, C.L.; Lewis, H.B.; Patient, C.; Davies, G.A.; Poitras, V.; Gray, C.; Jaramillo Garcia, A.; Barrowman, N.; Adamo, K.B.; Duggan, M.; et al. Diagnosis of gestational diabetes mellitus: Falling through the net. *Diabetologia* **2015**, *58*, 2003–2012. [CrossRef] [PubMed]
60. Wahabi, H.; Fayed, A.; Esmaeil, S.; Mamdouh, H.; Kotb, R. Prevalence and complications of pregestational and gestational diabetes in Saudi women: Analysis from Riyadh Mother and Baby cohort study (RAHMA). *Biomed. Res. Int.* **2017**, *2017*, 6878263. [CrossRef]
61. Avalos, G.E.; Owens, L.A.; Dunne, F.; ATLANTIC DIP Collaborators. Applying current screening tools for gestational diabetes mellitus to a European population: Is it time for change? *Diabetes Care* **2013**, *36*, 3040–3044. [CrossRef]
62. Anderberg, E.; Källén, K.; Berntorp, K. The impact of gestational diabetes mellitus on pregnancy outcome comparing different cut-off criteria for abnormal glucose tolerance. *Acta Obstet. Gynecol. Scand.* **2010**, *89*, 1532–1537. [CrossRef]
63. Gu, Y.; Lu, J.; Li, W.; Liu, H.; Wang, L.; Leng, J.; Li, W.; Zhang, S.; Wang, S.; Tuomilehto, J.; et al. Joint Associations of Maternal Gestational Diabetes and Hypertensive Disorders of Pregnancy with Overweight in Offspring. *Front. Endocrinol.* **2019**, *10*. [CrossRef]
64. Waters, T.P.; Dyer, A.R.; Scholtens, D.M.; Dooley, S.L.; Herer, E.; Lowe, L.P.; Oats, J.J.; Persson, B.; Sacks, D.A.; HAPO Cooperative Study Research Group; et al. Maternal and Neonatal Morbidity for Women Who Would Be Added to the Diagnosis of GDM Using IADPSG Criteria: A Secondary Analysis of the Hyperglycemia and Adverse Pregnancy Outcome Study. *Diabetes Care* **2016**, *39*, 2204–2210. [CrossRef] [PubMed]
65. Moses, R.; Griffiths, R. Can a diagnosis of gestational diabetes be an advantage to the outcome of pregnancy? *J. Soc. Gynecol. Investig.* **1995**, *2*, 523–525. [CrossRef]
66. Karmon, A.; Levy, A.; Holcberg, G.; Wiznitzer, A.; Mazor, M.; Sheiner, E. Decreased perinatal mortality among women with diet-controlled gestational diabetes mellitus. *Int. J. Gynaecol. Obstet.* **2009**, *104*, 199–202. [CrossRef]
67. Capula, C.; Chiefari, E.; Vero, A.; Arcidiacono, B.; Iiritano, S.; Puccio, L.; Pullano, V.; Foti, D.P.; Brunetti, A.; Vero, R. Gestational Diabetes Mellitus: Screening and Outcomes in Southern Italian Pregnant Women. *ISRN Endocrinol.* **2013**, *2013*, 1–8. [CrossRef]
68. Von Katterfeld, B.; Li, J.; McNamara, B.; Langridge, A.T. Maternal and neonatal outcomes associated with gestational diabetes in women from culturally and linguistically diverse backgrounds in Western Australia. *Diabet. Med.* **2012**, *29*, 372–377. [CrossRef] [PubMed]
69. López Stewart, G. *Diagnostic Criteria and Classification of Hyperglycaemia First Detected in Pregnancy: A World Health Organization Guideline*; World Health Organization: Geneva, Switzerland, 2014.
70. Bogdanet, D.; O'Shea, P.M.; Lyons, C.; Shafat, A.; Dunne, F. The Oral Glucose Tolerance Test—Is It Time for a Change?—A Literature Review with an Emphasis on Pregnancy. *J. Clin. Med.* **2020**, *9*, 3451. [CrossRef] [PubMed]
71. Ansarzadeh, S.; Salehi, L.; Mahmoodi, Z.; Mohammadbeigi, A. Factors affecting the quality of life in women with gestational diabetes mellitus: A path analysis model. *Health Qual. Life Outcomes* **2020**, *18*, 1–9. [CrossRef]
72. Hoffman, L.; Nolan, C.; Wilson, J.D.; Oats, J.J.N.; Simmons, D. Gestational diabetes mellitus—Management guidelines: The Australasian Diabetes in Pregnancy Society. *Med. J. Aust.* **1998**, *169*, 93–97. [CrossRef] [PubMed]
73. ACOG. *Gestational Diabetes Mellitus*; ACOG Practice Bulletin; ACOG: Washington, DC, USA, 2018.
74. Lash, R.W. Diabetes and Pregnancy—An Endocrine Society Clinical Practice Guideline Publication Note. *J. Clin. Endocrinol. Metab.* **2018**, *103*, 4042. [CrossRef] [PubMed]

75. Mission, J.F.; Ohno, M.S.; Cheng, Y.W.; Caughey, A.B. Gestational diabetes screening with the new IADPSG guidelines: A cost-effectiveness analysis. *Am. J. Obstet. Gynecol.* **2012**, *207*, 326.e1. [CrossRef]
76. Weile, L.K.; Kahn, J.G.; Marseille, E.; Jensen, D.M.; Damm, P.; Lohse, N. Global cost-effectiveness of GDM screening and management: Current knowledge and future needs. *Best Pract. Res. Clin. Obstet. Gynaecol.* **2015**, *29*, 206–224. [CrossRef]
77. Fitria, N.; Van Asselt, A.D.I.; Postma, M.J. Cost-effectiveness of controlling gestational diabetes mellitus: A systematic review. *Eur. J. Health Econ.* **2019**, *20*, 407–417. [CrossRef] [PubMed]
78. Moss, J.R.; Crowther, C.A.; Hiller, J.E.; Willson, K.J.; Robinson, J.S.; Australian Carbohydrate Intolerance Study in Pregnant Women Group. Costs and consequences of treatment for mild gestational diabetes mellitus–evaluation from the ACHOIS randomised trial. *BMC Pregnancy Childbirth* **2007**, *7*, 27. [CrossRef] [PubMed]
79. Ohno, M.S.; Sparks, T.N.; Cheng, Y.W.; Caughey, A.B. Treating mild gestational diabetes mellitus: A cost-effectiveness analysis. *Am. J. Obstet. Gynecol.* **2011**, *205*, 282.e1. [CrossRef]
80. Poncet, B.; Touzet, S.; Rocher, L.; Berland, M.; Orgiazzi, J.; Colin, C. Cost-effectiveness analysis of gestational diabetes mellitus screening in France. *Eur. J. Obstet. Gynecol. Reprod. Biol.* **2002**, *103*, 122–129. [CrossRef]
81. Kalra, S.; Baruah, M.P.; Gupta, Y.; Kalra, B. Gestational diabetes: An onomastic opportunity. *Lancet Diabetes Endocrinol.* **2013**, *1*, 91. [CrossRef]
82. Marchetti, D.; Carrozzino, D.; Fraticelli, F.; Fulcheri, M.; Vitacolonna, E. Quality of Life in Women with Gestational Diabetes Mellitus: A Systematic Review. *J. Diabetes Res.* **2017**, *2017*, 1–12. [CrossRef] [PubMed]
83. Kalra, B.; Gupta, Y.; Baruah, M.P. Renaming gestational diabetes mellitus: A psychosocial argument. *Indian J. Endocrinol. Metab.* **2013**, *17*, 593–595. [CrossRef]
84. Pantzartzis, K.A.; Manolopoulos, P.P.; Paschou, S.A.; Kazakos, K.; Kotsa, K.; Goulis, D.G. Gestational diabetes mellitus and quality of life during the third trimester of pregnancy. *Qual. Life Res.* **2019**, *28*, 1349–1354. [CrossRef]
85. Weissgerber, T.L.; Mudd, L.M. Preeclampsia and diabetes. *Curr. Diabetes Rep.* **2015**, *15*, 1–10. [CrossRef] [PubMed]
86. Naylor, C.D.; Sermer, M.; Chen, E.; Sykora, K. Cesarean Delivery in Relation to Birth Weight and Gestational Glucose Tolerance. *JAMA* **1996**, *275*, 1165–1170. [CrossRef] [PubMed]

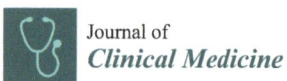

Article

Neutrophil to Lymphocyte Ratio in Maternal Blood: A Clue to Suspect Amnionitis

Joon-Hyung Lee [1], Chan-Wook Park [1,2,*], Kyung-Chul Moon [3], Joong-Shin Park [1] and Jong-Kwan Jun [1,2]

[1] Department of Obstetrics and Gynecology, Seoul National University College of Medicine, Seoul 03080, Korea; kontractubex12@gmail.com (J.-H.L.); jsparkmd@snu.ac.kr (J.-S.P.); jhs0927@snu.ac.kr (J.-K.J.)
[2] Institute of Reproductive Medicine and Population, Seoul National University Medical Research Center, Seoul 03080, Korea
[3] Department of Pathology, Seoul National University College of Medicine, Seoul 03080, Korea; blue7270@gmail.com
* Correspondence: hwpark0803@gmail.com; Tel.: +82-2-2072-0635

Abstract: There is no information about whether maternal neutrophil to lymphocyte ratios (NLRs) progressively increase with respect to the progression of acute histologic chorioamnionitis (acute-HCA) and increased maternal NLR is a risk factor for amnionitis, known as advanced acute-HCA, in pregnant women at risk for spontaneous preterm birth (PTB). The objective of the current study is to examine this issue. The study population included 132 singleton PTB (<34 weeks) due to either preterm labor or preterm-PROM with both placental pathology and maternal CBC results within 48 h before delivery. We examined maternal NLRs according to the progression of acute-HCA in extra-placental membranes (EPM) (i.e., group-0, inflammation-free EPM; group-1, inflammation restricted to decidua; group-2, inflammation restricted to the membranous trophoblast of chorion and the decidua; group-3, inflammation in the connective tissue of chorion but not amnion; group-4, amnionitis). Maternal NLRs significantly and progressively increased with the progression of acute-HCA (Spearman's rank correlation test, $\gamma = 0.363$, $p = 0.000019$). Moreover, the increased maternal NLR (≥ 7.75) (Odds-ratio 5.56, 95% confidence-interval 1.26-24.62, $p < 0.05$) was a significant independent risk factor for amnionitis even after the correction for potential confounders. In conclusion, maternal NLRs significantly and progressively increased according to the progression of acute-HCA and the increased maternal NLR (≥ 7.75) was an independent risk factor for amnionitis in spontaneous PTB. The evaluation of the performance of NLR should clearly require a prospective description of this parameter in a cohort of patients with either threatened PTL or preterm-PROM.

Keywords: amnionitis; maternal blood; neutrophil to lymphocyte ratio; preterm birth

Citation: Lee, J.-H.; Park, C.-W.; Moon, K.-C.; Park, J.-S.; Jun, J.-K. Neutrophil to Lymphocyte Ratio in Maternal Blood: A Clue to Suspect Amnionitis. *J. Clin. Med.* **2021**, *10*, 2673. https://doi.org/10.3390/jcm10122673

Academic Editor: Rinat Gabbay-Benziv

Received: 25 March 2021
Accepted: 15 June 2021
Published: 17 June 2021

Publisher's Note: MDPI stays neutral with regard to jurisdictional claims in published maps and institutional affiliations.

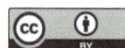

Copyright: © 2021 by the authors. Licensee MDPI, Basel, Switzerland. This article is an open access article distributed under the terms and conditions of the Creative Commons Attribution (CC BY) license (https://creativecommons.org/licenses/by/4.0/).

1. Introduction

Ascending intrauterine infection is one of the major physiologies in spontaneous preterm birth (PTB) (i.e., preterm labor and intact membranes (PTL) and preterm premature rupture of membranes (preterm-PROM)) [1,2]. Micro-organisms from the vaginal and cervical canal ascend to chorio-decidua and advance to the amnion in extra-placental membranes (EPM) [2]; this eventually results in fetal infection [1–3]. During the progression of ascending intrauterine infection, maternal neutrophils sequentially migrate from the decidua through the membranous trophoblast of chorion to the connective tissue of chorion and finally infiltrates into amnion in EPM [4]. Acute histologic chorioamnionitis (acute-HCA) generated by neutrophils infiltration into the EPM is considered a maternal inflammatory response because neutrophils in EPM are derived from maternal vessels of decidua parietalis [5,6].

It is well known that intra-amniotic inflammatory responses are closely associated with acute-HCA [7–10]. Moreover, our previous study reported that intra-amniotic inflammatory responses increase with outside-in neutrophils migration in the chorio-decidua (i.e., 'inflammation restricted to decidua', 'inflammation restricted to the membranous trophoblast of chorion', and 'inflammation in the connective tissue of chorion') [11]. Moreover, intra-amniotic and fetal inflammatory responses are more intense and the early-onset neonatal sepsis is more frequent in amnionitis (more advanced stage inflammation) than in inflammation restricted to chorio-decidua (less advanced stage inflammation) of EPM [12]. In general, intra-amniotic inflammatory response is gauged by several markers (i.e., white blood cell (WBC) count, matrix metalloproteinase-8 (MMP-8), and IL-6 in amniotic fluid (AF) obtained by amniocentesis. However, amniocentesis is an invasive procedure and may not be feasible in cases with decreased AF volume in the context of preterm-PROM. Therefore, numerous studies attempted to find potential markers in maternal blood but not in AF for the identification of acute-HCA in EPM (Table S1) [13–46]. However, acute-HCA remains unpredictable with the use of maternal inflammatory blood markers and, moreover, there are limitations in previous studies as follows (Table S1); (1) no previous studies examined maternal inflammatory blood markers according to the progression of acute-HCA in the sub-divisions of EPM (i.e., decidua, the membranous trophoblast of chorion, the connective tissue of chorion, and amnion) [13–42]; (2) a substantial number of studies did not adjust for gestational age (GA) at delivery or maternal blood sampling [13,14,16–20,23–28,30–42] and did not provide a meaningful temporal relationship between the maternal inflammatory blood tests and the placental pathologic examinations after delivery [16,17,22–25,27,31,32,41].

Recently, the neutrophil to lymphocyte ratio (NLR) as a biomarker for systemic inflammatory conditions in adults is known to be positively correlated with disease activity in rheumatic disease [47–53] and known to be associated with the prognosis (i.e., survival) of sepsis, systemic inflammatory response syndrome (SIRS), and septic shock [54–58] in patients. Moreover, some researchers demonstrated that increased neonatal NLR is a marker or predictor for significant neonatal morbidities (i.e., early-onset neonatal sepsis [EONS], broncho-pulmonary dysplasia (BPD), and necrotizing enterocolitis (NEC)) [59–61]. What is noteworthy is that maternal NLRs are reported to be elevated in cases with preeclampsia [62–64], which is associated with exaggerated inflammatory responses in the maternal vascular system [65]. However, there is no information on the relationship between maternal NLRs and the progression of acute-HCA among pregnant women at risk for PTB in the current body of research. We hypothesized that maternal NLRs progressively increase according to the progression of acute-HCA and increased maternal NLR is a risk factor for amnionitis known as advanced acute-HCA among pregnant women at risk for spontaneous PTB. We additionally examined maternal high-sensitivity C-reactive protein (hs-CRP) concentrations to demonstrate the usefulness of maternal NLR for the identification of amnionitis. The objective of the current study is to examine this issue.

2. Materials and Methods

2.1. Study Design and Patient Population

The study population included 132 singleton pregnant women who met the following criteria: (1) Korean; (2) GA at delivery between 20.6 weeks and 33.9 weeks; (3) PTB due to either PTL (63 cases) or preterm-PROM (69 cases); (4) available placental pathologic slides; (5) maternal complete blood count (CBC) profile available within 48 h before delivery. The last criterion was used to preserve a meaningful temporal relationship between maternal CBC profiles and placental pathologic findings at delivery. At our institution, the maternal CBC test and placental pathologic examination after delivery were routinely recommended and performed to all pregnant women hospitalized with either PTL or preterm-PROM. PTL and preterm-PROM were diagnosed in accordance with previously published criteria [8,9]. Written informed consent was obtained from the entire study population. The Institutional Review Board of our institute specifically approved the current study.

2.2. Clinical Characteristics and Pregnancy Outcomes

Clinical characteristics and pregnancy outcomes were investigated from medical records. Data included maternal age, parity, clinical history of antenatal vaginal bleeding or the evidence of placenta previa, cause of preterm delivery, gender of newborn, delivery mode, GA at delivery, birth weight, 1 min and 5 min Apgar scores, meconium staining, antenatal use of corticosteroids, antenatal use of antibiotics, and antenatal use of tocolytics.

2.3. Diagnosis of Acute Histologic Chorioamnionitis (Acute-HCA) in Extra-Placental Membranes (EPM)

Placental tissue samples for pathologic examination included EPM (i.e., chorio-decidua and amnion), chorionic plate, and the umbilical cord. These samples were fixed in 10% neutral buffered formalin and embedded in paraffin. Sections of prepared tissue blocks were stained with hematoxylin and eosin (H&E). Clinical information regarding the placental tissues was not disclosed to pathologists. Acute-HCA in EPM was defined as the presence of neutrophil infiltration in either chorio-decidua or amnion. Acute inflammation in chorio-decidua and amnion was diagnosed according to the previously published criteria: (1) Chorio-deciduitis was diagnosed in the presence of at least one focus of >5 neutrophils in chorio-decidua; (2) amnionitis was diagnosed in the presence of at least one focus of >5 neutrophils in amnion. The progression of acute-HCA in EPM was divided according to outside-in neutrophils migration in EPM as follows: (1) group-0, inflammation-free EPM; (2) group-1, inflammation restricted to decidua; (3) group-2, inflammation restricted to the membranous trophoblast of chorion and the decidua; (4) group-3, inflammation in the connective tissue of chorion but not amnion; (5) group-4, amnionitis.

2.4. Maternal Neutrophil to Lymphocyte Ratio (NLR)

Maternal blood was collected in ethylenediaminetetraacetic-acid (EDTA) tubes by venipuncture of the antecubital vein within 48 h before delivery and CBC with differential leukocyte count was performed. NLR is defined as absolute neutrophil count divided by absolute lymphocyte count. We additionally examined maternal hs-CRP concentrations within 48 h before delivery to demonstrate the usefulness of maternal NLR for the identification of amnionitis.

2.5. Statistical Analysis

Continuous and categorical variables were compared with the Kruskal–Wallis test and Pearson's chi-square test, respectively. Multiple comparisons of continuous and categorical variables between the groups according to the progression of acute-HCA in EPM were performed with 1-way ANOVA with post-hoc Tukey test and Fisher's exact test with Bonferroni's correction, respectively. Spearman's rank correlation test was used to examine the relationship between maternal NLRs and acute-HCA in EPM. The receiver operating characteristics (ROC) curve was used to estimate the best cut-off values (maximum sum of sensitivity and specificity) and to identify maternal NLRs as being raised or not raised for the detection of amnionitis. Using this cut-off value, we compared the frequency of increased maternal NLR according to the progression of acute-HCA in EPM with Pearson's chi-square test. Moreover, linear by linear association was used to investigate the trend about the frequency of increased maternal NLR (≥ 7.75) according to the progression of acute-HCA in EPM. Diagnostics indices (i.e., sensitivity, specificity, positive predictive value, negative predictive value, positive likelihood ratio, and negative likelihood ratio) were determined for increased maternal NLR for the identification of amnionitis. We performed multiple logistic regression analysis for the exploration of the relationship between various variables and amnionitis. We analyzed maternal hs-CRP with the same statistical methods to demonstrate the usefulness of maternal NLR for the identification of amnionitis. Statistical significance was defined as $p < 0.05$.

3. Results

3.1. Clinical Characteristics and Pregnancy Outcomes According to the Progression of Acute Histologic Chorioamnionitis (Acute-HCA) in Extra-Placental Membranes (EPM)

Group-0, group-1, group-2, group-3, and group-4 was present in 36.4% (48/132), 14.4% (19/132), 20.5% (27/132), 17.4% (23/132), and 11.4% (15/132) of study population, respectively (Table 1). Table 2 demonstrated that GA at delivery and birth weight were significantly decreased according to the progression of acute-HCA in EPM and there was a significant difference in the frequency of antenatal use of antibiotics among five groups according to the progression of acute-HCA in EPM (Table 2).

Table 1. Clinical characteristics and pregnancy outcomes according to the progression of acute histologic chorioamnionitis (acute-HCA) in extra-placental membranes (EPM).

	Group-0 [†]	Group-1 [†]	Group-2 [†]	Group-3 [†]	Group-4 [†]	p Value [a]
	36.4% (48/132)	14.4% (19/132)	20.5% (27/132)	17.4% (23/132)	11.4% (15/132)	
Maternal age, year (mean ± SD)	32.8 ± 4.6	32.9 ± 3.4	32.5 ± 3.9	34.7 ± 3.6	33.2 ± 4.6	NS (0.302)
Nulliparity	50.0% (24/48)	47.4% (9/19)	37.0% (10/27)	34.8% (8/23)	33.3% (5/15)	NS (0.610)
Either clinical history of antenatal vaginal bleeding or evidence of placenta previa	18.8% (9/48)	15.8% (3/19)	0% (0/27)	4.3% (1/23)	13.3% (2/15)	NS (0.107)
Preterm-PROM as a cause of PTB	50.0% (24/48)	31.6% (6/19)	59.3% (16/27)	69.6% (16/23)	46.7% (7/15)	NS (0.145)
Male Newborn	58.3% (28/48)	57.9% (11/19)	70.4% (19/27)	34.8% (8/23)	66.7% (10/15)	NS (0.125)
Cesarean delivery	41.7% (20/48)	31.6% (6/19)	18.5% (5/27)	34.8% (8/23)	33.3% (5/15)	NS (0.378)
Median GA at delivery, weeks (range)	31.6 (21.6–33.9)	30.3 (23.4–33.7)	30.3 (20.6–33.4)	28.0 (22.0–31.9) [b]	26.6 (21.3–31.4) [c, d]	<0.001
Birth weight, g (mean ± SD)	1572 ± 567	1478 ± 547	1444 ± 636	1129 ± 330 [e]	1057 ± 419 [e]	0.003
1 min Apgar score of <7	77.1% (37/48)	63.2% (12/19)	66.7% (18/27)	91.3% (21/23)	80.0% (12/15)	NS (0.193)
5 min Apgar score of <7	31.2% (15/48)	26.3% (5/19)	22.2% (6/27)	43.5% (10/23)	60.0% (9/15)	NS (0.101)
Meconium staining	8.3% (4/48)	0% (0/19)	0% (0/27)	17.4% (4/23)	6.7% (1/15)	NS (0.108)
Antenatal use of corticosteroids	81.2% (39/48)	68.4% (13/19)	77.8% (21/27)	82.6% (19/23)	86.7% (13/15)	NS (0.702)
Antenatal use of antibiotics	70.8% (34/48)	73.7% (14/19)	81.5% (22/27)	100% (23/23) [f]	93.3% (14/15)	0.029
Antenatal use of tocolytics	66.7% (32/48)	78.9% (15/19)	81.5% (22/27)	91.3% (21/23)	86.7% (13/15)	NS (0.145)

GA, gestational age; NS, not significant; preterm-PROM, preterm premature rupture of membranes; PTB, preterm birth; SD, standard deviation. [†] Group-0: inflammation-free extra-placental membranes (EPM). [†] Group-1: inflammation restricted to decidua. [†] Group-2: inflammation restricted to the membranous trophoblast of chorion and the decidua. [†] Group-3: inflammation in the connective tissue of chorion but not the amnion. [†] Group-4: amnionitis. [a] Intergroup difference by Chi-square test (categorical variables) and Kruskal–Wallis test (continuous variables). [b] $p < 0.05$ vs. group-0 (1-way ANOVA with post-hoc Tukey test). [c] $p < 0.005$ vs. group-0 (1-way ANOVA with post-hoc Tukey test). [d] $p < 0.05$ vs. group-1 (1-way ANOVA with post-hoc Tukey test). [e] $p < 0.05$ vs. group-0 (1-way ANOVA with post-hoc Tukey test). [f] $p < 0.05$ vs. group-0 (Fisher's exact test with Bonferroni's correction).

Table 2. Diagnostic indices, predictive values, and likelihood ratios of maternal NLR (neutrophil to lymphocyte ratio) ≥ 7.75 within 48 h before delivery for the identification of amnionitis in cases with either preterm labor and intact membranes (PTL) or preterm premature rupture of membranes (preterm-PROM) (The prevalence of amnionitis is 11.4% (15/132)).

	Sensitivity	Specificity	Positive Predictive Value	Negative Predictive Value	Positive LR (95% CI)	Negative LR (95% CI)
NLR ≥ 7.75	80.0% (12/15)	59.0% (69/117)	20.0% (12/60)	95.8% (69/72)	2.9487 (1.0597–8.2047)	0.5128 (0.3674–0.7158)

CI, confidence interval; LR, likelihood ratio; NLR, neutrophil to lymphocyte ratio.

3.2. Maternal Neutrophil to Lymphocyte Ratios (NLRs) According to the Progression of Acute Histologic Chorioamnionitis (Acute-HCA) in Extra-Placental Membranes (EPM)

Figure 1 shows maternal NLRs according to the progression of acute-HCA in EPM. Maternal NLRs significantly and progressively increased with the progression of acute-HCA (Kruskal–Wallis test, $p = 0.001$; and Spearman's rank correlation test, $\gamma = 0.363$, $p = 0.000019$) (Figure 1). Maternal hs-CRP (mg/dL) also significantly and progressively increased with the progression of acute-HCA (Kruskal–Wallis test, $p = 0.006$; and Spearman's rank correlation test, $\gamma = 0.298$, $p = 0.000900$) (Figure S1).

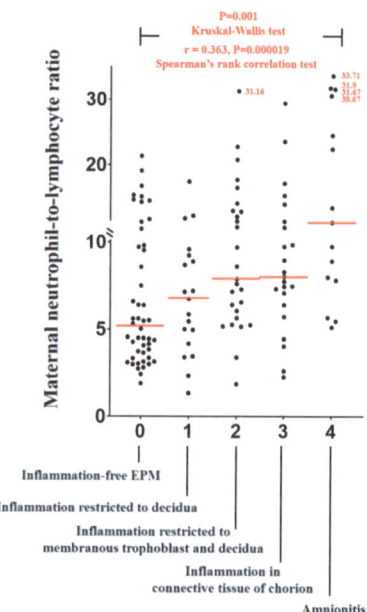

Figure 1. Maternal neutrophil to lymphocyte ratios (NLRs) according to the progression of acute histologic chorioamnionitis (acute-HCA) in extra-placental membranes (EPM). Maternal NLRs significantly and progressively increased with the progression of acute-HCA (group-0 vs. group-1 vs. group-2 vs. group-3 vs. group-4; median, range; 5.15 (1.90–21.30) vs. 6.70 (1.30–17.40) vs. 7.90 (1.90–31.20) vs. 8.00 (2.30–29.40) vs. 11.20 (5.10–33.70)). Each p value is shown in the graph.

3.3. Diagnostic Indices, Predictive Values, and Likelihood Ratios of Increased Maternal Neutrophil to Lymphocyte Ratio (NLR) for the Identification of Amnionitis

ROC curves were constructed to select the cut-off values for identifying maternal NLR (area under curve (AUC), 0.745; standard error (SE), 0.066; p = 0.002) as being raised or not raised for the identification of amnionitis and a cut-off value of 7.75 was chosen (Figure S2, red line). Moreover, for the comparison with maternal NLR, we constructed a ROC curve to choose the cut-off values for the discovery of maternal hs-CRP (AUC, 0.581; SE, 0.086; p = 0.323) as being raised or not raised for the diagnosis of amnionitis and a cut-off value of 1.035 mg/dL was chosen (Figure S2, blue line). Table 2 displays diagnostic indices, predictive values, and the likelihood ratios of increased maternal NLR ($\geq$7.75) within 48 h before delivery for the identification of amnionitis. Moreover, we demonstrated diagnostic indices, predictive values, and likelihood ratios of maternal hs-CRP $\geq$ 1.035 mg/dL within 48 h before delivery for the identification of amnionitis in cases with either PTL or preterm-PROM (Table S2). However, these positive and negative likelihood ratios were not significant (Table S2).

3.4. The Frequency of Increased Maternal Neutrophil to Lymphocyte Ratio (NLR) According to the Progression of Acute Histologic Chorioamnionitis (Acute-HCA) in Extra-Placental Membranes (EPM)

There was a significant stepwise increase in the frequency of increased maternal NLR ($\geq$7.75) according to the progression of acute-HCA in EPM (Pearson's chi-square test, p = 0.014; and linear by linear association, p = 0.000833) (Figure 2). Moreover, Table 3 demonstrated that increased maternal NLR ($\geq$7.75) was a significant independent risk factor for amnionitis even after the correction for potential confounding variables. We additionally demonstrated the frequency of increased maternal hs-CRP ($\geq$1.035 mg/dL) according to the progression of acute-HCA in EPM (Figure S3). However, increased maternal hs-CRP ≥ 1.013 mg/dL was not an independent risk factor for amnionitis (Table S3).

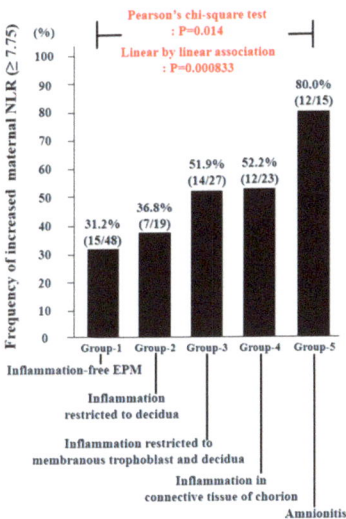

Figure 2. Frequency of increased maternal neutrophil to lymphocyte ratio (NLR) (≥ 7.75) according to the progression of acute histologic chorioamnionitis (acute-HCA) in extra-placental membranes (EPM). Each p value is shown in the graph.

Table 3. Relationship of various independent variables with amnionitis analyzed by overall logistic regression analysis.

	Odds Ratio	95% Confidence Interval	p Value
Increased maternal NLR (≥ 7.75)	5.559	1.255–24.621	0.024
Gestational age at delivery (on a daily basis)	0.716	0.562–0.912	0.007
Parity (≥ 1)	2.209	0.567–8.602	NS (0.253)
Preterm-PROM as a cause of PTB	1.258	0.311–5.091	NS (0.748)
Vaginal delivery	0.945	0.217–4.116	NS (0.940)
Antenatal corticosteroids use	9.474	0.989–90.794	NS (0.051)
Antenatal antibiotics use	0.980	0.076–12.607	NS (0.987)
Antenatal tocolytics use	1.367	0.193–9.665	NS (0.754)
Meconium staining	0.752	0.071–7.938	NS (0.813)
Male sex of newborn	1.765	0.486–6.406	NS (0.388)
Either clinical history of antenatal vaginal bleedingor the evidence of placenta previa	2.674	0.296–24.131	NS (0.381)

NLR, neutrophil to lymphocyte ratio; preterm-PROM, preterm premature rupture of membranes; PTB, preterm birth.

3.5. Histopathology and Schema of the Progression of Acute Histologic Chorioamnionitis (Acute-HCA) in Extra-Placental Membranes (EPM)

Figure 3 shows representative images for inflammation-free EPM (a, group-0), inflammation restricted to decidua (b, group-1), inflammation restricted to the membranous trophoblast of chorion and the decidua (c, group-2), inflammation in the connective tissue of chorion but not amnion (d, group-3), and amnionitis (e, group-4) in H&E stained histologic sections of EPM. Figure 3f is the schema depicting the progression of acute-HCA generated by outside-in neutrophils migration in the entire sub-divisions of EPM.

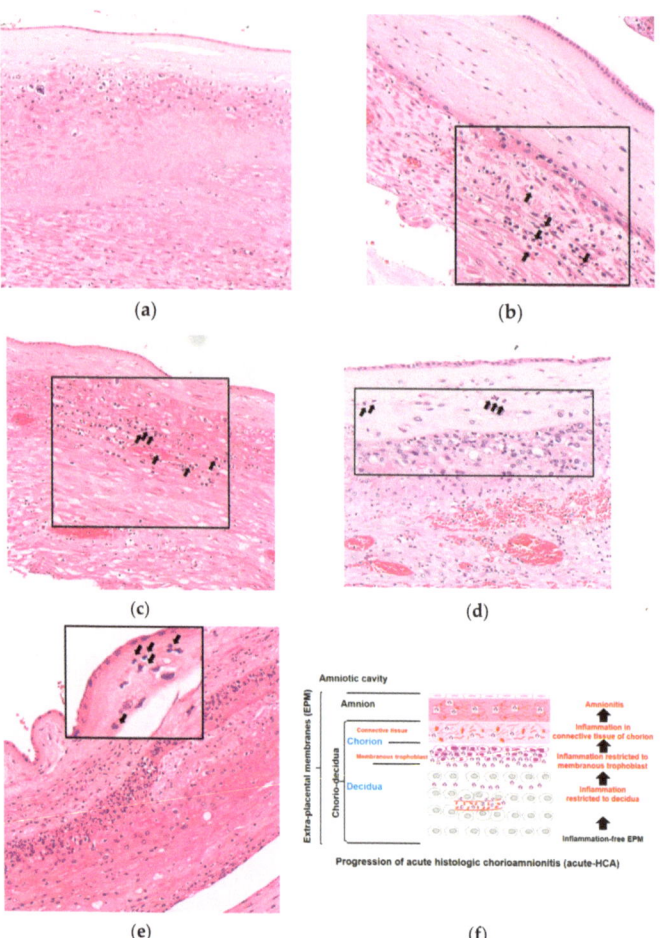

Figure 3. Histopathology and schema of the progression of acute histologic chorioamnionitis (acute-HCA). Hematoxylin and eosin stained histologic sections of extra-placental membrane (EPM) are shown as follows: (**a**) group-0, inflammation-free EPM; (**b**) group-1, inflammation restricted to decidua; (**c**) group-2, inflammation restricted to the membranous trophoblast of chorion and the decidua; (**d**) group-3, inflammation in the connective tissue of chorion but not amnion; (**e**) group-4, amnionitis. These images are based on the magnification setting ×200 and the insets of panels are based on the magnification setting ×400. Some neutrophils are shown in the decidua (group-1) (**b**), the membrane trophoblast of chorion (group-2) (**c**), the connective tissue of chorion (**d**), and amnion (**e**) (see the insets of panels). Black arrows in the insets of panels indicate neutrophils infiltrating into EPM (**b**–**e**). The schema of the progression of acute-HCA depicts outside-in neutrophils migration in the whole sub-divisions of EPM (**f**).

4. Discussion

4.1. Principal Findings of This Study

Maternal NLRs significantly and progressively increased according to the progression of acute-HCA (Figure 4) and increased maternal NLR (≥ 7.75) was an independent risk factor for amnionitis in spontaneous PTB. This finding suggests maternal NLR may be used as a non-invasive antenatal marker for amnionitis.

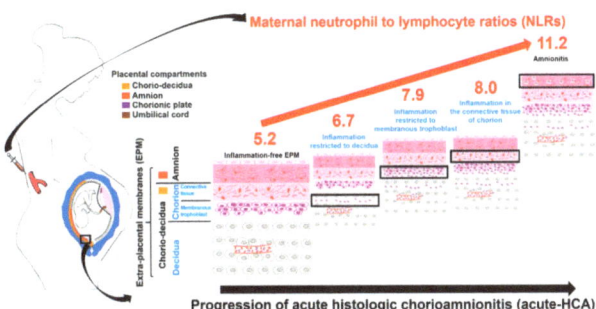

Figure 4. Schema of maternal neutrophil to lymphocyte ratios (NLRs) according to the progression of acute histologic chorioamnionitis (acute-HCA).

4.2. Limitations of Previous Studies Reporting the Relationship between Maternal Inflammatory Blood Markers and Acute Histologic Chorioamnionitis (Acute-HCA) in Extra-Placental Membranes (EPM)

There is a good chance that maternal inflammatory blood markers and immunologic responses develop when acute-HCA sequentially progresses in EPM resulting in either PTL or preterm-PROM. However, previous studies show inconclusive results and, moreover, possessed limitations in terms of the diagnosis of the progression of acute-HCA in EPM, which did not evaluate the whole sub-divisions of EPM (i.e., decidua, the membranous trophoblast of chorion, the connective tissue of chorion, and amnion) as follows (Table 1): (1) not available for the diagnostic criteria of acute-HCA in EPM [19,23,27,30,32]; (2) does not include the decidua [17–19,22,23,27,30,32,34,36,37,39,42]; (3) does not include chorion [19,23,27,30,32,42]; (4) does not include the chorio-decidua [19,23,27,30,32,42]; (5) does not include the membranous trophoblast of chorion [19,23,27,30,32,42]; (6) does not include the connective tissue of chorion [19,23,27,30,32,42]; (7) does not divide chorio-decidua into chorion and decidua [15,19–21,23,27–30,32,38,40,42]; (8) does not divide chorion into membranous trophoblast and connective tissue [13–16,19–21,23–33,35,36,38–42]; (9) does not differentiate the connective tissue of the chorion from amnion [16–19,22,23,27,30,32,34,37]; (10) does not consider amniotropic neutrophils migration as a progression of acute-HCA in EPM [19,23,27,30–32,42].

4.3. The Usefulness of Neutrophil to Lymphocyte Ratio (NLR) as a Maternal Inflammatory Blood Marker during Pregnancy

What is noteworthy is that the absolute count of each neutrophil and lymphocyte, but not the percentage of each neutrophil and lymphocyte as a relative ratio within leukocytes, should be interpreted cautiously because leukocytosis usually occurs during normal pregnancy [66] and the normal range of leukocyte count is widely variable among pregnant women [67–71]. Therefore, it is reasonable that the percentage of each neutrophil and lymphocyte, but not the absolute count of each neutrophil and lymphocyte in maternal blood, is used for the differentiation between inflammation-free placenta and acute-HCA during antenatal period.

4.4. Biologic Plausibility about Increased Maternal Inflammatory Blood Markers According to the Progression of Acute Histologic Chorioamnionitis (Acute-HCA) in Extra-Placental Membranes (EPM)

We previously demonstrated that intra-amniotic infection and inflammation recruits maternal neutrophils to the feto-maternal interface of chorio-decidua from maternal decidual vessels in both preterm rhesus model and human spontaneous PTB [72]; moreover, intra-amniotic inflammatory responses are more severe according to outside-in neutrophils migration in the chorio-decidua of EPM in human spontaneous PTB (i.e., 'inflammation restricted to decidua', 'inflammation restricted to the membranous trophoblast of chorion and the decidua', and 'inflammation in the connective tissue of chorion') [12]. Given that 'leukocyte integrin lymphocyte function-associated antigen 1 (LFA-1)' and its endothelial ligand 'intercellular adhesion molecule (ICAM)-1' play an important role in the endothelial adhesivity and transmigration of neutrophils in the capillaries of in vivo and in vitro inflammation models [73,74], we should find evidence about the expression of LFA-1/ICAM-1 in both maternal blood and EPM in the context of acute-HCA to explain the biological plausibility with respect to the positive correlation between maternal NLRs and the progression of acute-HCA generated by outside-in neutrophils migration in EPM. Indeed, maternal blood ICAM-1 was reported to be a reliable indicator of acute-HCA among cases with either PTL [28,42] or preterm-PROM [42] in spite of the above-mentioned limitations in those studies [28,42]. Moreover, EPM shows about a five-fold elevation of LFA-1 and about a three-fold elevation of ICAM-1 in mRNA sequencing profiles in preterm rhesus macaques delivered after 48 h following intra-amniotic lipopolysaccharides (LPS) infusion in our previous study (unpublished data). Therefore, one can expect that maternal NLRs significantly and progressively increased according to the progression of acute-HCA generated by outside-in neutrophils migration in EPM.

4.5. Major Strengths and Limitation of This Study

Firstly, the current study analyzed the progression of acute-HCA in the whole sub-divisions of EPM (i.e., decidua, the membranous trophoblast of chorion, the connective tissue of chorion, and amnion). Secondly, this study demonstrated that increased maternal NLR is an independent risk factor for amnionitis, known as advanced acute-HCA in EPM, even after the adjustment for the potential confounding variables including GA at delivery. Thirdly, this study recommended maternal NLR as a maternal inflammatory blood maker for the identification of acute-HCA with the use of a simple and widely available CBC in every medical institution. Although we did not compare the specificity and sensitivity for the identification of amnionitis between maternal NLR and other tests such as cytokines and chemokines, the measurements of cytokines and chemokines are not generally and widely available in every hospital. Limitation of this study is that the positive and negative LRs of maternal NLR cut-off 7.75 for the identification of amnionitis remained low. However, we did not find any non-invasive maternal blood biomarker for amnionitis (Table S1) and, therefore, maternal NLR may be promising for future trials for the identification of amnionitis.

4.6. Significance of This Study

This is the first human research reporting that maternal NLRs are significantly and positively correlated with the progression of acute-HCA in the whole sub-divisions of EPM (Figure 4) and that maternal NLRs are an independent risk factor for amnionitis, known as advanced acute-HCA, even after the correction for the potential confounding variables. This finding suggests maternal NLR may be used as a non-invasive antenatal marker for amnionitis.

4.7. Unanswered Questions and Proposals for Future Study

It is not yet known whether maternal inflammatory blood markers (i.e., NLR) can be used for the prediction for early acute-HCA in EPM (i.e., inflammation restricted to the decidua and inflammation restricted to the membrane trophoblast of chorion). This kind of study will improve the value of non-invasive maternal blood inflammatory markers for the early identification of pregnant women at risk for spontaneous PTB. However, the evaluation of the performance of NLR should clearly require a prospective description of this parameter in a cohort of patients with threatened PTL or preterm-PROM, including a part of patients remaining undelivered as is observed in real life.

5. Conclusions

Maternal NLRs significantly and progressively increased according to the progression of acute-HCA and increased maternal NLR (≥7.75) was an independent risk factor for amnionitis in spontaneous PTB.

Supplementary Materials: The following are available online at https://www.mdpi.com/article/10.3390/jcm10122673/s1, Figure S1: Maternal high sensitivity C-reactive protein (hs-CRP) (mg/dL) according to the progression of acute histologic chorioamnionitis (acute-HCA) in extra-placental membranes (EPM), Figure S2: A receiver operating characteristics (ROC) curve was constructed to select the cut-off values at which to identify maternal NLR, as being raised or not raised for the identification of amnionitis, Figure S3: Frequency of increased maternal high sensitivity C-reactive protein (hs-CRP) (≥1.035 mg/dL) according to the progression of acute histologic chorioamnionitis (acute-HCA) in extra-placental membranes (EPM), Table S1: Previous studies reporting the relationship between maternal inflammatory blood markers and acute histologic chorioamnionitis (acute-HCA) in ex-tra-placental membranes (EPM), Table S2: Diagnostic indices, predictive values, and likelihood ratios of maternal high sensitivity C-reactive protein (hs-CRP) ≥ 1.035 mg/dL within 48 h before delivery for the identification of amnionitis in cases with either preterm labor and intact membranes (PTL) or preterm premature rupture of membranes (preterm-PROM), Table S3: Relationship of various independent variables with amnionitis analyzed by overall logistic regression analysis.

Author Contributions: Conceptualization, C.-W.P. and J.-H.L.; methodology, C.-W.P.; software, C.-W.P.; validation, C.-W.P. and J.-H.L.; formal analysis, C.-W.P.; investigation, C.-W.P. and J.-H.L.; resources, C.-W.P.; data curation, C.-W.P.; writing—original draft preparation, C.-W.P. and J.-H.L.; writing—review and editing, C.-W.P., J.-H.L., K.-C.M., J.-S.P. and J.-K.J.; visualization, C.-W.P.; supervision, C.-W.P.; project administration, C.-W.P.; funding acquisition, C.-W.P. All authors have read and agreed to the published version of the manuscript.

Funding: This work was supported by the Research Resettlement Fund for the new faculty of Seoul National University (800-20160056).

Institutional Review Board Statement: The study was conducted according to the guidelines of the Declaration of Helsinki and the Institutional Review Board of Seoul National University Hospital specifically approved this study (IRB-No: 1910-126-1072, and 28 October 2019).

Informed Consent Statement: Written informed consent was obtained from the entire study population.

Conflicts of Interest: The authors declare no conflict of interest.

References

1. Goldenberg, R.L.; Hauth, J.C.; Andrews, W.W. Intrauterine Infection and Preterm Delivery. *N. Engl. J. Med.* **2000**, *342*, 1500–1507. [CrossRef] [PubMed]
2. Romero, R.; Mazor, M. Infection and Preterm Labor. *Clin. Obstet. Gynecol.* **1988**, *31*, 553–584. [CrossRef] [PubMed]
3. Gomez, R.; Romero, R.; Ghezzi, F.; Yoon, B.H.; Mazor, M.; Berry, S.M. The fetal inflammatory response syndrome. *Am. J. Obstet. Gynecol.* **1998**, *179*, 194–202. [CrossRef]
4. Kim, C.J.; Romero, R.; Chaemsaithong, P.; Chaiyasit, N.; Yoon, B.H.; Kim, Y.M. Acute chorioamnionitis and funisitis: Definition, pathologic features, and clinical significance. *Am. J. Obstet. Gynecol.* **2015**, *213*, S29–S52. [CrossRef]
5. Redline, R.W.; Faye-Petersen, O.; Heller, D.; Qureshi, F.; Savell, V.; Vogler, C. Amniotic Infection Syndrome: Nosology and Reproducibility of Placental Reaction Patterns. *Pediatr. Dev. Pathol.* **2003**, *6*, 435–448. [CrossRef]
6. Khong, T.Y.; Mooney, E.E.; Ariel, I.; Balmus, N.C.M.; Boyd, T.K.; Brundler, M.-A.; Derricott, H.; Evans, M.J.; Faye-Petersen, O.M.; Gillan, J.E.; et al. Sampling and Definitions of Placental Lesions: Amsterdam Placental Workshop Group Consensus Statement. *Arch. Pathol. Lab. Med.* **2016**, *140*, 698–713. [CrossRef]
7. Hyunyoon, B.; Kwanjun, J.; Hoonpark, K.; Chulsyn, H.; Gomez, R.; Romero, R. Serum C-reactive protein, white blood cell count, and amniotic fluid white blood cell count in women with preterm premature rupture of membranes. *Obstet. Gynecol.* **1996**, *88*, 1034–1040. [CrossRef]
8. Yoon, B.; Yang, S.; Jun, J.; Park, K.; Kim, C.; Romero, R. Maternal blood C-reactive protein, white blood cell count, and temperature in preterm labor: A comparison with amniotic fluid white blood cell count. *Obstet. Gynecol.* **1996**, *87*, 231–237. [CrossRef]
9. Yoon, B.H.; Romero, R.; Bin Moon, J.; Shim, S.-S.; Kim, M.; Kim, G.; Jun, J.K. Clinical significance of intra-amniotic inflammation in patients with preterm labor and intact membranes. *Am. J. Obstet. Gynecol.* **2001**, *185*, 1130–1136. [CrossRef]
10. Shim, S.-S.; Romero, R.; Hong, J.-S.; Park, C.-W.; Jun, J.K.; Kim, B.I.; Yoon, B.H. Clinical significance of intra-amniotic inflammation in patients with preterm premature rupture of membranes. *Am. J. Obstet. Gynecol.* **2004**, *191*, 1339–1345. [CrossRef]

11. Oh, J.-W.; Park, C.-W.; Moon, K.C.; Park, J.S.; Jun, J.K. Inflammation in the connective-tissue of chorion, but not inflammation restricted to the trophoblast-layer of chorion and the decidua, is associated with the development of amnionitis and more intense acute-histologic chorioamnionitis in the context of choriodeciduitis. *Placenta* **2017**, *57*, 327–328. [CrossRef]
12. Park, C.-W.; Moon, K.C.; Park, J.S.; Jun, J.K.; Romero, R.; Yoon, B.H. The Involvement of Human Amnion in Histologic Chorioamnionitis is an Indicator that a Fetal and an Intra-Amniotic Inflammatory Response is more Likely and Severe: Clinical Implications. *Placenta* **2009**, *30*, 56–61. [CrossRef]
13. Kidokoro, K.; Furuhashi, M.; Kuno, N.; Ishikawa, K. Amniotic fluid neutrophil elastase and lactate dehydrogenase: Association with histologic chorioamnionitis. *Acta Obstet. Gynecol. Scand.* **2006**, *85*, 669–674. [CrossRef]
14. Erdemir, G.; Kultursay, N.; Calkavur, S.; Zekioğlu, O.; Koroglu, O.A.; Cakmak, B.; Yalaz, M.; Akisu, M.; Sagol, S. Histological Chorioamnionitis: Effects on Premature Delivery and Neonatal Prognosis. *Pediatr. Neonatol.* **2013**, *54*, 267–274. [CrossRef]
15. Park, C.-W.; Yoon, B.H.; Park, J.S.; Jun, J.K. An elevated maternal serum C-reactive protein in the context of intra-amniotic inflammation is an indicator that the development of amnionitis, an intense fetal and AF inflammatory response are likely in patients with preterm labor: Clinical implications. *J. Matern. Neonatal Med.* **2013**, *26*, 847–853. [CrossRef]
16. Kim, M.-A.; Lee, Y.S.; Seo, K. Assessment of Predictive Markers for Placental Inflammatory Response in Preterm Births. *PLoS ONE* **2014**, *9*, e107880. [CrossRef]
17. Martinez-Portilla, R.J.; Hawkins-Villarreal, A.; Alvarez-Ponce, P.; Chinolla-Arellano, Z.L.; Moreno-Espinosa, A.L.; Sandoval-Mejia, A.L.; Moreno-Uribe, N. Maternal Serum Interleukin-6: A Non-Invasive Predictor of Histological Chorioamnionitis in Women with Preterm-Prelabor Rupture of Membranes. *Fetal Diagn. Ther.* **2018**, *45*, 168–175. [CrossRef]
18. Howman, R.A.; Charles, A.; Jacques, A.; Doherty, D.A.; Simmer, K.; Strunk, T.; Richmond, P.; Cole, C.H.; Burgner, D.P. Inflammatory and Haematological Markers in the Maternal, Umbilical Cord and Infant Circulation in Histological Chorioamnionitis. *PLoS ONE* **2012**, *7*, e51836. [CrossRef]
19. Zhu, X.; Xie, A.; Zhang, W.; Chen, M.; Wang, Y.; Wang, Y.; Zhou, Q. Related Factors and Adverse Neonatal Outcomes in Women with Preterm Premature Rupture of Membranes Complicated by Histologic Chorioamnionitis. *Med. Sci. Monit.* **2015**, *21*, 390–395. [CrossRef] [PubMed]
20. Kim, S.A.; Park, K.H.; Lee, S.M. Non-Invasive Prediction of Histologic Chorioamnionitis in Women with Preterm Premature Rupture of Membranes. *Yonsei Med. J.* **2016**, *57*, 461–468. [CrossRef]
21. Park, J.W.; Park, K.H.; Kook, S.Y.; Jung, Y.M.; Kim, Y.M. Immune biomarkers in maternal plasma to identify histologic chorioamnionitis in women with preterm labor. *Arch. Gynecol. Obstet.* **2019**, *299*, 725–732. [CrossRef]
22. Hackney, D.N.; MacPherson, T.; Dunigan, J.T.; Simhan, H.N. First-trimester maternal plasma concentrations of C-reactive protein in low-risk patients and the subsequent development of chorioamnionitis. *Am. J. Perinatol.* **2008**, *25*, 407–411. [CrossRef] [PubMed]
23. Wu, H.-C.; Shen, C.-M.; Wu, Y.-Y.; Yuh, Y.-S.; Kua, K.-E. Subclinical Histologic Chorioamnionitis and Related Clinical and Laboratory Parameters in Preterm Deliveries. *Pediatr. Neonatol.* **2009**, *50*, 217–221. [CrossRef]
24. Yamada, T.; Matsubara, S.; Minakami, H.; Ohkuchi, A.; Hiratsuka, M.; Sato, I. Relation between viability of vaginal polymorphonuclear leukocytes and presence of listologic chorioamnionitis. *Acta Obstet. et Gynecol. Scand.* **2000**, *79*, 818–823. [CrossRef]
25. Kurakazu, M.; Yotsumoto, F.; Arima, H.; Izuchi, D.; Urushiyama, D.; Miyata, K.; Kiyoshima, C.; Fukagawa, S.; Yoshikawa, K.; Kurakazu, M.; et al. The combination of maternal blood and amniotic fluid biomarkers improves the predictive accuracy of histologic chorioamnionitis. *Placenta* **2019**, *80*, 4–7. [CrossRef]
26. Maeda, K.; Matsuzaki, N.; Fuke, S.; Mitsuda, N.; Shimoya, K.; Nakayama, M.; Suehara, N.; Aono, T.; Mitsuda, N. Value of the Maternal Interleukin 6 Level for Determination of Histologic Chorioamnionitis in Preterm Delivery. *Gynecol. Obstet. Investig.* **1997**, *43*, 225–231. [CrossRef]
27. Kwak, D.-W.; Cho, H.Y.; Kwon, J.-Y.; Park, Y.-W.; Kim, Y.-H. Usefulness of maternal serum C-reactive protein with vaginal Ureaplasma urealyticum as a marker for prediction of imminent preterm delivery and chorioamnionitis in patients with preterm labor or preterm premature rupture of membranes. *J. Périnat. Med.* **2015**, *43*, 409–415. [CrossRef]
28. Steinborn, A. Serum intercellular adhesion molecule-1 levels and histologic chorioamnionitis. *Obstet. Gynecol.* **2000**, *95*, 671–676. [CrossRef]
29. Oh, K.; Park, K.; Kim, S.-N.; Jeong, E.; Lee, S.; Yoon, H. Predictive value of intra-amniotic and serum markers for inflammatory lesions of preterm placenta. *Placenta* **2011**, *32*, 732–736. [CrossRef]
30. Makino, I.; Makino, Y.; Yoshihara, F.; Nishikimi, T.; Kawarabayashi, T.; Kangawa, K.; Shibata, K. Decreased mature adrenomedullin levels in feto-maternal tissues of pregnant women with histologic chorioamnionitis. *Biochem. Biophys. Res. Commun.* **2003**, *301*, 437–442. [CrossRef]
31. Cho, H.Y.; Jung, I.; Kwon, J.-Y.; Kim, S.J.; Park, Y.W.; Kim, Y.-H. The Delta Neutrophil Index as a predictive marker of histological chorioamnionitis in patients with preterm premature rupture of membranes: A retrospective study. *PLoS ONE* **2017**, *12*, e0173382. [CrossRef] [PubMed]
32. Broumand, F.; Naji, S.; Seivani, S. Predictive values of maternal serum levels of procalcitonin, ESR, CRP, and WBC in the diagnosis of chorioamnionitis in mothers with preterm premature rupture of membrane. *Iranian J. Neonatol.* **2018**, *9*, 50–60. [CrossRef]
33. Shimoya, K.; Matsuzaki, N.; Taniguchi, T.; Okada, T.; Saji, F.; Murata, Y. Interleukin-8 level in maternal serum as a marker for screening of histological chorioamnionitis at term. *Int. J. Gynecol. Obstet.* **1997**, *57*, 153–159. [CrossRef]

34. Ahmed, W.A.S.; Ahmed, M.R.; Mohamed, M.L.; Hamdy, M.A.; Kamel, Z.; Elnahas, K.M. Maternal serum interleukin-6 in the management of patients with preterm premature rupture of membranes. *J. Matern. Neonatal Med.* **2015**, *29*, 3162–3166. [CrossRef]
35. Yoneda, S.; Shiozaki, A.; Ito, M.; Yoneda, N.; Inada, K.; Yonezawa, R.; Kigawa, M.; Saito, S. Accurate Prediction of the Stage of Histological Chorioamnionitis before Delivery by Amniotic Fluid IL-8 Level. *Am. J. Reprod. Immunol.* **2015**, *73*, 568–576. [CrossRef]
36. Gulati, S.; Bhatnagar, S.; Raghunandan, C.; Bhattacharjee, J. Interleukin-6 as a Predictor of Subclinical Chorioamnionitis in Preterm Premature Rupture of Membranes. *Am. J. Reprod. Immunol.* **2012**, *67*, 235–240. [CrossRef]
37. Caloone, J.; Rabilloud, M.; Boutitie, F.; Traverse-Glehen, A.; Allias-Montmayeur, F.; Denis, L.; Boisson-Gaudin, C.; Hot, I.J.; Guerre, P.; Cortet, M.; et al. Accuracy of several maternal seric markers for predicting histological chorioamnionitis after preterm premature rupture of membranes: A prospective and multicentric study. *Eur. J. Obstet. Gynecol. Reprod. Biol.* **2016**, *205*, 133–140. [CrossRef]
38. Cobo, T.; Kacerovsky, M.; Palacio, M.; Hornychova, H.; Hougaard, D.M.; Skogstrand, K.; Jacobsson, B. A prediction model of histological chorioamnionitis and funisitis in preterm prelabor rupture of membranes: Analyses of multiple proteins in the amniotic fluid. *J. Matern. Neonatal Med.* **2012**, *25*, 1995–2001. [CrossRef]
39. Gulati, S.; Agrawal, S.; Raghunandan, C.; Bhattacharya, J.; Saili, A.; Agarwal, S.; Sharma, D. Maternal serum interleukin-6 and its association with clinicopathological infectious morbidity in preterm premature rupture of membranes: A prospective cohort study. *J. Matern. Neonatal Med.* **2012**, *25*, 1428–1432. [CrossRef]
40. Škrablin, S.; Lovrić, H.; Banović, V.; Kralik, S.; Dijaković, A.; Kalafatic, D. Maternal plasma interleukin-6, interleukin-1β and C-reactive protein as indicators of tocolysis failure and neonatal outcome after preterm delivery. *J. Matern. Neonatal Med.* **2007**, *20*, 335–341. [CrossRef]
41. Ohyama, M.; Itani, Y.; Yamanaka, M.; Goto, A.; Kato, K.; Ijiri, R.; Tanaka, Y. Re-evaluation of chorioamnionitis and funisitis with a special reference to subacute chorioamnionitis. *Hum. Pathol.* **2002**, *33*, 183–190. [CrossRef]
42. Li, Z.; Huijun, Z.; Jianfang, Z.; Jianwen, Z. The value of the soluable intercellular adhesion molecule-1 levels in matermal serum for determination of occult chorioamnionitis in premature rupture of membranes. *Acta Acad. Med. Wuhan* **2004**, *24*, 154–157. [CrossRef]
43. Blanc, W.A. Pathology of the placenta, membranes, and umbilical cord in bacterial, fungal, and viral infections in man. *Monogr. Pathol.* **1981**, *22*, 67–132.
44. Yoon, B.H.; Romero, R.; Kim, C.J.; Jun, J.K.; Gomez, R.; Choi, J.-H.; Syu, H.C. Amniotic fluid interleukin-6: A sensitive test for antenatal diagnosis of acute inflammatory lesions of preterm placenta and prediction of perinatal morbidity. *Am. J. Obstet. Gynecol.* **1995**, *173*, 960–970. [CrossRef]
45. Blanc, W.A. Amniotic infection syndrome; pathogenesis, morphology, and significance in circumnatal mortality. *Clin. Obstet. Gynecol.* **1959**, *2*, 705–734. [CrossRef]
46. Salafia, C.M.; Weigl, C.; Silberman, L. The prevalence and distribution of acute placental inflammation in uncomplicated term pregnancies. *Obstet. Gynecol.* **1989**, *73*, 383–389. [CrossRef]
47. Abd-Elazeem, M.I.; Mohamed, R.A. Neutrophil-lymphocyte and platelet-lymphocyte ratios in rheumatoid arthritis patients: Relation to disease activity. *Egypt. Rheumatol.* **2018**, *40*, 227–231. [CrossRef]
48. Fu, H.; Qin, B.; Hu, Z.; Ma, N.; Yang, M.; Wei, T.; Tang, Q.; Huang, Y.; Huang, F.; Liang, Y.; et al. Neutrophil- and Platelet-to-Lymphocyte Ratios are Correlated with Disease Activity in Rheumatoid Arthritis. *Clin. Lab.* **2015**, *61*, 269–273. [CrossRef]
49. Wu, Y.; Chen, Y.; Yang, X.; Chen, L.; Yang, Y. Neutrophil-to-lymphocyte ratio (NLR) and platelet-to-lymphocyte ratio (PLR) were associated with disease activity in patients with systemic lupus erythematosus. *Int. Immunopharmacol.* **2016**, *36*, 94–99. [CrossRef]
50. Yang, W.; Wang, X.; Zhang, W.; Ying, H.; Xu, Y.; Zhang, J.; Min, Q.; Chen, J. Neutrophil-lymphocyte ratio and platelet-lymphocyte ratio are 2 new inflammatory markers associated with pulmonary involvement and disease activity in patients with dermatomyositis. *Clin. Chim. Acta* **2017**, *465*, 11–16. [CrossRef]
51. Qin, B.; Ma, N.; Tang, Q.; Wei, T.; Yang, M.; Fu, H.; Hu, Z.; Liang, Y.; Yang, Z.; Zhong, R. Neutrophil to lymphocyte ratio (NLR) and platelet to lymphocyte ratio (PLR) were useful markers in assessment of inflammatory response and disease activity in SLE patients. *Mod. Rheumatol.* **2016**, *26*, 372–376. [CrossRef]
52. Mercan, R.; Bitik, B.; Tufan, A.; Bozbulut, U.B.; Atas, N.; Ozturk, M.A.; Haznedaroglu, S.; Goker, B. The Association between Neutrophil/Lymphocyte Ratio and Disease Activity in Rheumatoid Arthritis and Ankylosing Spondylitis. *J. Clin. Lab. Anal.* **2016**, *30*, 597–601. [CrossRef] [PubMed]
53. Balkarli, A.; Kucuk, A.; Babur, H.; Erbasan, F. Neutrophil/lymphocyte ratio and mean platelet volume in Behçet's disease. *Eur. Rev. Med. Pharmacol. Sci.* **2016**, *20*, 3045–3050. [PubMed]
54. Huang, Z.; Fu, Z.; Huang, W.; Huang, K. Prognostic value of neutrophil-to-lymphocyte ratio in sepsis: A meta-analysis. *Am. J. Emerg. Med.* **2020**, *38*, 641–647. [CrossRef] [PubMed]
55. Hwang, S.Y.; Shin, T.G.; Jo, I.J.; Jeon, K.; Suh, G.Y.; Lee, T.R.; Yoon, H.; Cha, W.C.; Sim, M.S. Neutrophil-to-lymphocyte ratio as a prognostic marker in critically-ill septic patients. *Am. J. Emerg. Med.* **2017**, *35*, 234–239. [CrossRef]
56. Liu, X.; Shen, Y.; Wang, H.; Ge, Q.; Fei, A.; Pan, S. Prognostic Significance of Neutrophil-to-Lymphocyte Ratio in Patients with Sepsis: A Prospective Observational Study. *Mediat. Inflamm.* **2016**, *2016*, 1–8. [CrossRef]

57. Ni, J.; Wang, H.; Li, Y.; Shu, Y.; Liu, Y. Neutrophil to lymphocyte ratio (NLR) as a prognostic marker for in-hospital mortality of patients with sepsis: A secondary analysis based on a single-center, retrospective, cohort study. *Medicine* **2019**, *98*, e18029. [CrossRef]
58. Farkas, J.D. The complete blood count to diagnose septic shock. *J. Thorac. Dis.* **2020**, *12*, S16–S21. [CrossRef]
59. Can, E.; Hamilcikan, Ş.; Can, C. The Value of Neutrophil to Lymphocyte Ratio and Platelet to Lymphocyte Ratio for Detecting Early-onset Neonatal Sepsis. *J. Pediatr. Hematol.* **2018**, *40*, e229–e232. [CrossRef]
60. Ozdemir, A. Predictive value of serum neutrophil-to-lymphocyte ratio in bronchopulmonary dysplasia: A retrospective observational study. *Ann. Med. Res.* **2018**, *25*, 512. [CrossRef]
61. Lee, J.; Park, K.-H.; Kim, A.; Yang, H.-R.; Jung, E.-Y.; Cho, S.-H. Maternal and Placental Risk Factors for Developing Necrotizing Enterocolitis in Very Preterm Infants. *Pediatr. Neonatol.* **2017**, *58*, 57–62. [CrossRef]
62. Gezer, C.; Ekin, A.; Ertas, I.E.; Ozeren, M.; Solmaz, U.; Mat, E.; Taner, C.E. High first-trimester neutrophil-to-lymphocyte and platelet-to-lymphocyte ratios are indicators for early diagnosis of preeclampsia. *Ginekol. Polska* **2016**, *87*, 431–435. [CrossRef]
63. Kurtoglu, E.; Kökçü, A.; Celik, H.; Tosun, M.; Malatyalioglu, E. May ratio of neutrophil to lymphocyte be useful in predicting the risk of developing preeclampsia? A pilot study. *J. Matern. Neonatal Med.* **2015**, *28*, 97–99. [CrossRef]
64. Serin, S.; Avcı, F.; Ercan, O.; Köstü, B.; Bakacak, M.; Kıran, H. Is neutrophil/lymphocyte ratio a useful marker to predict the severity of pre-eclampsia? *Pregnancy Hypertens.* **2016**, *6*, 22–25. [CrossRef]
65. Redman, C.W.; Sacks, G.P.; Sargent, I.L. Preeclampsia: An excessive maternal inflammatory response to pregnancy. *Am. J. Obstet. Gynecol.* **1999**, *180*, 499–506. [CrossRef]
66. Canzoneri, B.J.; Lewis, D.F.; Groome, L.; Wang, Y. Increased Neutrophil Numbers Account for Leukocytosis in Women with Preeclampsia. *Am. J. Perinatol.* **2009**, *26*, 729–732. [CrossRef]
67. Karim, S.A.; Khurshid, M.; Rizvi, J.H.; Jafarey, S.N.; Rizwana, I. Platelets and leucocyte counts in pregnancy. *J. Pak. Med. Assoc.* **1992**, *42*, 86–87.
68. Balloch, A.J.; Cauchi, M.N. Reference ranges for haematology parameters in pregnancy derived from patient populations. *Int. J. Lab. Hematol.* **2008**, *15*, 7–14. [CrossRef]
69. Belo, L.; Santos-Silva, A.; Rocha, S.; Caslake, M.; Cooney, J.; Pereira-Leite, L.; Quintanilha, A.; Rebelo, I. Fluctuations in C-reactive protein concentration and neutrophil activation during normal human pregnancy. *Eur. J. Obstet. Gynecol. Reprod. Biol.* **2005**, *123*, 46–51. [CrossRef]
70. Lockitch, G. *Handbook of Diagnostic Biochemistry and Hematology in Normal Pregnancy*; CRC Press: Boca Baton, FL, USA, 1993.
71. Sanci, M.; Töz, E.; Ince, O.; Özcan, A.; Polater, K.; Inan, A.H.; Beyan, E.; Akkaya, E. Reference values for maternal total and differential leukocyte counts in different trimesters of pregnancy and the initial postpartum period in western Turkey. *J. Obstet. Gynaecol.* **2017**, *37*, 571–575. [CrossRef]
72. Presicce, P.; Park, C.-W.; Senthamaraikannan, P.; Bhattacharyya, S.; Jackson, C.; Kong, F.; Rueda, C.M.; DeFranco, E.; Miller, L.A.; Hildeman, D.A.; et al. IL-1 signaling mediates intrauterine inflammation and chorio-decidua neutrophil recruitment and activation. *JCI Insight* **2018**, *3*, 98306. [CrossRef]
73. Smith, C.W.; Marlin, S.D.; Rothlein, R.; Toman, C.; Anderson, D.C. Cooperative interactions of LFA-1 and Mac-1 with intercellular adhesion molecule-1 in facilitating adherence and transendothelial migration of human neutrophils in vitro. *J. Clin. Investig.* **1989**, *83*, 2008–2017. [CrossRef] [PubMed]
74. Shaw, S.K.; Ma, S.; Kim, M.B.; Rao, R.M.; Hartman, C.U.; Froio, R.M.; Yang, L.; Jones, T.; Liu, Y.; Nusrat, A.; et al. Coordinated Redistribution of Leukocyte LFA-1 and Endothelial Cell ICAM-1 Accompany Neutrophil Transmigration. *J. Exp. Med.* **2004**, *200*, 1571–1580. [CrossRef] [PubMed]

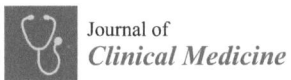

Article

Predictive Factors Involved in Postpartum Regressions of Cytological/Histological Cervical High-Grade Dysplasia Diagnosed during Pregnancy

Yvan Gomez [1,2,*], Vincent Balaya [1,3], Karine Lepigeon [1,2], Patrice Mathevet [1,2] and Martine Jacot-Guillarmod [1,2]

1. Colposcopy Unit, Women-Mother-Child Department, Lausanne University Hospital, 1011 Lausanne, Switzerland; v.balaya@hopital-foch.com (V.B.); karine.lepigeon@chuv.ch (K.L.); patrice.mathevet@chuv.ch (P.M.); Martine.jacot-guillarmod@chuv.ch (M.J.-G.)
2. Faculty of Biology and Medicine, University of Lausanne, 1015 Lausanne, Switzerland
3. Department of Gynecology and Obstetrics, Foch Hospital, 92150 Suresnes, France
* Correspondence: yvan.gomez1@gmail.com

Citation: Gomez, Y.; Balaya, V.; Lepigeon, K.; Mathevet, P.; Jacot-Guillarmod, M. Predictive Factors Involved in Postpartum Regressions of Cytological/ Histological Cervical High-Grade Dysplasia Diagnosed during Pregnancy. *J. Clin. Med.* **2021**, *10*, 5319. https://doi.org/10.3390/ jcm10225319

Academic Editor: Rinat Gabbay-Benziv

Received: 15 October 2021
Accepted: 12 November 2021
Published: 15 November 2021

Publisher's Note: MDPI stays neutral with regard to jurisdictional claims in published maps and institutional affiliations.

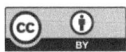

Copyright: © 2021 by the authors. Licensee MDPI, Basel, Switzerland. This article is an open access article distributed under the terms and conditions of the Creative Commons Attribution (CC BY) license (https:// creativecommons.org/licenses/by/ 4.0/).

Abstract: Objective: The aim of this study was to describe the evolution of high-grade cervical dysplasia during pregnancy and the postpartum period and to determine factors associated with dysplasia regression. Methods: Pregnant patients diagnosed with high-grade lesions were identified in our tertiary hospital center. High-grade lesions were defined either cytologically, by high squamous intraepithelial lesion/atypical squamous cells being unable to exclude HSIL (HSIL/ASC-H), or histologically, with cervical intraepithelial neoplasia (CIN) 2+ (all CIN 2 and CIN 3) during pregnancy. Postpartum regression was defined cytologically or histologically by at least a one-degree reduction in severity from the antepartum diagnosis. A logistic regression model was applied to determine independent predictive factors for high-grade cervical dysplasia regression after delivery. Results: Between January 2000 and October 2017, 79 patients fulfilled the inclusion criteria and were analyzed. High-grade cervical lesions were diagnosed by cytology in 87% of cases (69/79) and confirmed by histology in 45% of those (31/69). The overall regression rate in our cohort was 43% (34/79). Univariate analysis revealed that parity ($p = 0.04$), diabetes ($p = 0.04$) and third trimester cytology ($p = 0.009$) were associated with dysplasia regression. Nulliparity (OR = 4.35; 95%CI = (1.03–18.42); $p= 0.046$) was identified by multivariate analysis as an independent predictive factor of high-grade dysplasia regression. The presence of HSIL on third-trimester cervical cytology (OR = 0.17; 95%CI = (0.04–0.72); $p = 0.016$) was identified as an independent predictive factor of high-grade dysplasia persistence at postpartum. Conclusion: Our regression rate was high, at 43%, for high-grade cervical lesions postpartum. Parity status may have an impact on dysplasia regression during pregnancy. A cervical cytology should be performed at the third trimester to identify patients at risk of CIN persistence after delivery. However, larger cohorts are required to confirm these results.

Keywords: high-grade dysplasia; cervical cancer; cervical intraepithelial neoplasia; CIN; HSIL; ASC-H; pregnancy

1. Introduction

In current obstetrical practice, antenatal consultations are commonly considered as an opportunity to screen for cervical cancer. High-grade dysplasia is most frequently diagnosed during the childbearing years, with an incidence of 8.1/1000 women aged 25–29 years [1]. Cervical intraepithelial neoplasia (CIN) is diagnosed in 1–7% of pregnant women [2,3], among whom the prevalence of high-grade lesions (defined as CIN2+) is 0.5% [4]. The progression of high-grade lesions during pregnancy to microinvasive lesions ranges from 0% to 13% [5,6]. Human papilloma virus (HPV) infections appear to be more frequent among pregnant women, which may be related to the immunotolerance observed in pregnancy [7,8].

According to international criteria [9], pregnant patients with cytological abnormalities should be investigated by colposcopy in order to exclude a cancer by targeted biopsy. Although assessment of the cervix in pregnancy may be complicated due to pelvic congestion, colposcopic criteria remain the same as for non-pregnant women. In addition, the transformation zone is well visualized due to the eversion of the endocervix as pregnancy progresses. Cytology, colposcopy, and targeted biopsies are as reliable during pregnancy as for non-pregnant-women [10].

As regards the evolution of cervical dysplasia during pregnancy, the literature has shown a trend toward increased postpartum regression [11]. This regression is possibly related either to the return of the immune system or to a stimulation of it. A previous article suggested that during vaginal delivery, the cervical microlesions induced inflammation and, consequently, regression of the lesions. However, these results remain controversial.

Through a unicentric cohort of pregnant women diagnosed with high-grade cervical dysplasia during pregnancy, the aim of this study was to describe the evolution of high-grade cervical dysplasia during pregnancy and the postpartum period and to determine the factors that can be associated with dysplasia regression.

2. Materials and Methods

We retrospectively reviewed the medical records of pregnant women with high-grade lesions who were referred to the colposcopy unit of our tertiary hospital between January 2000 and September 2017. High-grade lesions were defined either cytologically by high squamous intraepithelial lesion/atypical squamous cells that cannot exclude HSIL (HSIL/ASC-H) or histologically with high-grade cervical intraepithelial neoplasia (CIN 2 and CIN 3), during pregnancy. All CIN 2 and CIN 3 high-grade histologic dysplasia were classified as CIN2+. Other data abstracted from the medical record included parity, tobacco use, diabetes, presence of HPV, first/second/third trimester feature, delivery route and postpartum feature.

Patients were excluded in cases of incomplete cytological or histological ante/postpartum data about the evolution of dysplastic lesions or in cases of the presence of a factor that could affect the patient's immunity (immunosuppressive treatment or acquired/innate immunodeficiency).

Cervical biopsies were not systematically performed but were required in cases of significant discordance between cervical cytology and colposcopic impression or those with colposcopic evidence of invasion. To ensure the expertise of the colposcopy assessment, all cases of high-grade lesions were supervised by a colposcopy expert (MJG), either by the image taken by the colpophotograph or directly during the colposcopy. The follow-up was based on a comparison with the images taken during the previous consultation.

When a diagnosis of high-grade dysplasia was confirmed in a pregnant woman, a quarterly follow-up was scheduled on the basis of typical obstetrical trimesters. At each visit, a cervical PAP smear and a colposcopy were performed, and an additional directed cervical biopsy was carried out in cases of suspected higher-grade lesions. The mode of delivery and other procedures were recorded as well.

In our cohort, the postpartum colposcopic follow-up was performed within six to eight weeks after childbirth. Postpartum regression was defined cytologically or histologically by a reduction of at least one-degree in severity from the antepartum diagnosis, such as HSIL regressed to LSIL/normal or CIN2+ regressed to CIN 1/normal. The histopathological findings in patients who underwent loop electrosurgical excision procedure (LEEP procedure) due to extensive lesions or cytology/colposcopic discordance were included to the analysis.

Qualitative data were compared by using the chi-square test and quantitative data by using the student t-test. Results are presented as 95% confidence intervals (95%CIs) or numbers (percentages). p values lower than 0.05 were retained as significant. Patients with CIN regression were compared to those with CIN persistence during the postpartum period. Relevant covariates associated with cervical dysplasia regressions that were significant ($p < 0.05$) in the univariate analysis were considered in a backward selection procedure to fit a multivariable model. A logistic regression model was applied to determine independent predictive factors for high-grade cervical dysplasia regression after delivery. All statistical analyses were carried out using XLStat Biomed software (AddInsoft V19.4, Paris, France). This study was approved by the ethical research committee of the canton de Vaud (25 July 2019, ID N 2017-01375).

3. Results

Ninety-four women diagnosed with high-grade dysplasia were identified. Among them, four patients with a cytological HSIL were excluded due to an extensive lesion during the antenatal period with colposcopic neoplasia suspicion, who subsequently underwent a LEEP procedure. Finally, only CIN 2+ lesions without invasive lesions were found in these four cases. No cases received corticosteroid treatment in our cohort; only one patient was known to have mother-to-child HIV infection with CD4+ in the normal range throughout her pregnancy. After exclusion of 15 patients, 79 patients fulfilled the inclusion criteria and were analyzed (Figure 1). The characteristics of the study population are presented in Tables 1 and 2.

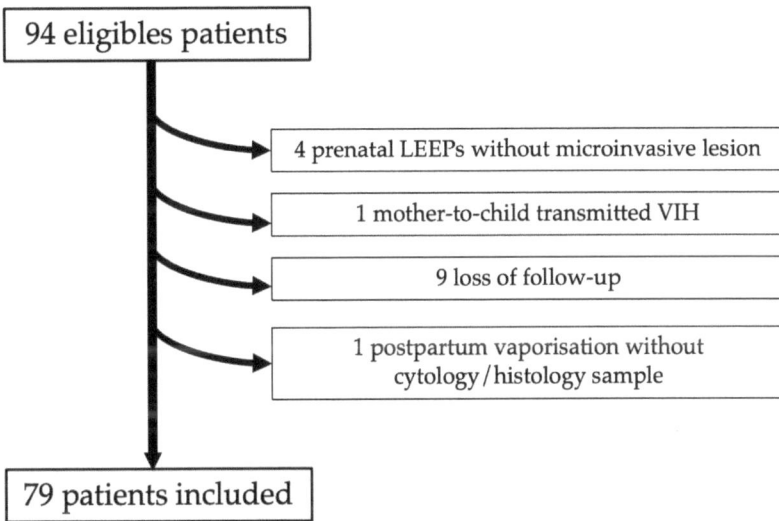

Figure 1. Flow-chart of population study.

Patients had at least two antenatal examinations in 90% of cases (71/79) and all had a postpartum evaluation. High-grade lesions were diagnosed by cytology in 87% of cases (69/79), of which 45% (31/69) were histologically confirmed, whereas the remaining 13% (10/79) were found on biopsies that revealed CIN2+ after initial LSIL cytology. During colposcopic follow-up, no cases of invasive lesions were found. Delivery routes were vaginal in 68% of cases (54/79) and by C-section in 32% of cases (25/79). Among the patients who had a vaginal delivery, 27 delivered spontaneously, 14 were induced for an obstetric indication and 13 were unspecified.

Table 1. General patient characteristics.

Predictive Variable	Overall Population n = 79	
	n Mean ± SD	(%) (Range)
Age (years)		
Mean	29.7 ± 4.8	(20–41)
Parity status		
Nulliparity	40	53.3
Multiparity	35	46.7
Not specified	4	
Tobacco use		
Yes	23	30.7
No	52	69.3
Not specified	4	
Gestational diabetes		
Yes	8	10.7
No	67	89.3
Not specified	4	
Presence of HPV		
Yes	18	22.8
No	61	77.2
Delivery route		
Vaginal delivery	54	68.4
C-section	25	31.6

Table 2. Colposcopy-related patient characteristics by trimester.

Predictive Variable	First Trimester		Second Trimester		Third Trimester		Postpartum Colposcopic Follow Up	
	Overall Population n = 79							
	n Mean ± SD	(%) (Range)	n Mean ± SD	(%) (Range)	n Mean ± SD	(%) (range)	n Mean ± SD	(%) (Range)
Colposcopy performed								
Yes	68	86.1	71	89.9	60	76.0	76	96.2
No	11	13.9	8	10.1	19	24.0	3	3.8
Gestational age (weeks)								
Median	10	(1–20)	20	(12–29)	32	(24–39)		
Aspect								
HSIL	21	65.6	41	67.2	34	68.0	36	65.5
LSIL	10	31.3	15	24.6	14	28.0	12	21.8
Normal	1	3.1	5	8.2	2	4.0	7	12.7
Not specified	36		10		10		21	

Table 2. Cont.

Predictive Variable	First Trimester		Second Trimester		Third Trimester		Postpartum Colposcopic Follow Up	
	Overall Population $n = 79$							
	n Mean ± SD	(%) (Range)	n Mean ± SD	(%) (Range)	n Mean ± SD	(%) (range)	n Mean ± SD	(%) (Range)
Cytology								
HSIL	44	66.7	24	53.3	25	51.0	26	42.6
LSIL	14	21.2	13	28.9	16	32.6	10	16.4
ASC-H	8	12.1	3	6.7	8	16.3	1	1.6
Normal			5	11.1			24	39.3
Not performed	2		26		11		15	
Biopsy								
HSIL	19	90.5	17	81.0	9	69.2	25	53.2
LSIL	2	9.5	2	9.5	2	15.4	12	25.5
Normal			2	9.5	2	15.4	10	21.3
Not performed	47		50		47		29	

At postpartum colposcopic follow up, all patients underwent colposcopy with cytology/histology except for three. These three cases underwent a LEEP procedure immediately postpartum due to CIN2+ extensive antenatal lesions, which was confirmed by the pathology. Of the 27 patients whose postpartum cytology revealed an HSIL, 18 (66.7%) histological samples confirmed a high-grade lesion (either by directed biopsy or conization result) and 6 (22%) samples did not. In the 34 cytological specimens showing an LSIL/ASCUS/normal lesion, only 20 (59%) histological specimens were collected, of which 10 (50%) confirmed a high-grade lesion. For patients who only underwent colposcopic evaluation (15/79), 13 histological samples were taken, 8 (62%) of which confirmed a HSIL lesion. Sixteen patients were only diagnosed cytologically and not histologically, of which only 3 (11%) were in the HSIL group. A total of 47 biopsies and 42 conizations were performed with a rate of 53% (25/47) and 79% (33/42), respectively, of persistent high-grade lesions. Seventy-one percent (56/79) of our cohort had a histological diagnosis at postpartum colposcopic follow up. The overall regression rate in our cohort was 43% (34/79).

Univariate analysis revealed that parity ($p = 0.04$), diabetes ($p = 0.04$) and third trimester cytology ($p = 0.009$) were associated with dysplasia regression. Age, smoking and delivery route did not impact on postpartum CIN regression rate (Tables 3 and 4). By multivariate analysis, nulliparity (OR = 4.35; 95%CI= (1.03–18.42); p= 0.046) and presence of HSIL at third-trimester cervical cytology (OR = 0.17; 95%CI = (0.04–0.72); $p = 0.016$) were identified as independent predictive factors for dysplasia regression (Table 5).

Table 3. Univariate analysis of general factors associated with postpartum CIN regression.

Predictive Variable	Persistence of CIN n = 45		Regression of CIN n = 34		p
	n Mean ± SD	(%) (Range)	n Mean ± SD	(%) (Range)	
Age (years)					
Mean	29.5 ± 4.8	(20–41)	30.1 ± 4.8	(21–41)	0.58
Parity status					
Nulliparity	19	43.2	21	67.7	
Multiparity	25	56.8	10	32.3	**0.04**
Not specified	1		3		
Tobacco use					
Yes	15	34.9	8	25.0	
No	28	65.1	24	75.0	0.36
Not specified	2		2		
Gestational diabetes					
Yes	2	4.5	6	19.4	
No	42	95.5	25	80.6	**0.04**
Not specified	1		3		
Presence of HPV					
Yes	10	22.2	8	23.5	
No	35	77.8	26	76.5	0.89
Delivery route					
Vaginal delivery	32	71.1	22	64.7	0.54
C-section	13	28.9	12	35.3	

Significant statistical values are marked with Bold.

Table 4. Univariate analysis of colposcopic factors by trimester associated with postpartum CIN regression.

	First Trimester Persistence of CIN n=45 n; (%) (Range)	First Trimester Regression of CIN n=34 n; (%) (Range)	p	Second Trimester Persistence of CIN n=45 n; (%) (Range)	Second Trimester Regression of CIN n=34 n; (%) (Range)	p	Third Trimester Persistence of CIN n=45 n; (%) (Range)	Third Trimester Regression of CIN n=34 n; (%) (Range)	p	Postpartum Colposcopic Follow Up Persistence of CIN n=45 n; (%) (Range)	Postpartum Colposcopic Follow Up Regression of CIN n=34 n; (%) (Range)	p
Colposcopy												
Yes	38 84.4	30 88.2	0.63	41 91.1	30 88.2	0.67	30 66.7	30 88.2	**0.03**	42 93.3	34 100	0.12
No	7 15.6	4 11.8		4 8.9	4 11.8		15 33.3	4 11.8		3 6.7	0 0	
Aspect												
HSIL	11 64.7	10 66.7	0.51	25 71.4	16 61.5	0.21	22 78.6	12 54.5	0.1	25 80.6	11 45.8	**0.01**
LSIL	6 35.3	4 26.7		9 25.7	6 23.1		6 21.4	8 36.4		5 16.1	7 29.2	
Normal	0 0.0	1 6.7		1 2.9	4 15.4		0 0.0	2 9.1		1 3.2	6 25	
Not specified	21	15		6	4		2	8		11	10	
Cytology												
HSIL	25 65.8	19 63.3	0.87	12 50.0	12 57.1	0.79	18 72.0	7 29.2	**0.009**	21 63.6	5 17.9	**0.003**
LSIL	7 18.4	7 23.3		8 33.3	5 23.8		4 16.0	12 50.0		3 9.1	7 25.0	
ASC-H	4 10.5	4 13.3		2 8.3	1 4.8		3 12.0	5 20.8		0 0	1 3.6	
Normal	2			2 8.3	3 14.3		5	6		9 27.3	15 53.6	
Not performed	2			17	9					9	6	
Biopsy												
HSIL	8 88.9	11 91.7	0.83	14 87.5	3 60	0.39	7 77.8	2 50.0	0.06	25 78.1	0 0	**<0.0001**
LSIL	1 11.1	1 8.3		1 6.2	1 20		2 22.2	0 0		4 12.5	8 53.3	
Normal				1 6.2	1 20		0 0	2 50.0		3 9.4	7 46.7	
Not performed	29	18		25	25		21	26		10	19	

Significant statistical values are marked with Bold.

Table 5. Multivariate analysis of factors associated with postpartum CIN regression.

Variable	Odds Ratio (95% CI)	p
Parity status		
Multiparity	1	
Nulliparity	4.35 (1.03–18.42)	**0.046**
Gestational diabetes		
No	1	
Yes	6.00 (0.45–79.46)	0.17
Third trimester cervical cytology		
LSIL or ASC-H	1	
HSIL	0.17 (0.04–0.72)	**0.016**

Significant statistical values are marked with Bold.

4. Discussion

The aim of this study was to assess the clinical interest in knowing which factors would allow targeting patients at potential risk of maintaining a high-grade lesion or progressing to a cancerous lesion in the postpartum period and avoiding loss to follow up for adequate treatment.

In our cohort, we reported a regression rate of high-grade lesion at 43% and no case of invasive lesions at postpartum colposcopy follow up. This rate is similar to those reported in the literature of 17–69% [4,5,12,13]. However, these studies show large disparities in terms of diagnostic criteria and therapeutic management. Considering all grades of dysplasia, caution should be paid to the interpretation of these data, since overall regression may design initial high-grade or low-grade lesions [6,11,14–18].

The correlation between cytology and final diagnosis within one degree of severity in pregnant woman has been found to be 78% [10], with cytology having an 88% positive predictive value for high-grade lesions [10]. Regarding colposcopic impressions, the results are consistent with final diagnoses in 73% of cases within one degree of severity [19]. In our cohort, we found a prenatal biopsy rate of 45% due to suspicion of cancerous lesion. This is due to overestimation of lesions related to colposcopic changes in pregnancy, which often leads to systematic sampling despite the examiner's experience. This is described by Fader et al. [20], in their large study based on correlations between colposcopic impression and final diagnosis by colposcopy experts; out of 62 samples taken for colposcopic suspicion of CIN2+/neoplasia, only 55% confirmed a high grade lesion. The overestimation of the severity of lesions when performing colposcopies among pregnant women is the main reason for the non-concordance [19]. In our cohort, 34 of the 45 patients with diagnoses of persistent HSIL/CIN2+ at postpartum colposcopy follow up had a LEEP procedure confirming high-grade non-invasive dysplastic lesions.

In our univariate analysis, there was a statistically significant result for the variable gestational diabetes; however, this should be interpreted with caution due to the small patient cohort (eight patients). In contrast, our results support the idea that the parity status may have an impact on HSIL/CIN regression rate during pregnancy. This finding is concordant with the findings reported by Hong et al. [21]. The authors highlighted that the persistence of high-grade lesions was more frequent in multiparous patients (OR: 10.52; 95%CI: 1.36–81.01; p = 0.004) [21]. Compared to multiparous patients, nulliparous patients would also have longer exposure estrogen impregnation related to cervical ripening [22], as well as related proinflammatory cytokine signaling, leading to increased local vascularization and a recrudescence of immune cells such as myeloid-derived immune cells and lymphocyte cells. These cells may participate in inflammation and recovery processes [23]. The density of CD4+ T-lymphocytes was shown to increase by 4-fold in pregnant patients who are not in labor and by 10-fold in pregnant patients in labor [24].

There is some evidence that persistent, high-risk HPV infections in the postpartum period may be an underlying factor in patients with either persistent or progressing lesions [21]. Pregnancy leads to physiological changes that induce temporary immunomodulatory effects in downregulating the expression of inflammatory chemokines [25] increasing susceptibility to HPV infection. Hong et al. [21] showed that the persistence of high-grade lesions were more frequent in patients with persistent, high-grade HPV infections (OR = 5.25; 95%CI: 2.26–12.18; $p < 0.001$).

However, no differences were found between both groups in terms of presence of high-risk HPV. As for non-pregnant women, it would be interesting to investigate other markers, such as P16 and Ki67, and to assess their prognostic value for more accurately identifying patients at risk of developing invasive lesions. Nonetheless, there is no consensus on the use of P16 and Ki67 during pregnancy, and the influences of hormones and immunity on these proteins remain unknown. The literature is scarce with only one study that has been published; furthermore, it was based on a small series of cases [26].

Some authors raised the hypothesis that cervical desquamation related to vaginal delivery resulted in an inflammatory response that leads to increased regressions of cervical intraepithelial lesions in the postpartum period [11]. However, the role of the delivery route is still subject to debate and remains controversial. As suggested by our results, the route of delivery had no influence on HSIL/CIN 2+ regression rate. This result is concordant with that reported by Yost et al. [5], who reported no difference in regression rates according to mode of delivery in a prospective study of 153 histologically diagnosed high-grade dysplasia.

This study has several limitations. First, the retrospective design and the small sample size lead to insufficient power to extrapolate these results. Second, our study is mainly based on colposcopic and cytological criteria, histological samplings being carried out only when a lesion is suspected of being cancerous. Although cytology has a positive predictive value of 88% for high-grade lesions in pregnant women, histology remains the gold standard for the diagnosis of high-grade lesions, thus excluding high-grade cytological lesions lacking histological confirmation [4–6,12,14,15,21,27]. This implies that if the sample does not contain the high-grade lesion, this minimizes the risk and results in these patients not being monitored during pregnancy and postpartum [28]. However, the results of the current study underlined that cytological regression at the third trimester was predictive of HSIL/CIN regression after delivery. In addition, Ueda et al. reported the same observations as those underlined in our study, with a spontaneous regression in a quarter of their cohort in the second and third trimester before delivery. Persistent HPV infection is necessary for the development of precancers and cancers. Although our study does not report HPV typing, there is a ripening of the cervix due to hormonal change and, consequently, a return of the inflammatory system in the third trimester. We support the idea that this process allows clearance of the HPV infection and, consequently, a regression of the lesion. Cytology in the third trimester will allow this change to be observed and, therefore, predict the evolution of the lesions.

5. Conclusions

In conclusion, our study follows the ASCCP (American Society of Colposcopy and Cervical Pathology) guidelines. Although assessment of high-grade dysplastic lesions may be postponed in the postpartum period, our observations revealed that the clinical value of surveillance for high-grade dysplasia during pregnancy is to identify lesions with a potential risk of progression to cervical carcinoma in the postpartum period. Our results highlighted that parity status may have an impact on the regression of dysplasia during pregnancy. Cervical cytology should be performed in the third trimester to identify patients at risk of persistent CIN after delivery. Therefore, larger cohorts are required to confirm these results. A prospective study, including biomarkers such as P16 and Ki67, as well as immune cell characteristics/density and HPV typing would be relevant to gain more knowledge and increase the accuracy of diagnosis and management of high-grade cervical lesions during pregnancy and postpartum.

Author Contributions: Y.G.: data acquisition, conception, design, analysis and interpretation, drafting, critical revision. M.J.-G.: conception, design, analysis and interpretation, drafting, critical revision. V.B.: analysis and interpretation, critical revision. K.L.: analysis and interpretation, critical revision. P.M.: conception, interpretation, critical revision. All authors have read and agreed to the published version of the manuscript.

Funding: This research received no external funding.

Institutional Review Board Statement: The study was conducted according to the guidelines of the Declaration of Helsinki, and approved by the Ethics Committee of the canton de Vaud, Switzerland, (25 July 2019, ID N 2017-01375).

Informed Consent Statement: Informed consent was obtained from all subjects involved in the study.

Data Availability Statement: All data analyzed during this study are included in this article. Further enquiries can be directed to the corresponding author.

Acknowledgments: The authors want to acknowledge the support of Mia Cespedes from Réseau Hospitalier Neuchâtelois Pourtalès for collecting clinical data and Stefan Gerber, former head of the colposcopy unit.

Conflicts of Interest: The authors declare no conflict of interest.

References

1. Insinga, R.P.; Glass, A.G.; Rush, B.B. Diagnoses and outcomes in cervical cancer screening: A population-based study. *Am. J. Obstet. Gynecol.* **2004**, *191*, 105–113. [CrossRef]
2. Douvier, S.; Filipuzzi, L.; Sagot, P. Management of cervical intra-epithelial neoplasm during pregnancy. *Gynecol. Obstet. Fertil.* **2003**, *31*, 851–855. [CrossRef]
3. Selleret, L.; Mathevet, P. Precancerous cervical lesions during pregnancy: Diagnostic and treatment. *J. Gynecol. Obstet. Biol. Reprod.* **2008**, *37* (Suppl. 1), S131–S138. [CrossRef]
4. Coppolillo, E.F.; DE Ruda Vega, H.M.; Brizuela, J.; Eliseth, M.C.; Barata, A.; Perazzi, B.E. High-grade cervical neoplasia during pregnancy: Diagnosis, management and postpartum findings. *Acta Obstet. Gynecol. Scand.* **2013**, *92*, 293–297. [CrossRef] [PubMed]
5. Yost, N.P.; Santoso, J.T.; McIntire, D.D.; Iliya, F.A. Postpartum regression rates of antepartum cervical intraepithelial neoplasia II and III lesions. *Obstet. Gynecol.* **1999**, *93*, 359–362. [CrossRef] [PubMed]
6. Ackermann, S.; Gehrsitz, C.; Mehlhorn, G.; Beckmann, M.W. Management and course of histologically verified cervical carcinoma in situ during pregnancy. *Acta Obstet. Gynecol. Scand.* **2006**, *85*, 1134–1137. [CrossRef]
7. Fife, K.H.; Katz, B.P.; Roush, J.; Handy, V.D.; Brown, D.R.; Hansell, R. Cancer-associated human papillomavirus types are selectively increased in the cervix of women in the first trimester of pregnancy. *Am. J. Obstet. Gynecol.* **1996**, *174*, 1487–1493. [CrossRef]
8. Domža, G.; Gudlevičienė, Z.; Didžiapetrienė, J.; Valuckas, K.P.; Kazbarienė, B.; Drąsutienė, G. Human papillomavirus infection in pregnant women. *Arch. Gynecol. Obstet.* **2011**, *284*, 1105–1112. [CrossRef]
9. Perkins, R.B.; Guido, R.S.; Castle, P.E.; Chelmow, D.; Einstein, M.H.; Garcia, F.; Huh, W.K.; Kim, J.J.; Moscicki, A.-B.; Nayar, R.; et al. 2019 ASCCP Risk-Based Management Consensus Guidelines for Abnormal Cervical Cancer Screening Tests and Cancer Precursors. *J. Low. Genit. Tract Dis.* **2020**, *24*, 102–131. [CrossRef] [PubMed]
10. Baldauf, J.J.; Dreyfus, M.; Ritter, J.; Philippe, E. Colposcopy and directed biopsy reliability during pregnancy: A cohort study. *Eur. J. Obstet. Gynecol. Reprod. Biol.* **1995**, *62*, 31–36. [CrossRef]
11. Ahdoot, D.; Van Nostrand, K.M.; Nguyen, N.J.; Tewari, D.S.; Kurasaki, T.; DiSaia, P.J.; Rose, G.S. The effect of route of delivery on regression of abnormal cervical cytologic findings in the postpartum period. *Am. J. Obstet. Gynecol.* **1998**, *178*, 1116–1120. [CrossRef]
12. Kärrberg, C.; Brännström, M.; Strander, B.; Ladfors, L.; Rådberg, T. Colposcopically directed cervical biopsy during pregnancy; minor surgical and obstetrical complications and high rates of persistence and regression. *Acta Obstet. Gynecol. Scand.* **2013**, *92*, 692–699. [CrossRef]
13. Mailath-Pokorny, M.; Schwameis, R.; Grimm, C.; Reinthaller, A.; Polterauer, S. Natural history of cervical intraepithelial neoplasia in pregnancy: Postpartum histo-pathologic outcome and review of the literature. *BMC Pregnancy Childbirth* **2016**, *16*, 74. [CrossRef] [PubMed]
14. Ueda, Y.; Enomoto, T.; Miyatake, T.; Yoshino, K.; Fujita, M.; Miyake, T.; Fujiwara, K.; Muraji, M.; Kanagawa, T.; Kimura, T. Postpartum outcome of cervical intraepithelial neoplasia in pregnant women determined by route of delivery. *Reprod. Sci.* **2009**, *16*, 1034–1039. [CrossRef]

15. Chung, S.M.; Son, G.H.; Nam, E.J.; Kim, Y.H.; Kim, Y.T.; Park, Y.W.; Kwon, J.Y. Mode of delivery influences the regression of abnormal cervical cytology. *Gynecol. Obstet. Investig.* **2011**, *72*, 234–238. [CrossRef] [PubMed]
16. Kaplan, K.J.; Dainty, L.A.; Dolinsky, B.; Rose, G.S.; Carlson, J.; McHale, M.; Elkas, J.C. Prognosis and recurrence risk for patients with cervical squamous intraepithelial lesions diagnosed during pregnancy. *Cancer* **2004**, *102*, 228–232. [CrossRef]
17. Kaneshiro, B.E.K.; Acoba, J.D.; Holzman, J.; Wachi, K.; Carney, M.E. Effect of delivery route on natural history of cervical dysplasia. *Am. J. Obstet. Gynecol.* **2005**, *192*, 1452–1454. [CrossRef] [PubMed]
18. Schuster, S.; Joura, E.; Kohlberger, P. Natural History of Squamous Intraepithelial Lesions in Pregnancy and Mode of Delivery. *Anticancer Res.* **2018**, *38*, 2439–2442. [CrossRef]
19. Economos, K.; Perez Veridiano, N.; Delke, I.; Collado, M.L.; Tancer, M.L. Abnormal cervical cytology in pregnancy: A 17-year experience. *Obstet. Gynecol.* **1993**, *81*, 915–918.
20. Fader, A.N.; Alward, E.K.; Niederhauser, A.; Chirico, C.; Lesnock, J.L.; Zwiesler, D.J.; Guido, R.S.; Lofgren, D.J.; Gold, M.A.; Moore, K.N. Cervical dysplasia in pregnancy: A multi-institutional evaluation. *Am. J. Obstet. Gynecol.* **2010**, *203*, 113.e1–113.e6. [CrossRef]
21. Hong, D.K.; Kim, S.A.; Lim, K.T.; Lee, K.H.; Kim, T.J.; So, K.A. Clinical outcome of high-grade cervical intraepithelial neoplasia during pregnancy: A 10-year experience. *Eur. J. Obstet. Gynecol. Reprod. Biol.* **2019**, *236*, 173–176. [CrossRef] [PubMed]
22. Andersson, S.; Minjarez, D.; Yost, N.P.; Word, R.A. Estrogen and progesterone metabolism in the cervix during pregnancy and parturition. *J. Clin. Endocrinol. Metab.* **2008**, *93*, 2366–2374. [CrossRef]
23. Yellon, S.M. Immunobiology of Cervix Ripening. *Front. Immunol.* **2019**, *10*, 3156. [CrossRef]
24. Bokström, H.; Brännström, M.; Alexandersson, M.; Norström, A. Leukocyte subpopulations in the human uterine cervical stroma at early and term pregnancy. *Hum. Reprod.* **1997**, *12*, 586–590. [CrossRef]
25. Nancy, P.; Tagliani, E.; Tay, C.-S.; Asp, P.; Levy, D.E.; Erlebacher, A. Chemokine gene silencing in decidual stromal cells limits T cell access to the maternal-fetal interface. *Science* **2012**, *336*, 1317–1321. [CrossRef]
26. Ciavattini, A.; Sopracordevole, F.; Di Giuseppe, J.; Moriconi, L.; Lucarini, G.; Mancioli, F.; Zizzi, A.; Goteri, G. Cervical intraepithelial neoplasia in pregnancy: Interference of pregnancy status with p16 and Ki-67 protein expression. *Oncol. Lett.* **2017**, *13*, 301–306. [CrossRef] [PubMed]
27. Coppola, A.; Sorosky, J.; Casper, R.; Anderson, B.; Buller, R.E. The clinical course of cervical carcinoma in situ diagnosed during pregnancy. *Gynecol. Oncol.* **1997**, *67*, 162–165. [CrossRef]
28. Benedet, J.L.; Selke, P.A.; Nickerson, K.G. Colposcopic evaluation of abnormal Papanicolaou smears in pregnancy. *Am. J. Obstet. Gynecol.* **1987**, *157*, 932–937. [CrossRef]

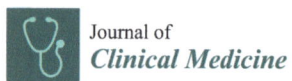

Article

Facilitators and Strategies for Breaking the News of an Intrauterine Death—A Mixed Methods Study among Obstetricians

Dana Anais Muin [1,*], Janina Sophie Erlacher [1], Stephanie Leutgeb [2] and Anna Felnhofer [3]

[1] Department of Obstetrics and Gynecology, Division of Fetomaternal Medicine, Comprehensive Center for Pediatrics Medical University of Vienna, Waehringer Guertel 18-20, 1090 Vienna, Austria; n01621749@students.meduniwien.ac.at

[2] Austrian Society of Obstetrics and Gynecology, Frankgasse 8, 1090 Vienna, Austria; stephanie.leutgeb@oeggg.at

[3] Department of Pediatrics and Adolescent Medicine, Division of Pediatric Pulmonology, Allergology and Endocrinology, Comprehensive Center for Pediatrics Medical University of Vienna, Waehringer Guertel 18-20, 1090 Vienna, Austria; anna.felnhofer@meduniwien.ac.at

* Correspondence: dana.muin@meduniwien.ac.at; Tel.: +43-1-40400-28210

Citation: Muin, D.A.; Erlacher, J.S.; Leutgeb, S.; Felnhofer, A. Facilitators and Strategies for Breaking the News of an Intrauterine Death—A Mixed Methods Study among Obstetricians. *J. Clin. Med.* **2021**, *10*, 5347. https://doi.org/10.3390/jcm10225347

Academic Editor: Rinat Gabbay-Benziv

Received: 1 October 2021
Accepted: 16 November 2021
Published: 17 November 2021

Publisher's Note: MDPI stays neutral with regard to jurisdictional claims in published maps and institutional affiliations.

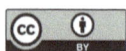

Copyright: © 2021 by the authors. Licensee MDPI, Basel, Switzerland. This article is an open access article distributed under the terms and conditions of the Creative Commons Attribution (CC BY) license (https://creativecommons.org/licenses/by/4.0/).

Abstract: (1) Background: The death of a baby in utero is a very sad event for both the affected parents and the caring doctors. By this study, we aimed to assess the tools, which may help obstetricians to overcome this challenge in their profession. (2) Methods: We conducted a cross-sectional online survey in 1526 obstetricians registered with the Austrian Society of Obstetrics and Gynecology between September and October 2020. (3) Results: With a response rate of 24.2% (n = 439), our study shows that diagnosing fetal death was associated with a moderate to high degree of stress, regardless of position ($p = 0.949$), age ($p = 0.110$), gender ($p = 0.155$), and experience ($p = 0.150$) of physicians. Coping strategies for delivering the news of intrauterine death to affected parents were relying on clinical knowledge and high levels of self-confidence (55.0%; 203/369), support from colleagues (53.9%; 199/369), and debriefing (52.8%; 195/369). In general, facilitators for breaking bad news were more commonly cultivated by female obstetricians [OR 1.267 (95% CI 1.149–1.396); $p < 0.001$], residents [$\chi^2(3;369) = 9.937$; $p = 0.019$], and obstetricians of younger age [41 (34–50) years vs. 45 (36–55) years; $p = 0.018$]. External facilitators were most frequently mentioned, including professional support, training, professional guidance, time, parents' leaflets, follow-up consultations, a supporting consultation atmosphere, and preparation before delivering the bad news. Internal facilitators included knowledge, empathy, seeking silence, reflection, privacy, and relief of guilt. (4) Conclusions: Communicating the diagnosis of fetal death evokes moderate to high levels of stress among obstetricians. Resources from both the professional and private environment are required to deal with this professional challenge on a personal level.

Keywords: stillbirth; fetal death; intrauterine death; breaking bad news; resilience; stress; coping strategies

1. Introduction

In high-income countries, the rate of antepartum stillbirth, or intrauterine fetal death (IUFD) above 22 weeks of gestation, ranges between 2.6 to 9.1 per 1000 births [1]. Despite its relatively small and stable prevalence in high-income countries, fetal death has an immeasurable and profound impact on the personal and intimate life of affected parents. In addition, from the perspective of the caring physician, detecting and/or communicating the diagnosis of intrauterine death has a personal impact with regard to stress and burden [2]. In semi-structured in-depth qualitative interviews with eight consultants, Nuzum et al. found that two super-ordinate themes dominate obstetricians' state following the diagnosis of stillbirth: the weight of experienced professional responsibility, and their personal human response to stillbirth [3]. Clearly, stillbirth was identified as one of the most difficult parts of their jobs, whilst, paradoxically, none of the physicians had received any specialist training in perinatal bereavement care, as all learned "on the job" and from senior colleagues during their training years. Physicians also noted that recalling these particular situations during the interview opened up "painful and vivid memories". Additionally, the burden of stillbirth experience was found to be unwaveringly high over time, with lasting resentments expressed as "sadness, fear, anger, disappointment and personal grief" [3,4].

Causes of intrauterine death are diverse, and in the majority of cases, unclear at the time of diagnosis [5]. Circumstances that lead women to seek the doctor's or midwife's office may be acute, such as bleeding or pain, or within the frame of a routine check-up. Often, however, women feel that "something is wrong", either by intuition, or by reduced or increased fetal movements [6,7]. Diagnosis of fetal death is usually made by real-time ultrasonography and confirmed upon absent fetal heart beats and blood circulation in the umbilical cord. For the attending physician, breaking news of fetal death requires a sensitive approach and an empathetic communication towards the affected parents [8]. The physician's confrontation with fetal death and care for the bereaved may be overwhelming, especially in case of perceived lack of training and limited support.

By means of this mixed methods study among Austrian obstetricians, we, therefore, sought to assess the level of stress which obstetricians experience when diagnosing fetal death and delivering the news to the parents. We, furthermore, aimed to explore factors that may facilitate this situation of breaking such bad news. Lastly, we set out to identify physicians' individual strategies that support them in coping with these and other professional challenges in obstetrics.

2. Materials and Methods

2.1. Data Collection

An online survey was conducted via SurveyMonkey (https://www.surveymonkey.de/ (accessed on 4 November 2020)), a standard tool for online surveys, which allows for collecting data anonymously without storing sensitive background information (i.e., IP-address). The target population was 1526 Austrian obstetricians and gynecologists registered with the Austrian Society of Obstetrics and Gynecology (Oesterreichische Gesellschaft fuer Gynaekologie und Geburtshilfe; OEGGG). The survey link was sent out with an invitation email via the OEGGG email-server between 21 September 2020 and 31 October 2020. Authorized access to the survey data source and email-list was solely and confidentially provided to the OEGGG secretary (S.L.). Two friendly reminders were sent out by weeks 2 and 3. No incentives were offered, and participants were informed that the data would be published and presented at the annual meeting of the society.

The survey questionnaire was conceived by the study team (D.A.M., J.S.E., A.F.) and approved by the Medical Board of the OEGGG as well as the Ethics Committee of the Medical University of Vienna. Usability and technical functionality of the electronic questionnaire were tested among the study team and with five voluntary participants before fielding the questionnaire. Reliability was established by an oral interview of the five participants after the completion of the survey, in which the survey questions were repeated. The variance between written and oral responses was 0.1%.

Participants were informed about the purpose of the study, the investigators, the anonymity of their data and the approximate length of the survey (15 min). The survey adhered to the Declaration of Helsinki, and an online informed consent by a tick-box was obtained upon digital participation.

The total online questionnaire entailed seven pages with four to five questions per page. Respondents were able to review and change their answers via a return button. Consistency or completeness checks were not included before signing-off. The closed survey was protected against un-authorized access. All received responses were anonymous, and no direct personal information were collected or stored. No cookies were used in this survey. Duplicate entries were avoided by preventing users' access to the survey twice.

Time to fill in a questionnaire was not assessed by the investigators. No methods were used to adjust for potential non-representative samples. Only completed questionnaires were analyzed. Collected data were transferred into an Excel file sheet and checked for integrity and consistency.

2.2. Measures

For this survey, we constructed a mixed methods research design, integrating quantitative and qualitative data derived from an online 16-item questionnaire, which included three validated questionnaires, overarching in total eight domains: (a) demographic data, (b) experience, (c) stress coping [9,10], (d) coping strategies, (e) open-answer textbox regarding facilitators, (f) trait empathy [11,12], (g) locus of control [12,13] and (h) affect. For the purpose of this study, we extracted data from domains (a–e) only. Data and results of the other domains are presented elsewhere (Muin et al., manuscript under revision).

Demographics

The following key demographic variables were assessed as categorical variables: gender, age, children, marital status, current position, year of residence, and current workplace (e.g., university hospital vs. private practice).

Experience

Participating obstetricians were asked to categorize their level of experience in having previously diagnosed and delivered the news of fetal deaths to affected parents (i.e., "0", "<5", "6–10", "11–30" and ">31" times).

Stress Perception

Participants were asked to rate the question "The situation was stressful for me" (i.e., perceived stress) when delivering the diagnosis of fetal death, on a 5-point-Likert-scale (1 = does not apply, 5 = fully applies) [9,10].

Coping Strategies

Obstetricians were asked to grade which strategies (i.e., activities or attitudes) were most useful to them for coping (a) with the circumstance of diagnosing or breaking news of fetal death, and (b) with challenging obstetrical situations in general.

The selection of variables was based upon the conceptual model of resilience in health-care professionals, encompassing the following values and items: social culture, personal life, individual identity, professional identity, professional community, and medical culture [14].

The participants could choose between the categories (a) "Clinical knowledge and self-confidence", "Team based decisions", "Psychological support", "Psychological debriefing after adverse events", "Balint groups", "Supervision", "Support from your supervisor/head of department", "Support from colleagues", "No strategy", and "Others", and (b) "Conversation with colleagues", "Conversation with my partner", "Follow-up consultations with parents", "Balint groups", "Distraction or avoidance", "Psychotherapy", "Antidepressant medication", "No strategy", and "Others", respectively.

Open Responses

Finally, a single text box for open responses was placed at the end of the questionnaire to the question "What do you think may help to facilitate this situation for you?" The answers from this open-ended question were collected, harmonized into main themes and divided into two categories by inductive approach for further analyses [15,16]. Individual items were counterchecked for plausibility and accuracy by all co-authors.

Facilitators were defined as factors, which help an individual to overcome a situation, rebuild and regain their strength for further professional performance and mitigate stress. Internal facilitators were defined as endogenic factors, i.e., values, attitudes or habits derived from within and cultivated by an individual person. External facilitators were defined as outer circumstances that can be either provided or acquired by the environment or by one-self in order to support an experience, such as the workflow, procedures or professional habits.

2.3. Definitions

Residents in obstetrics and gynecology are part-time or full-time working hospital doctors in specialist training for the duration of six to eight years in Austria. Routine duties include seeing patients in outpatient clinic, participating in ward rounds, theatre and delivery units, as well as doing on-calls and nights shifts.

Specialty doctors in obstetrics and gynecology working full- or part-time in hospital are considered equivalent to consultants. Their duties range from leading ward rounds, deliveries, theatres and outpatient clinics according to their special fields of interest, as well as doing on-calls and night shifts. They may have an additional part-time private practice outside the hospital; however, they were considered as "specialist doctors in hospitals" only.

Departmental heads are leading specialty doctors who are in charge of a department of obstetrics and/or gynecology and/or reproductive medicine, who usually work full-time in hospital and are on standby for emergencies during nights. They often lead outpatient clinics and may see their own patients in an affiliated private clinic or in hospital.

Specialty doctors working only in private or public funded practice are hospital-independent obstetricians and gynecologists with flexible working hours and an individual emphasis on obstetrics and/or gynecology. They are the first to be consulted by women with a gynecological problem or emergencies outside hospital. They also provide annual gynecological check-ups, carry out regular routine scans in pregnant women, and fetal and maternal well-being examinations.

2.4. Statistical Analyses

Distribution of data was analyzed using the Kolmogorov–Smirnov test. Categorical data are given as absolute (n) and relative frequencies (%). Continuous data are given as mean (M) and standard deviation (SD) or median and 25th and 75th percentile. Categorical data were compared with Chi^2 and Fisher's Exact test, respectively. Continuous data were compared with a Kruskal–Wallis test with Dunn's multiple comparison test. Univariate Analyses of Variance (ANOVAs) were used to analyze group-differences with ordinal variables. All reported p-values are two-sided, and a p-value < 0.05 was considered as statistically significant. Statistical tests were performed with SPSS Statistics Version 26 (IBM Corporation, Armonk, NY, USA). Figures were designed by GraphPad Prism 9 for macOS (GraphPad Software, LLC, San Diego, CA, USA). The Venn diagram was manually designed using Graphic for Mac to illustrate a theme cloud: The circle sizes correlate with the frequency of a mentioned element in the open-ended questions, and the circle colors represent the predominant professional group to mention this element.

3. Results

3.1. Baseline Characteristics

In total, 439 obstetricians and gynecologists completed the online survey (Figure 1).

For this study and due to missing responses, we included 369 participants (n = 88 residents; n = 129 hospital specialist doctors; n = 21 departmental heads; n = 131 specialist doctors working in private or public practice), all of who answered the question regarding coping strategies. Seventy-four were included into the qualitative assessment of facilitators for breaking news of fetal death. Median age of participants was 44 (36–54) years with a female participants' rate of 76.4%. The baseline characteristics of all participants are shown in Table 1.

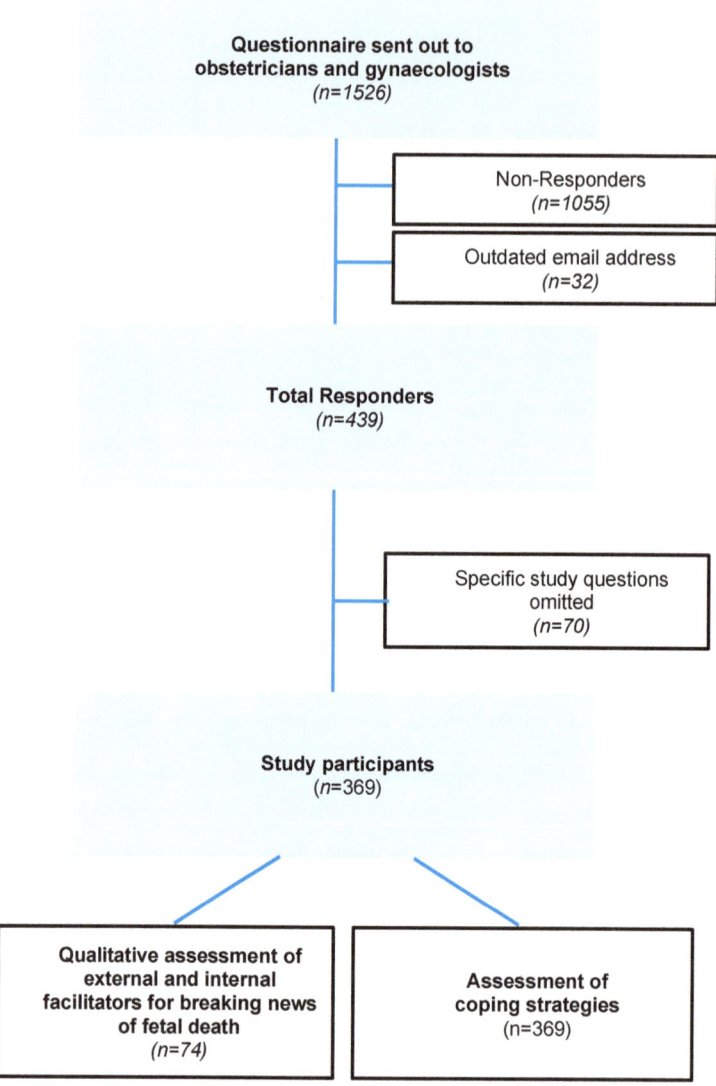

Figure 1. Flowchart illustrating the enrolment of participants (n = 369) to the survey conducted by the Austrian Society of Obstetrics and Gynecology between 21 September 2020 and 31 October 2020.

3.2. Main Parameters

3.2.1. Experience

Most participants indicated to have diagnosed and delivered the news of fetal death up to five times (n = 164/369; 44.4%, and n = 151/369; 40.9%, respectively), whereas departmental heads showed to have acquired significantly more experience compared to other professional groups [$F(3, 365)$ = 3.893, p = 0.009; and $F(3, 365)$ = 3.769, p = 0.011, respectively; Table 1)].

Table 1. Baseline characteristics of obstetricians who participated in the online survey conducted by the Austrian Society of Obstetrics and Gynecology between 21 September 2020 and 31 October 2020 ($n = 369$).

		Total ($n = 369$)	Resident ($n = 88$)	Specialist Doctor in Hospital ($n = 129$)	Departmental Head ($n = 21$)	Specialist Doctor in Private/Public Practice ($n = 131$)	p-Value
Age ($n = 351$)	(Median; min-max; in years)	44 (24–67)	31 (24–42)	43 (26–66)	57 (45–64)	52 (26–67)	
Sex ($n = 369$)	Female	282 (76.4%)	80 (90.9%)	99 (76.7%)	5 (23.8%)	98 (74.8%)	
	Male	87 (23.6%)	8 (9.1%)	30 (23.3%)	16 (76.2%)	33 (25.2%)	
Marital status ($n = 364$)	Single	52 (14.3%)	17 (19.5%)	24 (19.2%)	2 (9.5%)	9 (6.9%)	
	Coupled	71 (19.5%)	34 (39.1%)	19 (15.2%)	1 (4.8%)	17 (13%)	
	Married	228 (62.6%)	35 (40.2%)	77 (61.6%)	18 (85.7%)	98 (74.8%)	
	Divorced	13 (3.6%)	1 (1.1%)	5 (4.0%)	0 (0.0%)	7 (5.3%)	
Parent ($n = 367$)	Yes	253 (68.9%)	31 (35.2%)	97 (75.8%)	19 (90.5%)	106 (81.5%)	
	No	114 (31.1%)	57 (64.8%)	31 (24.2%)	2 (9.5%)	24 (18.5%)	
Diagnosed IUFD (n)	0	39 (10.6%)	27 (30.7%)	7 (5.4%)	0 (0.0%)	5 (3.8%)	χ^2 (12; $N = 369$) = 114.821; $p < 0.001$
	<5	164 (44.4%)	51 (58%)	51 (39.5%)	3 (14.3%)	59 (45.0%)	
	6–10	76 (20.6%)	9 (10.2%)	31 (24%)	1 (4.8%)	35 (26.7%)	
	11–30	53 (14.4%)	1 (1.1%)	22 (17.1%)	9 (42.9%)	21 (16%)	
	>31	37 (10%)	0 (0%)	18 (14%)	8 (38.1%)	11 (8.4%)	
Delivered diagnoses of IUFD (n)	0	42 (11.4%)	34 (38.6%)	5 (3.9%)	0 (0.0%)	3 (2.3%)	χ^2 (12; $N = 369$) = 147.043; $p < 0.001$
	<5	151 (40.9%)	45 (51.1%)	47 (36.4%)	2 (9.5%)	57 (43.5%)	
	6–10	82 (22.2%)	7 (8.0%)	36 (27.9%)	2 (9.5%)	37 (28.2%)	
	11–30	53 (14.4%)	2 (2.3%)	21 (16.3%)	8 (38.1%)	22 (16.8%)	
	>31	41 (11.1%)	0 (0.0%)	20 (15.5%)	9 (42.9%)	12 (9.2%)	

Abbreviations: IUFD, intrauterine fetal death.

3.2.2. Stress

Figure 2 illustrates the distribution of self-reported stress levels among obstetricians per position and shows that diagnosing fetal death is associated with moderate to high degrees of stress among all participants, regardless of position [M = 3.08, SD = 0.903; $F(4, 326) = 0.180$, $p = 0.949$], age [M = 45.91, SD = 10.88; $F(4, 311) = 1.901$, $p = 0.110$], gender [M = 1.26, SD = 0.438; $F(4, 326) = 1.676$, $p = 0.155$], and experience [M = 3.55, SD = 1.697; $F(4, 326) = 1.698$, $p = 0.150$].

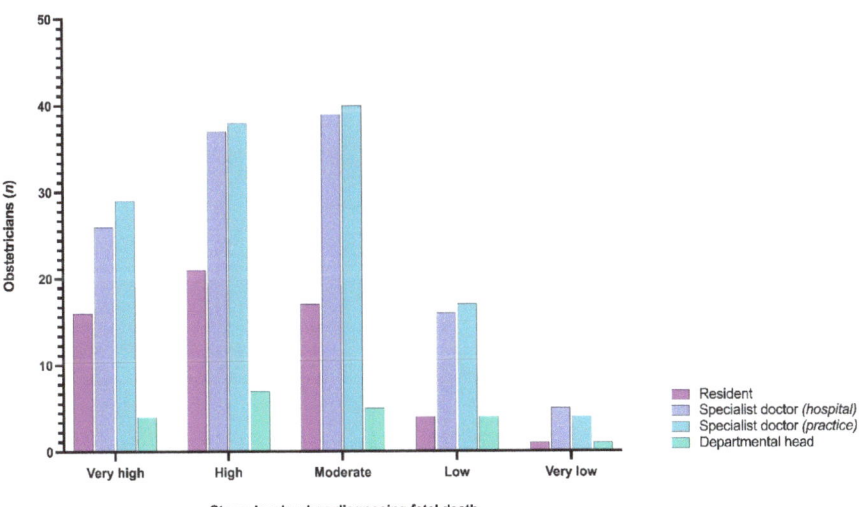

Figure 2. Clustered bar chart on stress levels (i.e., very high; high; moderate; low; very low) in obstetricians when diagnosing fetal death.

3.2.3. Coping Strategies for Breaking News of Fetal Death

The majority of obstetricians consider clinical knowledge and self-confidence the most useful strategy for coping with delivering the news of fetal death (*n* = 203/369; 55.0%). The second and third most prevalent coping tools were support from colleagues (*n* = 199/369; 53.9%), and debriefing (*n* = 195/369; 52.8%; Figure 3).

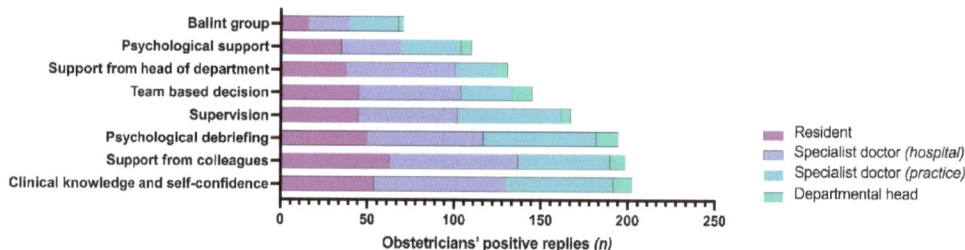

Figure 3. Clustered bar chart on the frequency of coping strategies among obstetricians for breaking news of fetal death.

3.2.4. Coping Strategies in Stressful Obstetrical Events

As to coping with professional challenges in obstetrics in general, the majority of obstetricians consider talking to colleagues as the most useful strategy (*n* = 325/369; 88.1%), followed by talking to one's spouse or partner (*n* = 229/369; 62.1%), and a follow-up consultation with parents (*n* = 198/369; 53.7%). A minority of obstetricians indicated to consume antidepressants or have no strategy at all (each *n* = 3/369; 0.8%; Figure 4).

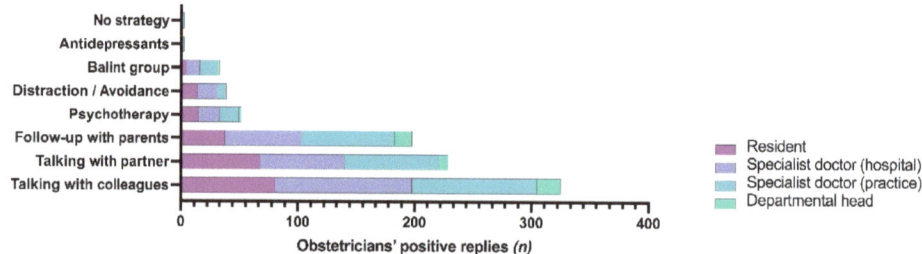

Figure 4. Clustered bar chart on the frequency of strategies among obstetricians for coping with stressful obstetric events.

3.2.5. Facilitators for Delivering News of Fetal Death

Facilitators were more commonly present in women [OR 1.267 (95% CI 1.149–1.396); $p < 0.001$] and residents [$\chi^2(3) = 9.937$; $p = 0.019$] and therefore obstetricians of younger median age [41 (34–50) years vs. 45 (36–55) years; $p = 0.018$]. From 74 responses, we distilled professional and personal values into a theme cloud of both external and internal facilitators to help break the news of fetal death for obstetricians (Figure 5).

In total, external facilitators most frequently resonated with participants, especially among residents. These entailed the values in professional culture, i.e., professional support, training, professional guidance, time, parents' leaflets, follow-up consultations, a supporting consultation atmosphere, and lastly, preparation before delivering the bad news. Sample narratives are presented in Table 2 to illustrate each theme.

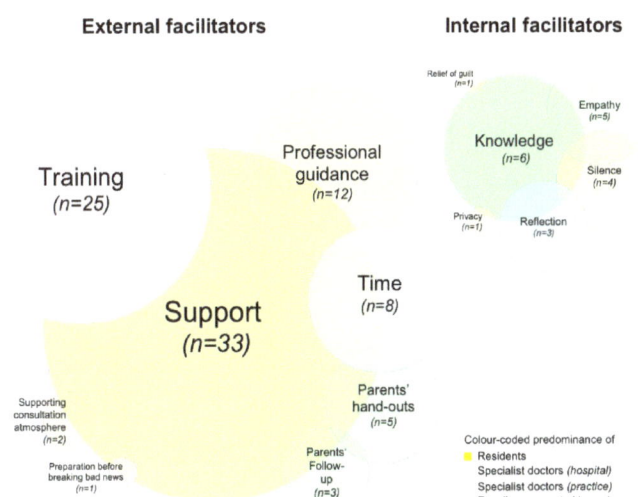

Figure 5. Graphical theme cloud illustrating obstetricians' external and internal facilitators for breaking news of fetal death to affected parents. The size of the circles directly correlates with the number of positive replies by obstetricians. The color of the circles represents the respective professional group, which predominantly quoted this element in the open response (i.e., residents; specialist doctors in hospital and practice, respectively; departmental heads).

Table 2. Sample narratives by obstetricians expressing their spectrum of external facilitators when delivering news of fetal death.

External Facilitator (Listed per Frequency)	Exemplar Quotes (Translated from German to English)
Support	*"To have the opportunity to talk to my colleagues regarding this situation"* (Female resident, 24 y/o, single, diagnosed IUFDs < 5 times)
	"To have support from experienced colleagues and professionals dealing with crisis-intervention" (Female 3rd year resident, 34 y/o, single, never diagnosed IUFD)
	"To know within the team what and how to break the bad news (with all residents, specialist doctors, midwives) and also debrief in this team after the consultation" (Female specialist doctor in private practice, 53 y/o, coupled; diagnosed IUFDs 6–10 times)
Training	*"To have continuous trainings and skills-and-drills simulation practice"* (Female specialist doctor in private practice, 45 y/o, married; diagnosed IUFDs 11–30 times)
	"This situation will always be terrible, whatever the circumstance. However, frequent courses help and foster reflective practice" (Female specialist doctor in public practice, 42 y/o; married, diagnosed IUFDs < 5 times)
	"To gain knowledge on how to handle these consultations by learning from experienced colleagues, psychologists, etc. You will never feel good during these consultations. It would be advisable to have predefined intern standards, on what needs to be checked post-mortem" (Male specialist doctor in public practice, 50 y/o, coupled; diagnosed IUFDs < 5 times)
Professional guidance	*"It would be helpful to have a short guidance or checklist with all points that have to be raised within such consultation and what needs to be considered"* (Female 1st year resident, married, never diagnosed IUFD)
Time	*"To have time during clinics, to be there for the patient and also for oneself to debrief after such consultation"* (Female consultant, diagnosed IUFDs > 31 times)

Table 2. Cont.

External Facilitator (Listed per Frequency)	Exemplar Quotes (Translated from German to English)
Parents' handouts	"Professional handouts and leaflets for the parents" (Female specialist doctor in pubic practice, 43 y/o; divorced, diagnosed IUFDs 6–19 times)
Parents' follow-up	"It would be helpful to receive feedback from affected women to understand what went well or not so well during these consultations, and what they wished to be different next time" (Female consultant, 55 y/o; married, diagnosed IUFDs < 5 times)
Supporting consultation atmosphere	"To lead this consultation with another colleague, to be stronger together" (Female 6th year resident, 35 y/o; married, diagnosed IUFDs 6–10 times)
Preparation	"Briefing and debriefing: Being mentally and verbally prepared what to say and how to act" (Female specialist doctor in public practice, 35 y/o; married, diagnosed IUFDs 6–10 times)

Internal facilitators, that support breaking bad news of fetal death, entailed the motives surrounding personal culture, i.e., knowledge/wisdom, empathy, silence, reflection, privacy and relief of guilt. Sample narratives are presented in Table 3 to illustrate each theme.

Table 3. Sample narratives by obstetricians expressing their spectrum of internal facilitators when delivering news of fetal death.

Internal Facilitator (Listed per Frequency)	Exemplar Quotes (Translated from German to English)
Knowledge	"To know and understand what needs to be done after fetal death (e.g., genetic testing), to know what, when and how to take all necessary samples and tissues. To know how to advice and consult parents after the diagnosis." (Female 2nd year resident, 31 y/o; coupled, diagnosed IUFDs < 5 times)
Empathy	"To be fully empathetic with the patient and be medically well trained and skilled" (Male specialist doctor in private practice, 62 y/o; married, diagnosed IUFDs 11–30 times)
Silence	"Time, silence and willingness to reflect for oneself after such event. Be centered and mindful." (Female specialist doctor in public practice, 42 y/o; married, diagnosed IUFDs < 5 times)
Reflection	"This situation will always be terrible; regular training and reflection are helpful" (Female consultant, 42 y/o; married, diagnosed IUFDs 6–10 times)
Privacy	"Privacy; to have my other half by my side" (Female 1st year resident, 26 y/o; Single, diagnosed IUFDs < 5 times)
Relief of professional guilt	"Somebody to tell me that I am not responsible for the adverse outcome" (Female consultant, 38 y/o; coupled, diagnosed IUFDs > 31 times)

4. Discussion

4.1. Main Findings

In this cross-sectional online survey, we found that diagnosing fetal death evokes moderate to high levels of stress in obstetricians, regardless of experience, position, age, or gender. When trying to cope with stress of breaking news of fetal death, obstetricians orient their needs towards different sources depending on their level of experience and position: Whilst residents more commonly turn to colleagues for help and support, departmental heads cope with stress by team debriefing. Specialist doctors in hospital and private or public practice, however, ground their stability through acquisition of expertise and clinical knowledge. Likewise, with regards to facilitators, the needs are individually directed as per role and position: In general, more externally-mediated facilitators were identified, with the most prevalent ones being "support" and "professional guidance", which, yet again, were most commonly requested by residents.

4.2. Results in the Context of What Is Known

Experiencing stillbirth as a bereaved parent is a traumatic event that requires careful and empathetic communication [17,18]. Previous studies have shown that stillbirth has an unacknowledged impact on obstetricians as well, which has been neglected in education and psychological support at the workplace [3]. Our findings support previous qualitative survey studies highlighting the need for additional training and the value of peer support from colleagues [3,19,20]. In 2008, Gold et al. explored experiences and attitudes about perinatal death, as well as coping strategies and training by an online survey among 804 obstetricians in the United States (U.S.) [20]. The authors found that the majority of respondents agreed that detecting stillbirth "took a large emotional toll" on them personally. Adequate training to cope with fetal death was noted to significantly mitigate the feelings of guilt, worries about legal actions, and the consideration of giving up obstetrics all together. In addition, most common coping strategies were found to be "talking to colleagues" (87%) or one's "friends" (56%).

These results are also in accordance with the findings of Farrow et al., who conducted a U.S. questionnaire survey on the psychological impact of stillbirth and the influence of epidemiological factors in stillbirth reactions among 499 obstetricians in 2013 [19]. The authors specifically explored the spectrum of physicians' psychological responses towards a pregnancy, which ended in stillbirth, and found that, overall, grief was the most common emotional response to stillbirth (53.7%), followed by self-doubt (17.2%). Of note, the authors found that older physicians ($\geq$51 years of age) and physicians in solo and private practice were more likely to suffer from depression, as they might feel more isolated and experience greater lack of support from colleagues to process stillbirth [19].

4.3. Clinical Implications

To our knowledge, our study is the first to specifically explore obstetricians' attitude and coping strategies when confirming and delivering the burdensome diagnosis of fetal death. More so, our data together with the findings from the previous surveys conducted by Gold and Farrow et al. [19,20] suggest that the psychological impact of fetal death on physicians is not to be ignored and that a sustainable social and peer network are of importance for coping with professional challenges.

"Obstetrics" is a term that emerged in the mid 18th century, derived from the modern Latin word *obstetrix*, meaning '*midwife*' and *obstare* 'to be *present*'. Indeed, obstetrics, as taught today at medical schools in the western world, primarily focuses on the science and knowledge regarding maternal and fetal care before, during and after childbirth. The prime intention of reproduction and pregnancy is to help to give birth to a healthy infant, with all its biological, social, cultural roles and expectations attached to and surrounded by [21]. The anticipation of a vital new-born—as grounded in our human nature by parental archetypes—marks a strong drive within the medical profession of obstetrics and midwifery, so that the contrary of such—the delivery of a dead infant—seems to erratically run against human instincts and causes disturbance and rejection on deep layers of medical professionalism and psychological identification of the individuals involved in its care. This phenomenon is reflected not only by the lack of relevant chapters on fetal death in numerous obstetric textbooks, yet also in the lack of consideration of respective teaching elements within the medical curriculum and during specialty training on how to break news of fetal death. The results of our study reflect this lack by flagging up the degree of stress in this population and the need for better training and education in that subject, biologically, psychologically and in terms of patient- and topic-centered-communication skills.

The design and introduction of a specific learning tool for clinicians "IMproving Perinatal Mortality Review and Outcomes Via Education" (IMPROVE; https://learn.stillbirthcre.org.au (accessed on 1 October 2021) showed to increase confidence and knowledge of healthcare professionals in managing perinatal deaths [22]: It delivers a structured and integrated clinical and problem-oriented learning on all domains of stillbirth (communication, post-mortem examination, classification, audit and bereavement care).

4.4. Research Implications

Learning tools, such as the IMPROVE workshop [22], may also support clinicians with managing stress surrounding diagnosis and communication. Specific training programs ought to be revised and implemented at institutions, which care for bereaved parents after fetal loss, the content of which should entail the medical, social and psychological impact of stillbirth, as well as techniques for enhancing communication skills and obstetricians' resilience encountering death in medicine. Subsequent steps to quantitatively and qualitatively assess parents' and physicians' experiences would close the audit loop and allow further improvement.

4.5. Strengths and Limitations

The paucity of data regarding the impact of diagnosing and delivering the diagnosis of fetal death on health care professionals, and the scarce body of evidence regarding resilience among obstetricians, justify our study and provide validity to our data to add to the current literature. In addition, our study is unique to have specifically examined the level of self-reported stress among attending physicians and their means of coping and facilitators at diagnosing and delivering the news of fetal death. The response rate of about 24.2% of participants is consistent with current trends for social science surveys administered through the internet [23]. The range of demographic and professional characteristics in responders reflects the diversity of physicians involved in stillbirth care.

After all, our study is not devoid of limitations inherent to the failure to control for recall bias of responders and thus data accuracy from returned questionnaires. We also acknowledge a potential response and selection bias by obstetricians with either greater interest in stillbirth or previous unfavorable experiences in diagnosing or communicating fetal death. Furthermore, our study did not assess the amount of time, which had elapsed since the responder's last experience of stillbirth, which might have made a difference with regards to the individual perception of stress. In addition, we retrospectively assessed the levels of stress and coping strategies, relying on the participants' memory. Hence, we cannot preclude a certain recall bias. Finally, our survey was conducted in a European high-income country. We, therefore, note that our data might not be fully generalizable due to potential fundamental differences in health care systems and governance, thus medical conduct and practice, cultural and social behavior, as well as teaching systems at medical school and during residency. After all, this limitation highlights the need for further data generation on that matter.

5. Conclusions

Our study shows that engagement in stillbirth evokes moderate to high levels of stress among obstetricians regardless of prior experiences, professional position, age, and gender. Handling these situations requires resources from both the professional and private environment, the context of which differs with the grade of professional experience and role.

Author Contributions: Conceptualization, D.A.M., J.S.E., S.L., A.F.; methodology, D.A.M., S.L., A.F.; software, S.L.; validation, D.A.M., A.F.; formal analysis, D.A.M., A.F.; investigation, D.A.M., J.S.E., S.L., A.F.; resources, D.A.M., S.L., A.F.; data curation, D.A.M., J.S.E., S.L., A.F.; writing—original draft preparation, D.A.M.; writing—review and editing, D.A.M., J.S.E., S.L., A.F.; visualization, D.A.M.; supervision, A.F.; project administration, S.L. All authors have read and agreed to the published version of the manuscript.

Funding: This research received no external funding.

Institutional Review Board Statement: The study was conducted according to the guidelines of the Declaration of Helsinki, and approved by the Institutional Review Board approved by the Medical Board of the OEGGG as well as the Ethics Committee of the Medical University of Vienna (2020).

Informed Consent Statement: Informed consent was obtained from all subjects involved in the study.

Data Availability Statement: The data that support the findings of this study are available from the corresponding author, D.A.M., upon reasonable request.

Acknowledgments: The authors are grateful to all participants in this online survey. The authors thank the board of the Austrian Society of Obstetrics and Gynecology for their critical intellectual input to the questionnaire and approving to the study. D.A.M. is thankful to J.C. Huber for his enduring support.

Conflicts of Interest: The authors declare no conflict of interest. No funding was received for conduction of this study.

References

1. Mohangoo, A.D.; Buitendijk, S.E.; Szamotulska, K.; Chalmers, J.; Irgens, L.M.; Bolumar, F.; Nijhuis, J.G.; Zeitlin, J. Gestational age patterns of fetal and neonatal mortality in Europe: Results from the Euro-Peristat project. *PLoS ONE* **2011**, *6*, e24727. [CrossRef] [PubMed]
2. Nuzum, D.; Meaney, S.; O'Donoghue, K. The impact of stillbirth on bereaved parents: A qualitative study. *PLoS ONE* **2018**, *13*, e0191635. [CrossRef]
3. Nuzum, D.; Meaney, S.; O'Donoghue, K. The impact of stillbirth on consultant obstetrician gynaecologists: A qualitative study. *BJOG Int. J. Obstet. Gynaecol.* **2014**, *121*, 1020–1028. [CrossRef]
4. Nuzum, D.; Meaney, S.; O'Donoghue, K. The Place of Faith for Consultant Obstetricians Following Stillbirth: A Qualitative Exploratory Study. *J. Relig. Health* **2016**, *55*, 1519–1528. [CrossRef]
5. Korteweg, F.J.; Gordijn, S.J.; Timmer, A.; Erwich, J.J.; Bergman, K.A.; Bouman, K.; Ravise, J.M.; Heringa, M.P.; Holm, J.P. The Tulip classification of perinatal mortality: Introduction and multidisciplinary inter-rater agreement. *BJOG Int. J. Obstet. Gynaecol.* **2006**, *113*, 393–401. [CrossRef] [PubMed]
6. Sharp, I.; Adeyeye, T.; Peacock, L.; Mahdi, A.; Farrant, K.; Sharp, A.N.; Greenwood, S.L.; Heazell, A.E.P. Investigation of the outcome of pregnancies complicated by increased fetal movements and their relation to underlying causes—A prospective cohort study. *Acta Obstet. Et Gynecol. Scand.* **2021**, *100*, 91–100. [CrossRef] [PubMed]
7. Ter Kuile, M.; Erwich, J.; Heazell, A.E.P. Stillbirths preceded by reduced fetal movements are more frequently associated with placental insufficiency: A retrospective cohort study. *J. Perinat. Med.* **2021**. [CrossRef]
8. Heazell, A.E.; McLaughlin, M.J.; Schmidt, E.B.; Cox, P.; Flenady, V.; Khong, T.Y.; Downe, S. A difficult conversation? The views and experiences of parents and professionals on the consent process for perinatal postmortem after stillbirth. *BJOG Int. J. Obstet. Gynaecol.* **2012**, *119*, 987–997. [CrossRef] [PubMed]
9. Gaab, J.; Rohleder, N.; Nater, U.M.; Ehlert, U. Psychological determinants of the cortisol stress response: The role of anticipatory cognitive appraisal. *Psychoneuroendocrinology* **2005**, *30*, 599–610. [CrossRef] [PubMed]
10. Kirschbaum, C. Mental stress follows mental rules. *J. Clin. Endocrinol. Metab.* **1999**, *84*, 4292. [CrossRef] [PubMed]
11. Davis, M.H. A Multidimensional Approach to Individual Differences in Empathy. *JSAS Cat. Sel. Doc. Psychol.* **1980**, *10*, 85–104.
12. Jakoby, N.J. Messung von internen und externen Kontrollüberzeugungen in allgemeinen Bevölkerungsumfragen. *ZUMA Nachr.* **1999**, *23*, 61–71.
13. Rotter, J.B. Generalized expectancies for internal versus external control of reinforcement. *Psychol. Monogr.* **1966**, *80*, 1–28. [CrossRef] [PubMed]
14. Winkel, A.F.; Robinson, A.; Jones, A.A.; Squires, A.P. Physician resilience: A grounded theory study of obstetrics and gynaecology residents. *Med. Educ.* **2019**, *53*, 184–194. [CrossRef] [PubMed]
15. Braun, V.; Clarke, V. What can "thematic analysis" offer health and wellbeing researchers? *Int. J. Qual. Stud. Health Well-Being* **2014**, *9*, 26152. [CrossRef] [PubMed]
16. Braun, V.; Clarke, V. Novel insights into patients' life-worlds: The value of qualitative research. *Lancet Psychiatry* **2019**, *6*, 720–721. [CrossRef]
17. Kelley, M.C.; Trinidad, S.B. Silent loss and the clinical encounter: Parents' and physicians' experiences of stillbirth-a qualitative analysis. *BMC Pregnancy Childbirth* **2012**, *12*, 137. [CrossRef]
18. Nuzum, D.; Meaney, S.; O'Donohue, K. Communication skills in Obstetrics: What can we learn from bereaved parents? *Ir. Med. J.* **2017**, *110*, 512.
19. Farrow, V.A.; Goldenberg, R.L.; Fretts, R.; Schulkin, J. Psychological impact of stillbirths on obstetricians. *J. Matern.-Fetal Neonatal Med. Off. J. Eur. Assoc. Perinat. Med. Fed. Asia Ocean. Perinat. Soc. Int. Soc. Perinat. Obs.* **2013**, *26*, 748–752. [CrossRef]
20. Gold, K.J.; Kuznia, A.L.; Hayward, R.A. How physicians cope with stillbirth or neonatal death: A national survey of obstetricians. *Obstet. Gynecol.* **2008**, *112*, 29–34. [CrossRef]
21. World Health Organization. Sexual and Reproductive Health and Research Including the Special Programme HRP. 2021. Available online: www.who.int/teams/sexual-and-reproductive-health-and-research/areas-of-work/maternal-and-perinatal-health/antenatal-care (accessed on 28 August 2021).

Keywords: kidney injury; preeclampsia; chronic kidney disease; microangiopathy; maternal-perinatal

1. Introduction

Preeclampsia (PE) is a syndrome characterised by the de novo appearance in a woman more than 20 weeks pregnant of hypertension (HT) associated with proteinuria and/or other manifestations of organ dysfunction. It is included within the category of hypertensive disorders of pregnancy (HDP), a term that refers to a set of entities whose link is the presence of arterial HT in a pregnant woman [1,2].

There are clinical and analytical conditions that confer severity upon preeclampsia and further increase the risk of maternal-perinatal morbidity and mortality [3,4]. Among them are systolic blood pressure $\geq$ 160 mmHg and/or diastolic blood pressure $\geq$ 110 mmHg; proteinuria $\geq$ 2 g; oliguria; renal failure; neurological or visual alterations; acute pulmonary oedema or cyanosis; pain in the epigastrium or right hypochondrium; liver dysfunction; haematological alterations or placental involvement, with foetal manifestations such as delayed intrauterine growth.

At present, we are witnessing an increase in the incidence of preeclampsia and SP; it is a frequently encountered obstetric complication and one of the main causes of maternal-perinatal morbidity and mortality [5–11]. In pregnancy, the glomerular filtration rate (GFR) increases by 40–60% compared to normal levels, which leads to a decrease in plasma creatinine levels (normal levels in pregnant women are 0.4–0.6 mg/dL) [12–14]. The formulas used to estimate the GFR with creatinine are not validated for pregnancy, which makes the diagnosis of acute kidney injury (AKI) difficult in this clinical situation [13]. As a result of these factors, there is controversy regarding the definition of AKI during pregnancy, which has led to different ways of defining it in the literature [14,15]. AKI, generally defined as a decrease in the GFR within hours or days, is a frequent complication in the hospital setting, especially in cases of previous chronic kidney disease (CKD) and chronic renal failure (CRF), defined as GFR < 60 mL/min/1.73 m^2 It is classically defined as a rare complication within the maternal clinical manifestations of PE. When it occurs in this context, it is associated with a worse maternal and perinatal prognosis [16]. In fact, as previously mentioned, it is one of the clinical criteria that defines severe preeclampsia (SP) and necessitates important considerations, such as whether to terminate the pregnancy, as it has a decisive influence on maternal and perinatal prognoses [3,4].

The objective of this study is to compare the maternal and perinatal clinical and analytical variables in patients with SP who develop AKI vs. those who do not develop this condition.

2. Materials and Methods

Design and patients: An observational study was conducted with a retrospective, hospital-based cohort of patients with SP treated at a tertiary centre between January 2007 and December 2018 to compare maternal-perinatal variables between patients who develop AKI and those who do not. SP was diagnosed according to the criteria of the American College of Obstetricians and Gynecologists Practice Guidelines for Gestational Hypertension and Preeclampsia [16] in patients with preeclampsia who met some of the following severity criteria: Systolic blood pressure (SBP) $\geq$ 160 mmHg and/or Diastolic blood pressure (DBP) $\geq$ 110 mmHg confirmed at 15 min; proteinuria $\geq$ 2 g measured in 24-h urine or estimated by the protein/creatinine ratio in urine; oliguria $\leq$ 500 mL/24 h or diuresis rate < 0.5 mL/kg/h for 2 h; renal insufficiency: serum creatinine > 1.1 mg/dL, or double the value of serum creatinine in the absence of other renal disease; neurological or visual alterations, including severe headache that does not subside with analgesics, blurred vision, diplopia or amaurosis; acute lung oedema or cyanosis; pain in the epigastrium or right hypochondrium; hepatic dysfunction: transaminase levels elevated to double the normal value; haematological alterations, including thrombocytopenia (<100,000 mm^3), disseminated intravascular coagulation (DIC) or haemolysis; placental involvement with foetal manifestations including intrauterine growth restriction (IGR), abnormal umbilical artery Doppler results and foetal death [3,4]. In this study, we considered the presence of a serum creatinine level greater than 1.1 mg/dL, which is a criterion for the severity of preeclampsia [16]. This cut-off point takes into account the Kidney Disease: Improving Global Outcomes (KDIGO) definition and attempts to avoid overestimating the incidence of AKI by including mild forms of renal function impairment.

In patients with pre-existing CKD, AKI was considered when the baseline serum creatinine level was 1.5 times higher than the baseline level. Oliguria was considered at a diuresis rate of less than 500 mL in 24 h or less than 0.5 mL/kg/h for 2 consecutive hours [16]. If AKI was accompanied by oliguria, it was defined as oliguric AKI. CKD was defined according to the criteria of the National Kidney Foundation-Kidney Disease Outcomes Quality Initiative (NKF-KDOQI) guidelines [17]. Also for CKD we included patients with proteinuria at <20 weeks HELLP (H: hemolysis, EL: elevated liver enzymes and LP: low platelets) syndrome was diagnosed according to the Sibai criteria: haemolysis (schistocytes in smear, $LDH \geq 600$ IU/L or bilirubin ≥ 1.2 mg/dL), platelet count < 100,000 cells/µL and $GPT \geq 70$ U/L [18]. Thrombotic microangiopathy (TMA) was clinically defined by the presence of microangiopathic haemolytic anaemia, thrombocytopenia and organ dysfunction, with primary involvement of the kidneys [19].

The study protocol was approved by the centres Ethics Committee for Medical Research, and patient follow-up was performed from the point at which the women were diagnosed with SP during either pregnancy, childbirth or postpartum, mainly until the normalisation of blood pressure (without the need for antihypertensive medication) and proteinuria; the maximum postpartum follow-up duration was 12 weeks in cases of specialised postpartum consultation for at-risk patients.

The study variables were collected at the following time points: pre-gestational; gestational; at the time of the preeclampsia diagnosis; peripartum; perinatal; upon discharge from the hospital; and at the 12-weeks postpartum consultation.

The study data were stored in a database created for this purpose until the statistical analysis. The variables were analysed using the statistical package IBM Corp. Released 2015. IBM SPSS Statistics for Windows, Version 23.0. Armonk, NY: IBM Corp. are presented as means and SDs for quantitative variables and as number and percentages for qualitative variables. For the comparison of the variables between the study groups, we conducted a univariate analysis by logistic regression to determine the probability ratio, odds ratio (OR) and 95% confidence interval (CI). After univariate analysis, variables with clinical relevance or a p-value equal to or less than 0.20 were included in the multivariate logistic regression analysis. Results with p less than 0.05 were accepted as significant.

3. Results

During the study period, 76,828 births took place at the centre; of these, 303 were to women diagnosed with SP. The annual incidence increased gradually over the study period, reaching 1.79% births/year in 2018. During the study period, no cases of maternal death were recorded among patients with SP. AKI occurred in 75 patients (24.8%), of whom 34.66% had oliguria, with a mean serum creatinine of 1.53 ± 0.73 mg/dL and a mean urea of 58.39 ± 25.83 mg/dL. In 32% of cases, AKI was caused by CKD, and in 5.33% (4 patients), it was caused by CRF. In the AKI group, 25.33% (19 patients) developed AKI in the context of HELLP syndrome, and in 3 developed AKI in the context of haemolytic uraemic syndrome secondary to pregnancy. Twenty-one patients who developed AKI (28%) required the transfusion of packed red blood cells; 12 of these patients also had HELLP syndrome, and 3 also had haemolytic uraemic syndrome secondary to pregnancy. Only 1 patient required temporary dialysis to recover renal function.

Tables 1–7 summarise the descriptive statistics of the study variables for all patients diagnosed with SP (n = 303), those who developed AKI (n = 75) and those who did not develop AKI (n = 228). As Table 1 shows, the comparative analysis found significant differences in personal history of CKD, CRF, mean baseline serum creatinine and mean pregestational proteinuria. Table 2 show that in AKI patients there were a significantly higher percentage of patients who became pregnant through in vitro fertilisation (IVF) and patients who had proteinuria before 20 weeks of gestation.

Table 1. Comparative analysis of the distribution of pre-pregnancy variables in all patients with pre-eclampsia and in the study groups (AKI vs Non AKI). Cr: creatinine; Obesity: body mass index (BMI) $\geq$ 30 Kg/m^2. Overweight BMI $\geq$ 25 Kg/m^2.

	Total n = 303		AKI (n = 75)		No AKI (n = 228)		
	N; Mean ± S.T	%	Mean ± S.T	%	Mean ± S.T	%	p
Maternal age	33.94 ± 6.29		35.09 ± 6.99		33.56 ± 6.02		0.068
Nationality							0.570
Spanish	179	59.1		60		58.8	
South American	91	29.6		33.3		28.9	
African	14	4.5		4		4.8	
European not Spanish	14	4.5		2.7		5.3	
Other	5	1.5		0		2.2	
HT	49	16.2		18.7		15.4	0.499
Diabetes Mellitus	7	2.3		1.3		2.6	0.516
Hypothyroidism	30	9.9		9.3		10.1	0.480
BMI (Kg/m^2)	26.23 ± 5.27		26.05 ± 5.44		26.29 ± 5.23		0.742
Obesity	66	24.0		21.1		25	0.510
Overweight	153	56.3		53.6		57.1	0.611
Autoimmune disease	7	2.3		4		1.8	0.261
CKD	24	7.9		17.3		4.8	0.001
CRF	5	1.7		5.3		0.4	0.004
Cr baseline serum (mg/dL)	0.64 ± 0.20		0.78 ± 0.31		0.60 ± 0.11		<0.001
Pregestational proteinuria	12	4		9.3		2.2	0.006
Number of pregnancies	2.01 ± 1.38		1.87 ± 1.31		2.06 ± 1.40		0.290
Nulliparity	153	50.5		54.7		49.1	0.405
Abortion History	107	35.3		26.7		38.2	0.071
Number of abortions	0.52 ± 0.87		0.44 ± 0.90		0.54 ± 0.81		0.352
History of preeclampsia	26	8.6		10.7		7.9	0.457
Family History of HT	116	38.3		39.7		39.4	0.957
Family history of preeclampsia	22	7.3		4		8.3	0.210

Table 2. Comparative analysis of the distribution of gestational variables in all patients with preeclampsia and in the study groups (AKI vs non AKI). UTI: urinary tract infection.

	Total n = 303		AKI (n = 75)		No AKI (n = 228)		
	n	%	n	%	n	%	p
IVF	63	20.8	24	32	39	17.1	0.006
Multiple pregnancy	55	18.2	19	25.3	36	15.8	0.063
HT before 20 weeks of follow-up	53	17.5	15	20	38	16.7	0.510
Gestational HT	78	25.7	14	18.7	64	28.1	0.106
Gestational Diabetes	30	9.9	8	10.7	22	9.6	0.798
Gestational hypothyroidism	33	10.9	11	14.7	22	9.6	0.480
Proteinuria < 20 weeks	12	4	7	9.3	5	2.2	0.006
UTI during pregnancy	97	32.1	25	33.3	72	31.6	0.778
Alphamethyldopa treatment	59	19.5	15	20	44	19.3	0.894
Calcium antagonist treatment	11	3.6	2	2.7	9	3.9	0.607
Labetalol treatment	40	13.2	18	23.5	22	17	0.758

Table 3. Comparative analysis of the distribution of the variables that refer to the time of diagnosis of severe preeclampsia in all the patients and in the study groups (AKI vs. non AKI). CrCl: Creatinine clearance.

	Total n = 303		AKI (n = 75)		No AKI (n = 228)		
	N; Mean ± SD	%	Mean ± SD	%	Mean ± SD	%	p
SBP mmHg	178.97 ± 16.52		179.04 ± 20.13		178.95 ± 15.20		0.971
DBP mmHg	103.84 ± 11.82		102.52 ± 13.81		104.28 ± 11.09		0.263
Gestational age at diagnosis	34.03 ± 4.37		33.31 ± 3.99		34.27 ± 4.46		0.098
Gestational age at diagnosis <28 weeks 28–36.6 weeks ≥37 weeks	25 175 103	8.3 57.8 34		8 72 20		8.3 53.1 36.6	0.010
Early initiation of SP	125	41.3		49.3		38.6	0.101
Puerperal PE	66	21.8		14.7		24.1	0.085
Proteinuria (g/24 h)	2.8 ± 2.78		3.18 ± 2.92		2.67 ± 2.72		0.170
Creatinine (mg/dL)	0.89 ± 0.53		1.53 ± 0.73		0.68 ± 0.14		<0.001
Urea (mg/dL)	37.88 ± 21.48		58.39 ± 25.83		29.68 ± 12.08		<0.001
CrCl (mL/min)	112.24 ± 42.65		81.64 ± 41.58		127.39 ± 34.37		<0.001
Uric acid (mg/dL)	6.80 ± 1.68		8.13 ± 1.54		6.36 ± 1.48		<0.001
Maximum uric acid level (mg/dL)	7.37 ± 1.74		8.87 ± 1.74		6.88 ± 1.45		<0.001
GOT (U/L)	110.28 ± 298.74		220.87 ± 488.14		60.880 ± 126.00		0.010
GPT (U/L)	68.50 ± 143.03		139.63 ± 244.96		45.10 ± 73.72		0.001
Platelets ($\times 10^3/\mu L$)	165.25 ± 72.12		138.21 ± 78.15		174.25 ± 67.15		<0.001
LDH (U/L)	356.81 ± 340.91		534.15 ± 588.81		298.47 ± 166.71		0.001
Hemoglobin (g/dl)	10.66 ± 1.76		9.89 ± 2.05		10.91 ± 1.58		<0.001
Magnesium (mg/dL)	4.20 ± 2.59		5.28 ± 2.47		3.77 ± 2.52		<0.001
C3 level (mg/dL)	141.26 ± 39.46		131.59 ± 45.20		145.35 ± 36.15		0.025
C4 level (mg/dL)	26.34 ± 10.25		24.90 ± 11.15		26.96 ± 9.81		0.156

Table 3. Cont.

	Total n = 303		AKI (n = 75)		No AKI (n = 228)		
	N; Mean ± SD	%	Mean ± SD	%	Mean ± SD	%	p
IgG level (mg/dL)	810.97 ± 283.01		756.81 ± 291.17		833.81 ± 277.23		0.056
IgA level (mg/dL)	202.78 ± 77.91		197.15 ± 80.34		205.16 ± 76.99		0.472
IgM level (mg/dL)	128.06 ± 63.05		119.10 ± 60.21		131.85 ± 64.02		0.157
Antiphospholipid 1st	9	3.4		4.4		3	0.575
ANA	16	6.7		5.6		7.1	0.670
antiDNA	4	1.7		1.4		1.8	0.853
Albumin (g/dL)	3.41 ± 0.68		3.21 ± 0.77		3.53 ± 0.60		0.004
Triglycerides (mg/dL)	194.30 ± 94.80		227.01 ± 95.35		180.80 ± 91.45		<0.001
Cholesterol (mg/dL)	247.51 ± 73.28		228.27 ± 64.76		255.25 ± 75.23		0.009
Magnesium sulfate treatment	208	68.6		82.7		64	0.003
Labetalol treatment	247	81.5		82.7		81.1	0.768
Treatment with hydralazine	98	32.3		8.9		23.4	0.435
Diuretic treatment	15	5		10.7		3.1	0.009
Oliguria	32	10.6		34.7		2.6	<0.001
HELLP syndrome	31	10.2		25.3		5.3	<0.001
TMA (includes HELLP)	35	11.6		29.3		5.7	<0.001
Eclampsia	10	3.3		0		4.4	0.065

Table 4. Comparative analysis of the distribution of intrapartum and immediate postpartum variables in all patients with pre-eclampsia and in the study groups (AKI vs non AKI). ARB: angiotensine receptor blockers.

	Total n = 303		AKI (n = 75)		Non AKI (n = 228)		
	Mean ± SD	%	Mean ± SD	%	Mean ± SD	%	p
Delivery follow-up	34.46 ± 3.86		33.80 ± 3.60		34.68 ± 3.92		0.089
Gestational age at diagnosis							
<28 weeks	16	5.3		5.3		5.3	
28–36.6 weeks	178	58.7		73.3		53.9	0.008
≥37 weeks	109	36		21.3		40.8	
Birth initiation method:							
Spontaneous	25	8.3		4		9.6	
Induced	135	44.6		38.7		46.5	0.077
Elective caesarean section	143	47.2		57.3		43.9	
Completion of delivery:							
Vaginal	107	35.3		17.3		41.2	<0.001
Caesarean	196	64.7		82.7		58.8	
HT at delivery	260	85.8		86.7		85.5	0.806
Transfusion	30	9.9		6.9		3	<0.001
Postpartum Labetalol	292	96.4		96		96.5	0.844
Postpartum hydralazine	147	48.5		56		46.3	0.143
Postpartum Enalapril	275	90.8		80		94.3	<0.001
ARB II postpartum	17	5.6		8.1		4.8	0.291
Postpartum calcium antagonists	202	66.7		66		70.2	0.031
Postpartum furosemide	102	33.7		44		30.3	0.082

Table 5. Comparative analysis of the distribution of perinatal variables in all patients with pre-eclampsia and in the study groups (AKI vs non AKI). SGA: small for their gestational age. Newborn: NB.

	Total n = 303/351		AKI (n = 75)		No AKI (n = 228)		
	Mean ± SD	%	Mean ± SD	%	Mean ± SD	%	p
Follow-up at birth	34.46 ± 3.86		33.80 ± 3.60		34.68 ± 3.92		0.089
Lung maturation	146	48.2		60		44.3	0.018
Intrauterine growth restriction (IUGR)	71	20.2		18.7		25	0.261
SGA 1st Newborn (non IUGR)	62	17.7		10.8		23.9	0.036
Sex 1st Newborn Male Female	138 165	45.5 54.5		41.3 58.7		46.9 53.1	0.399
Sex 2nd Newborn Male Female	20 28	41.7 58.3		41.2 58.8		41.9 58.1	0.959
Weight 1st Newborn (grams)	2.128.24 ± 864.29		2.023.81 ± 851.33		2.162.59 ± 867.61		0.228
Weight 2nd Newborn (grams)	1.919.86 ± 504.70		2.052.22 ± 433.28		1.845.41 ± 532.71		0.167
Apgar Test value 1st min	7.52 ± 1.76		6.96 ± 1.82		7.73 ± 1.67		0.002
Apgar Test Value 1st min 2nd NB	7.94 ± 1.23		7.72 ± 1.36		8.06 ± 1.16		0.355
Apgar Test Value 5 min 1st NB	8.44 ± 1.70		8.5 ± 1.43		9.02 ± 1.18		0.006
Apgar test value 5 min 2nd NB	9.16 ± 0.86		9.11 ± 0.90		9.19 ± 0.85		0.768
1st NB cord pH	7.24 ± 0.09		7.23 ± 0.11		7.25 ± 0.08		0.310
2nd NB cord pH	7.29 ± 0.08		7.28 ± 0.11		7.29 ± 0.07		0.513
Exitus perinatal	18	5.1		2.7		7	0.165
Admission to Neonatal Intensive Care Unit	96	27.4		42.7		28.1	0.018
Cause of admission Heart disease Distres Intubation difficulty Prematurity IUGR	15 37 10 13 21	15.6 38.5 10.4 13.5 21.9		9.4 50.0 15.6 12.5 12.5		18.8 32.8 7.8 14.1 26.6		0.20

Table 6. Comparative analysis of the distribution of variables at hospital discharge in all patients with pre-eclampsia and in the study groups (AKI vs non AKI).

	Total *n* = 303		AKI (*n* = 75)		No AKI (*n* = 228)		
	Mean ± SD	%	Mean ± SD	%	Mean ± SD	%	*p*
HT	288	95		86.7		97.8	<0.001
Number of Antihypertensive treatment							
0	16	5.3		13.3		2.6	
1	130	43.9		46.7		41.7	0.002
2	132	43.6		33.3		46.9	
≥3	25	8.3		6.7		8.8	
Proteinuria	219	72.3		71.6		75.1	0.552
Creatinine (mg/dL)	0.68 ± 0.26		0.88 ± 0.42		0.62 ± 0.12		<0.001
Urea (mg/dL)	33.15 ± 13.59		41.18 ± 18.73		29.90 ± 9.07		<0.001
Ccr (mL/min)	123.49 ± 34.58		104.35 ± 37.38		130.71 ± 30.61		<0.001
Uric acid (mg/dL)	5.73 ± 1.44		6.21 ± 1.72		5.58 ± 1.30		0.005
Proteinuria (g/24 h)	1.04 ± 1.17		1.36 ± 1.51		0.93 ± 1.02		0.026
GOT (U/L)	31.87 ± 23.60		36.22 ± 27.54		29.95 ± 21.46		0.075
GPT (U/L)	30.17 ± 25.08		39.56 ± 36.01		27.08 ± 19.38		0.005
Platelets at discharge ($\times 10^3$/μL)	288.45 ± 101.82		294.00 ± 115.21		286.02 ± 97.18		0.574
LDH (U/L)	245.75 ± 82.36		268.36 ± 122.88		238.28 ± 62.17		0.045
Haemoglobin (g/dL)	11.22 ± 1.45		10.87 ± 1.48		11.33 ± 1.43		0.016

Table 7. Comparative analysis of the distribution of variables at discharge from the risk puerperium consultation in all patients with pre-eclampsia and in the study groups (AKI vs non AKI).

	Total *n* = 303		AKI (*n* = 75)		No AKI (*n* = 228)		
	Mean ± SD	%	Mean ± SD	%	Mean ± SD	%	*p*
Persistent hypertension	72	23.8		24.3		25.8	0.797
Persistent proteinuria	31	11.1		21.4		7.6	0.001
Renal insufficiency	7	2.3		9.9		0	<0.001
Proteinuria (mg/mg)	0.19 ± 0.47		0.38 ± 0.88		0.13 ± 0.21		0.032
Serum creatinine (mg/dL)	0.69 ± 0.21		0.85 ± 0.35		0.65 ± 0.11		<0.001
CrCl (mL/min)	115.17 ± 29.8		99.61 ± 27.57		121.68 ± 28.37		<0.001
Evolution							
Referral to family doctor	203	67		64		68	
Referral to Nephrology	72	23.8		29.3		21.9	0.341
Loss of follow-up	28	9.2		6.7		10.1	

Regarding the variables measured at the time of SP diagnosis, presented in Table 3, the occurrence of AKI was positive associated with the gestational week at which SP was diagnosed, OR 1.67 (CI 95%: 1.07–2.61). Statistically significant differences were found in the mean levels of some biochemical variables in maternal blood. The difference in uric acid was especially notable, with an OR 2.11 (CI 95%: 1.70–2.60) in AKI group. The mean levels of platelets, haemoglobin and albumin were significantly lower in the AKI group, as were the plasma levels of C3. The AKI group had a significantly higher percentage of patients with HELLP, and patients treated with diuretics and magnesium sulfate than the group without AKI.

Regarding variables measured intrapartum and immediately postpartum, shown in Table 4, we found a significantly higher percentage of patients in the AKI group who had a caesarean section, OR: 3.35 (CI 95%: 1.74–6.43), or required a transfusion. Regarding the week of gestation at the time of delivery, the group with AKI had a higher percentage of premature delivery (<37 weeks of gestation) OR: 3.4 (CI 95%: 1.7–6.4). There were also significant differences in the type of antihypertensive treatment used during the immediate postpartum period: a lower percentage of patients in the AKI group were treated with enalapril, and a higher percentage were treated with calcium antagonists. No significant differences were found for the rest of the variables.

A perinatal mortality rate of 5.1% was found for all 351 neonates. A total of 64% were premature (<37 weeks of gestation), and 5.3% were extremely premature at less than 28 weeks of gestation at birth. The mean gestational age at delivery was 34 weeks. Table 5 presents the perinatal variables and shows that a significantly higher percentage of the neonates born to the AKI group required foetal lung maturation with steroids, OR 1.89 (CI 95%: 1.11–3.21) and ICU admission. The mean Apgar scores at 1 min and 5 min of life were significantly lower in the AKI group than in the non-AKI group, OR 0.74 (CI 95%: 0.61–0.91). Regarding IGR, no differences were found between the groups. In contrast, the percentage of infants who were small for their gestational age (SGA) was higher in the non-AKI group.

Regarding the variables measures at the time of hospital discharge, shown in Table 6, there was a lower percentage of hypertensive patients in the AKI group than in the no-AKI group, OR 0.15 (CI 95%: 0.05–0.44), and there were statistically significant differences in the number of antihypertensive drugs being taken at discharge. There were no differences in the percentage of patients with proteinuria at discharge, although the mean proteinuria level at discharge was significantly higher in the group with AKI. There were also significant differences in the mean GPT, uric acid, LDH and haemoglobin values at discharge.

After hospital discharge, 9.2% of the participants were lost to follow-up. At discharge from the postpartum risk consultation, as shown in Table 7, the highest percentage of patients lost to follow-up were in the no-AKI group. On the other hand, there were statistically significant differences between groups in the percentage of patients with persistent proteinuria at 12 weeks postpartum, OR 3.31 (CI 95%: 1.54–7.11), and in the mean value of proteinuria in the AKI group than in the no-AKI group.

After a maximum follow-up of 12 weeks postpartum, 25 patients (9%) without a previous history of chronic HT remained hypertensive. Similarly, 19 patients (7%) without pregestational proteinuria showed persistent postpartum proteinuria (protein/creatinine index greater than 0.3 mg/mg), and 7 patients (2.3%) had persistent AKI, including 2 who had previous CRF. After 12 weeks postpartum, 72 patients were referred to the nephrology consultation for persistent HT, proteinuria or renal failure.

In the multivariate logistic regression analysis (Figure 1), previous CKD and IVF predicted an increased risk of AKI onset. The pre-AKI uric acid level was the strongest biochemical marker of the onset of AKI. TMA was a cause of AKI in SP. Indications for caesarean section were associated with the onset of AKI in SP.

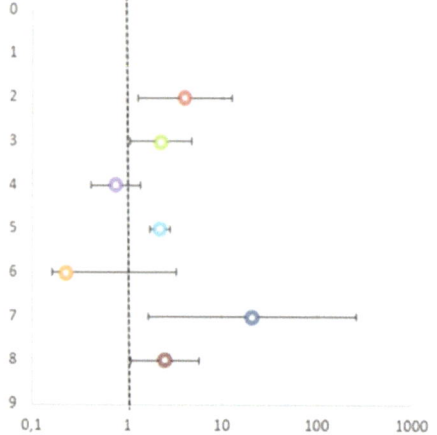

	OR	CI 95%		P
		lower	higher	
CKD	3.99	1.27	12.50	0.017
IVF	2.25	1.06	4.75	0.034
GAD	0.75	0.41	1.37	0.348
Ac. Uric	2.17	1.70	2.76	0.000
HELLP	0.23	0.16	3.21	0.273
TMA	20.52	1.64	256.15	0.019
Caesarean	2.49	1.08	5.70	0.032

Figure 1. Association study of maternal-perinatal variables with acute renal failure in the group of pregnant women with severe pre-eclampsia. Multivariate logistic regression analysis (variables included in the model). Pre-pregnancy CKD; IVF in vitro fertilization; GAD gestational age at diagnosis of AKI; Ac. Uric pre AKI; HELLP syndrome; TMA thrombotic micro angiopathy; indication for caesarean section.

4. Discussion

Our results describe a high frequency of AKI in our series of pregnant women with SP stands out: it affects 25% of these patients and 9.76/10,000 births in our hospital-based population. In SP cases, AKI occur in the third trimester and in the immediate postpartum period, and HDP, mainly preeclampsia and HELLP syndrome, are the main causes [13,20,21]. Other maternal and perinatal variables associated with AKI cases were a history of CRF, pregnancies after assisted reproductive techniques use, higher maternal blood of uric acid and creatinine levels, higher rate of preterm delivery, c-section and postpartum complications such as haemorrhage the need for red blood cell transfusion. Despite a higher rate of preterm and admission in neonatal ICU, neonatal mortality rate was significantly lower in AKI cases.

Comparing to the literature, in a series of pregnancy-associated AKI in India, the researchers observed that 17% of patients with preeclampsia and 60% of patients with HELLP syndrome developed AKI [20]. In any case, it is important to consider other causes of AKI associated with pregnancy, which, although infrequent, are very serious. Examples include forms of TMA that can occur in the final phase of pregnancy or immediately postpartum and that are often difficult to differentiate from SP or HELLP syndrome. In fact, both SP and HELLP syndrome are currently considered types of TMA [22]. Our incidence is clearly higher than that described in the literature, including the incidences of 2.68/10,000 births in a Canadian study [23] and 4.5/10,000 births in a US series [24].

Seventy-five percent of cases of AKI occur in the third trimester and in the immediate postpartum period, and HDP, mainly preeclampsia and HELLP syndrome, are the main causes [13,20,21]. Preeclampsia involves histological changes at the renal level that are characterised by glomerular endotheliosis, podocyturia and proteinuria; functional changes, such as decreased renal tubular secretion of uric acid; and haemodynamic alterations consisting of intrarenal vasoconstriction, decreased renal plasma flow and a GFR reduction of between 30 and 40% [25]. These conditions lead to susceptibility to renal ischaemic injury and the onset of AKF.

In the general population, one of the main risk factors for AKI is a history of CRF and, above all, its severity [26]. The results of our study are consistent with these data, showing an OR 12.79 (CI 95%: 1.41–116.28), $p = 0.02$, for CRF. This result is supported by the findings of other authors [27,28].

Regarding pregnancy-related variables, a higher frequency of assisted reproductive techniques and IVF use was found among the SP patients who developed AKI than in those without AKI (32 vs. 17.1%). The risk of developing AKI was 2.28 times higher among patients with SP who underwent IVF. To date, we have not found any studies that that relate AKI to the use of assisted reproductive techniques in patients with SP, although there are studies that describe the relationship between AKI and assisted reproduction techniques in pregnant women in general [29,30]. What is well established is that preeclampsia is the most frequent cause of AKI in developed countries [13,21,23,24,31,32], and it is very likely that the established relationship between preeclampsia and assisted reproductive techniques justifies our results [33–36].

When analysing the association between the development of AKI and variables measured at the time of SP diagnosis, it was found that the mean uric acid value was significantly higher in the group with SP and AKI than in the group without AKI, 8.87 ± 1.74 vs. 6.88 ± 1.45 mg/dL, $p < 0.001$. This result is explained by the fact that uric acid is eliminated mainly by the kidneys and therefore, when SP develops and the GFR and tubular secretion decrease, uric acid levels increase [37]. Hyperuricaemia is correlated with the severity of glomerular endotheliosis, and in pregnant women with SP, the level of uric acid is an early marker of kidney damage and maternal-foetal prognosis [38–42]. In this sense, Le TM et al. [40] found that a uric acid level of 6.6 mg/dL is a good predictor of the severity of preeclampsia/eclampsia, OR 5.19 (CI 95%: 2.79–9.65). A possible line of study is the use of this and other markers of the progression of renal damage in SP.

In our series, HELLP syndrome, a form of TMA associated with pregnancy [22,43,44], occurred significantly more frequently in the group of women with SP who developed AKI than in those who did not develop AKI (25.3% vs. 5.3%, respectively). Many studies have established the role of HELLP syndrome in AKI associated with pregnancy [15,20–22,44–47]. In the series by Jai Prakash et al. [21] that included 132 pregnant women with AKI, HELLP syndrome was responsible for 6.8% of all cases. This percentage is even higher in the series of Huang C et al. [47], in which HELLP syndrome was responsible for 60% of AKI cases. It is important to note that these authors defined AKI as serum creatinine levels greater than 0.8 mg/dL. In the meta-analysis of Liu Y et al. [15], in which a group of 834 patients with pregnancy-associated AKI was compared to 5334 pregnant women without AKI, the pregnant women with AKI had a 1.86-fold higher risk of having HELLP syndrome than the pregnant women without AKI. We mention this work to highlight the relevance of the temporality of the analysis of the causal association between AKI and HELLP syndrome. In our study, we considered AKI a consequence of HELLP syndrome, with an OR of 6.11 (CI 95%: 2.8–13.33), $p < 0.01$. In contrast, the aforementioned authors considered that AKI determines the risk of developing HELLP syndrome [15]. Although we demonstrated an association, we understand the clinical difficulty of determining which pathology precedes the other. The sudden onset of both clinical pictures makes it difficult to obtain definitive conclusions in one direction or another.

Regarding the measurement of variables at the time of delivery, we observed a statistically significant association between the development of AKI and gestational age at the time of delivery, with a higher percentage of preterm births (<37 weeks of gestation) to patients with AKI. In the meta-analysis of Liu Y et al. [15] mentioned above, the gestational age at the time of delivery was 0.7 weeks lower in the group of pregnant women with AKI. In our cohort of pregnant women with SP, the gestational age at the time of delivery was 1 week lower in the group of patients with AKI than in the group of patients without AKI: 33.8 vs. 34.7 weeks. This finding can be explained, at least in part, by the fact that AKI is severity criterion in pregnant women with preeclampsia and often determines the completion of childbirth [48].

The risk of caesarean section was 3.35 times higher in the SP group with AKI than in the group without AKI (CI 95%: 1.74–6.46, $p < 0.01$). This value is higher than that reported in the meta-analysis of Liu Y et al. [15], who found a 1.49 times higher risk of caesarean section in the AKI group (OR 1.49 (CI 95%: 1.37–1.61)). In this case, it is important to emphasise that our study included only women with SP, a group that was not included in the AKI group in the meta-analysis by Liu Y et al. [15]. In the study by Huang C et al. [47], the incidence of AKI in patients with SP who underwent caesarean section was as high as 60%. The clinical situation of the patient, the heterogeneity for AKI definition used by the authors and the intraoperative management of blood volume can decisively influence the incidence of AKI associated with caesarean section [49–51]. In our series, we relate caesarean section to the association between AKI in the SP patients however, since we did not record the time at which AKI appears in patients, before or after cesarean section, we cannot attribute a causal association of it to the development of AKI. In AKI cases after cesarean section, it could be explained that cesarean section involves greater volume loss, compared to vaginal delivery, with possible acute hemodynamic changes that lead to AKI. On the contrary, in the case in which a patient develops AKI during pregnancy and with the intention of improving the maternal-fetal prognosis, the termination of the pregnancy is decided by caesarean section due to unfavorable obstetric conditions.

There was also a statistical association between the development of AKI and the need for red blood cell transfusion, with transfused patients presenting a 9.46 times higher risk of developing AKI (OR 9.46, CI 95%: 4.10–21.83). Peripartum haemorrhage is a frequent cause of AKI associated with pregnancy and is even more common than preeclampsia in some developing countries [52–54]. Severe cases that require transfusion present an ischaemia-reperfusion model that can explain the development of acute tubular necrosis as a cause of AKI associated with childbirth [55].

Regarding the perinatal variables, it should first be noted that the need for steroids for foetal lung maturation was 1.89 times more frequent in the SP with AKI group OR 1.89 (CI 95%: 1.1–3.21, $p < 0.05$). The higher need for treatments for foetal lung maturation is probably linked to the greater number of newborns with a gestational age between 28 and 37 weeks in the AKI group. In our study, there was a higher percentage of SGA infants in the SP group without AKI (23.9% vs. 10.8% in the AKI group). However, no significant differences were found in the percentage of IGR. These somewhat contradictory results are reflected in the literature: the meta-analysis of Liu Y et al. [15] found that neonates born to mothers with AKI had a lower birth weight than those born to mothers without AKI, and Cooke et al. [54], in a series of 26 patients with AKI from a cohort of 322 pregnant women, found that AKI had no substantial impact on perinatal prognosis. The risk of new-borns requiring admission to the neonatal ICU was 1.9 times higher in the group with AKI (OR 1.90; CI 95%: 1.11–3.28, p 0.002); however, perinatal mortality in the group of pregnant women with SP and AKI was 2.7%, significantly lower than that of the group with SP without AKI (7%). This result is in disagreement with the report of Liu Y et al. [15], who found that the risk of perinatal mortality in pregnant women with AKI was 3.39 times higher than that in pregnant women without AKI. Along this line, we must say that more studies are necessary to weigh the impact of AKI on neonates born to women with SP.

In the multivariate analysis performed to predict the risk of AKI, only a history of CKD, IVF, TMA (including HELLP syndrome), uric acid level and caesarean section were independently associated with the development of AKI in pregnant women with SP. CRF and pregestational proteinuria, which had a high magnitude of effect in the univariate analysis, lost their statistical significance in the multivariate analysis because both are related to CKD. When HELLP syndrome was considered in isolation outside of TMA, it also lost the ability to predict AKI, despite its important association with AKI in the univariate analysis. A likely explanation is the small sample size ($n = 31$). Uric acid, as a marker of renal risk, was maintained as a predictor of AKI, but the average haemoglobin, platelet and LDH values were not. The relationship of these analytical variables with TMA, defined as microangiopathic haemolytic anaemia and thrombocytopenia, probably justifies the loss of their statistical association with AKI, (Although in the opinion of the authors, due to the fact that a high IQ range is described, this value should be taken with caution despite its statistical association). Finally, caesarean section maintained its statistical significance, but the need for transfusion did not. The association of transfusion with TMA and postpartum haemorrhage, which is more common with caesarean delivery, may explain this result. Liu Y et al. [15] conducted a systematic review on the subject and found that pregnancy-associated AKI carries a significantly higher risk of caesarean section, postpartum haemorrhage, abruptio placentae, DIC and maternal death. At this point, we want to highlight that patients who resort to IVF are patients with more frequent previous pathologies that predispose to developing hypertensive pathology during pregnancy and endothelial lesion included at the renal level in early gestational ages [56]. Despite the fact that pregnant women with IVF have a higher rate of cesarean section, in our series we found an independent statistical association for the development of AKI.

At the same time, they found a significantly higher risk of perinatal mortality, prematurity and SGA. Regarding the renal prognosis, they observed a 2.4% incidence of the evolution to terminal renal failure with the need for renal replacement therapy.

The prognosis of AKI associated with preeclampsia is relatively good as long as there are no other associated complications, such as sepsis, DIC or severe bleeding, and most patients resume normal renal function postpartum [29,50]. Persistent renal dysfunction and the need for dialysis is more common in patients with previous CKD [20,57]. However, several authors have shown that pregnant women with preeclampsia have a higher risk of developing CKD than normotensive pregnant women [58,59]. Therefore, short- and long-term monitoring of renal function is necessary in women with a history of hypertensive disorders during pregnancy, childbirth and puerperium [60].

The study has limitations that are important to take into consideration when interpreting the data including a lack of other variables that were not the focus of this study, and that could provide additional information, such as ethnicity, body mass index or weight gain during pregnancy. In addition, we must clarify that since some study variables, such as the c-section, can occur before or after the appearance of AKI, as well as before or after the appearance of SP, the established causal associations must be analyzed with caution due to the fact that the temporality of the cause and effect is not fulfilled in all cases. In relation to the strengths of the study, although our results are not novel and support those obtained previously by the various studies already described in the discussion, with a large number of SP patients. All these patients were attended in a tertiary hospital in Madrid, one of the reference hospitals for obstetrics in Spain with more than 70,000 deliveries, attended over more than 11 years. Furthermore, our study analyses and compared the maternal and perinatal variables between AKI and No AKI groups.

5. Conclusions

Severe preeclampsia is constantly increasing in developing countries and in those patients, AKI is a common complication, especially among those with a history of CKD, those who became pregnant using assisted reproduction techniques and in cases of caesarean section. Among biochemical and haematological markers, the uric acid level prior to the development of AKI has a direct and significant correlation with the risk of AKI in patients with preeclampsia, as does the development of TMA. Therefore, the need for strict monitoring of renal function in cases of preeclampsia should be noted.

Author Contributions: Conceptualization, P.R.-B., I.A.M., M.A.O., J.A.D.L.-L.; methodology, I.A.M., P.R.-B., C.O.B., M.A.O., J.A.D.L.-L.; validation, J.A.D.L.-L.; formal analysis P.R.-B.; investigation, I.A.M., P.R.-B., C.O.B., Y.C.L., F.Y., P.P.R., C.B.A., M.Á.-M., M.A.O., J.A.D.L.-L.; resources, M.A.O., J.A.D.L.-L.; data curation, P.R.-B., I.A.M., C.O.B., J.A.D.L.-L.; writing—original draft preparation, I.A.M., P.R.-B., C.O.B., Y.C.L., F.Y., P.P.R., C.B.A., M.Á.-M., M.A.O., J.A.D.L.-L.; writing—review and editing, I.A.M., P.R.-B., C.O.B., Y.C.L., F.Y., P.P.R., C.B.A., M.Á.-M., M.A.O., J.A.D.L.-L.; supervision, M.A.O., J.A.D.L.-L.; project administration, M.A.O.; funding acquisition, M.Á.-M., M.A.O., J.A.D.L.-L. All authors have read and agreed to the published version of the manuscript.

Funding: This study (FIS-PI18/00912) was supported by the Instituto de Salud Carlos III (Plan Estatal de I + D + i 2013–2016) and co-financed by the European Regional Development Fund "A Road to Europe" (ERDF), as well as B2017/BMD-3804 MITIC-CM, B2020/MITICAD-CM and Halekulani S.L.

Institutional Review Board Statement: For the use of the delivery room data, authorization was obtained from the hospital's ethics committee with protocol establish (PEG19). In addition, a dissociated database was created so that it is not possible to identify the medical records of the patients in the study.

Informed Consent Statement: This is a retrospective cohort study, so written consent from the patient is not necessary.

Data Availability Statement: Data from this study are available at the obstetrics service of the Hospital General Universitario Gregorio Marañón in Madrid and will be made available upon request.

Conflicts of Interest: The authors declare no conflict of interest.

References

1. Brown, M.A.; Magee, L.A.; Kenny, L.C.; Karumanchi, S.A. International Society for the Study of Hypertension in Pregnancy (ISSHP). Hypertensive Disorders of Pregnancy: ISSHP Classification, Diagnosis, and Management Recommendations for International Practice. *Hypertension* **2018**, *72*, 24–43. [CrossRef] [PubMed]
2. National Guideline Alliance (UK). Hypertension in Pregnancy: Diagnosis and Management (NG133). 2019. Available online: https://www.nice.org.uk/guidance/ng133 (accessed on 9 March 2021).
3. Sibai, B.M. Publications Committee, Society for Maternal-Fetal Medicine. Evaluation and management of severe preeclampsia before 34 weeks' gestation. *Am. J. Obs. Gynecol.* **2011**, *205*, 191–198. [CrossRef] [PubMed]
4. von Dadelszen, P.; Payne, B.; Li, J.; Ansermino, J.M. Prediction of adverse maternal outcomes in pre-eclampsia: Development and validation of the full PIERS model. PIERS Study Group. *Lancet* **2011**, *377*, 219–227. [CrossRef]
5. Hucheon, J.A.; Lisonkova, S.; Joseph, K.S. Epidemiology of preeclampsia and the other hypertensive disorders of pregnancy. *Best Pract. Res. Clin. Obstet. Gynaecol.* **2011**, *25*, 391–403. [CrossRef]
6. Abalos, E.; Cuesta, C.; Grosso, A.L.; Chou, D. Global and regional estimates of preeclampsia and eclampsia: A systematic review. *Eur. J. Obs. Gynecol. Reprod. Biol.* **2013**, *170*, 1–7. [CrossRef] [PubMed]
7. Lo, J.O.; Mission, J.F.; Caughey, A.B. Hypertensive disease of pregnancy an maternal mortality. *Curr. Opin. Obs. Gynecol.* **2013**, *25*, 124–132. [CrossRef] [PubMed]
8. Khan, K.S.; Wojdyla, D.; Say, L.; Gülmezoglu, A.M. WHO analysis of causes of maternal death: A systematic review. *Lancet* **2006**, *367*, 1066–1074. [CrossRef]
9. Wallis, A.B.; Saftlas, A.F.; Hsia, J.; Atrash, H.K. Secular trends in the rates of preeclampsia, eclampsia, and gestational hypertension, United States, 1987–2004. *Am. J. Hypertens.* **2008**, *21*, 521–526. [CrossRef]
10. Ananth, C.V.; Keyes, K.M.; Wapner, R.J. Pre-eclampsia rates in the United States, 1980–2010: Age-period-cohort analysis. *BMJ* **2013**, *347*, f6564. [CrossRef]
11. Umesawa, M.; Kobashi, G. Epidemiology of hypertensive disorders in pregnancy: Prevalence, risk factors, predictors and prognosis. *Hypertens. Res.* **2017**, *40*, 213–220. [CrossRef] [PubMed]
12. Gonzalez Suarez, M.L.; Kattah, A.; Grande, J.P.; Garovic, V. Renal disorders in pregnancy: Core curriculum 2019. *Am. J. Kidney Dis.* **2019**, *73*, 119–130. [CrossRef] [PubMed]
13. Prakash, J.; Ganiger, V.C. Acute kidney injury in pregnancy-specific disorders. *Indian J. Nephrol.* **2017**, *27*, 258–270. [CrossRef]
14. Hall, D.R.; Conti-Ramsden, F. Acute kidney injury in pregnancy including renal disease diagnosed in pregnancy. *Best Pract. Res. Clin. Obstet. Gynaecol.* **2019**, *57*, 47–59. [CrossRef]
15. Liu, Y.; Ma, X.; Zheng, J.; Liu, X. Pregnancy outcomes in patients with acute kidney injury during pregnancy: A systematic review and meta-analysis. *BMC Pregnancy Childbirth* **2017**, *17*, 1–9. [CrossRef] [PubMed]
16. Goetzl, L.M. American College of Obstetricians and Gynecologists' Committee on Practice Bulletins—Obstetrics. ACOG Practice Bulletin No. 222: Gestational Hypertension and Preeclampsia. *Obstet. Gynecol.* **2020**, *135*, 237–260.
17. Johnson, C.A. National Kidney Foundation. (K/DOQI) clinical practice guidelines for chronic kidney disease: Evaluation, classification, and stratification. *Am. J. Kidney Dis.* **2002**, *39*, S1–S266.
18. Sibai, B.M. Diagnosis, controversies, and management of the syndrome of hemolysis, elevated liver enzymes, and low platelet count. *Obstet. Gynecol.* **2004**, *103*, 981–991. [CrossRef]
19. Campistol, J.M.; Arias, M.; Ariceta, G.; Blasco, M. An update for atypical haemolytic uraemic syndrome: Diagnosis and treatment. A consensus document. *Nefrologia* **2013**, *33*, 27–34. [CrossRef]
20. Mahesh, E.; Puri, S.; Varma, V.; Madhyastha, P.R. Pregnancy-related acute kidney injury: An analysis of 165 cases. *Indian J. Nephrol.* **2017**, *27*, 113–137. [CrossRef]
21. Prakash, J.; Ganiger, V.C.; Prakash, S.; Iqbal, M. Acute kidney injury in pregnancy with special reference to pregnancy specific disorders: A hospital-based study (2014–2016). *J. Nephrol.* **2018**, *31*, 79–85. [CrossRef]
22. Fakhouri, F.; Vercel, C.; Frémeaux-Bacchi, V. Obstetric Nephrology: AKI and thrombotic microangiopathies in pregnancy. *Clin. J. Am. Soc. Nephrol.* **2012**, *7*, 2100–2106. [CrossRef]
23. Mehrabadi, A.; Liu, S.; Bartholomew, S.; Hutcheon, J.A. Hypertensive disorders of pregnancy and the recent increase in obstetric acute renal failure in Canada: Population based retrospective cohort study. *BMJ* **2014**, *349*, g4731. [CrossRef]

24. Callaghan, W.M.; Creanga, A.A.; Kuklina, E.V. Severe maternal morbidity among delivery and postpartum hospitalizations in the United States. *Obstet. Gynecol.* **2012**, *120*, 1029–1036. [CrossRef]
25. Pankiewicz, K.; Szczerba, E.; Maciejewski, T.; Fijałkowska, A. Non-obstetric complications in preeclampsia. *Prz. Menopauzalny.* **2019**, *18*, 99–109. [CrossRef] [PubMed]
26. Chawla, L.S.; Eggers, P.W.; Star, R.A.; Kimmel, P.L. Acute kidney injury and chronic kidney disease as interconnected syndromes. *N. Engl. J. Med.* **2014**, *371*, 58–66. [CrossRef]
27. Piccoli, G.B.; Cabiddu, G.; Attini, R.; Vigotti, F.N.; Maxia, S.; Lepori, N. Risk of adverse pregnancy outcomes in women with CKD. *J. Am. Soc. Nephrol.* **2015**, *26*, 2011–2022. [CrossRef]
28. Alkhunaizi, A.; Melamed, N.; Hladunewich, M.A. Pregnancy in advanced chronic kidney disease and end-stage renal disease. *Curr. Opin. Nephrol. Hypertens.* **2015**, *24*, 252–259. [CrossRef]
29. Abou Arkoub, R.; Xiao, C.W.; Claman, P.; Clark, E.G. Acute kidney injury due to ovarian hyperstimulation syndrome. *Am. J. Kidney Dis.* **2019**, *73*, 416–420. [CrossRef]
30. Timmons, D.; Montrief, T.; Koyfman, A.; Long, B. Ovarian hyperstimulation syndrome: A review for emergency clinicians. *Am. J. Emerg. Med.* **2019**, *37*, 1577–1584. [CrossRef]
31. Prakash, J.; Niwas, S.; Parekh, A.; Pandey, L.K. Acute kidney injury in late pregnancy in developing countries. *Renal Fail.* **2010**, *32*, 309–313. [CrossRef] [PubMed]
32. Prakash, J.; Pant, P.; Prakash, S.; Sivasankar, M. Changing picture of acute kidney injury in pregnancy: Study of 259 cases over a period of 33 years. *Indian J. Nephrol.* **2016**, *26*, 262–267. [CrossRef] [PubMed]
33. Almasi-Hashiani, A.; Omani-Samani, R.; Mohammadi, M.; Amini, P. Assisted reproductive technology and the risk of preeclampsia: An updated systematic review and meta-analysis. *BMC Pregnancy Childbirth* **2019**, *19*, 149. [CrossRef]
34. Omani-Samani, R.; Alizadeh, A.; Almasi-Hashiani, A.; Mohammadi, M. Risk of preeclampsia following assisted reproductive technology: Systematic review and meta-analysis of 72 cohort studies. *J. Matern. Fetal Neonatal Med.* **2020**, *33*, 2826–2840. [CrossRef]
35. Thomopoulos, C.; Salamalekis, G.; Kintis, K.; Andrianopoulou, I. Risk of hypertensive disorders in pregnancy following assisted reproductive technology: Overview and meta-analysis. *J. Clin. Hypertens.* **2017**, *19*, 173–183. [CrossRef]
36. Chih, H.J.; Elias, F.T.S.; Gaudet, L.; Velez, M.P. Assisted reproductive technology and hypertensive disorders of pregnancy: Systematic review and meta-analyses. *BMC Pregnancy Childbirth* **2021**, *21*, 449. [CrossRef] [PubMed]
37. Goicoechea, M. Ácido úrico y Enfermedad Renal Crónica. Nefrología al Día. Available online: https://www.nefrologiaaldia.org/200 (accessed on 1 November 2021).
38. Ugwuanyi, R.U.; Chiege, I.M.; Agwu, F.E.; Eleje, G.U. Association between serum uric acid levels and perinatal outcome in women with preeclampsia. *Obs. Gynecol. Int.* **2021**, 6611828. [CrossRef]
39. Rajalaxmi, K.; Radhakrishna, N.; Manjula, S. Serum uric acid level in preeclampsia and its correlation to maternal and fetal outcome. *Int. J. Biomed. Res.* **2014**, *5*, 22–24.
40. Le, T.M.; Nguyen, L.H.; Phan, N.L.; Le, D.D. Maternal serum uric acid concentration and pregnancy outcomes in women with pre-eclampsia/eclampsia. *Int. J. Gynaecol. Obstet.* **2019**, *144*, 21–26. [CrossRef] [PubMed]
41. Osakwe, C.R.; Ikpeze, O.C.; Ezebialu, I.U.; Osakwe, J.O. The predictive value of serum uric acid for the occurrence, severity and outcomes of pre-eclampsia among parturients at Nnewi, Nigeria. *Niger. J. Med.* **2015**, *24*, 192–200.
42. Liu, D.; Li, C.; Huang, P.; Fu, J. Serum levels of uric acid may have a potential role in the management of immediate delivery or prolongation of pregnancy in severe preeclampsia. *Hypertens. Pregnancy* **2020**, *39*, 260–266. [CrossRef]
43. Fakhouri, F. Pregnancy-related thrombotic microangiopathies: Clues from complement biology. *Transfus. Apher. Sci.* **2016**, *54*, 199–202. [CrossRef] [PubMed]
44. Meibody, F.; Jamme, M.; Tsatsaris, V.; Provot, F. Post-partum acute kidney injury: Sorting placental and non-placental thrombotic microangiopathies using the trajectory of biomarkers. *Nephrol. Dial. Transplant.* **2020**, *35*, 1538–1546. [CrossRef] [PubMed]
45. Eswarappa, M.; Rakesh, M.; Sonika, P.; Snigdha, K. Spectrum of renal injury in pregnancy-induced hypertension: Experience from a single center in India. *Saudi J. Kidney Dis. Transpl.* **2017**, *28*, 279–284. [CrossRef]
46. Liu, Q.; Ling, G.J.; Zhang, S.Q.; Zhai, W.Q.; Chen, Y.J. Effect of HELLP syndrome on acute kidney injury in pregnancy and pregnancy outcomes: A systematic review and metaanalysis. *BMC Pregnancy Childbirth* **2020**, *20*, 657. [CrossRef] [PubMed]
47. Huang, C.; Chen, S. Acute kidney injury during pregnancy and puerperium: A retrospective study in a single center. *BMC Nephrol.* **2017**, *18*, 146. [CrossRef]
48. Chappell, L.C.; Brocklehurst, P.; Green, M.E.; Hunter, R. Planned early delivery or expectant management for late preterm pre-eclampsia (PHOENIX): A randomised controlled trial. *Lancet* **2019**, *394*, 1181–1190. [CrossRef]
49. Silva, W.A.D.; Varela, C.V.A.; Pinheiro, A.M.; Scherer, P.C. Restrictive versus liberal fluid therapy for post-cesarean acute kidney injury in severe preeclampsia: A pilot randomized clinical trial. *Clinics* **2020**, *75*, e1797. [CrossRef] [PubMed]
50. Mazda, Y.; Tanaka, M.; Terui, K.; Nagashima, S. Postoperative renal function in parturients with severe preeclampsia who underwent cesarean delivery: A retrospective observational study. *J. Anesth.* **2018**, *32*, 447–451. [CrossRef]
51. Park, S.K.; Hur, M.; Kim, W.H. Acute kidney injury in parturients with severe preeclampsia. *J. Anesth.* **2018**, *32*, 787. [CrossRef] [PubMed]
52. Davis, E.F.; Lazdam, M.; Lewandowski, A.J.; Worton, S.A. Cardiovascular risk factors in children and young adults born to preeclamptic pregnancies: A systematic review. *Pediatrics* **2012**, *129*, 1552–1561. [CrossRef] [PubMed]

53. Kabbali, N.; Tachfouti, N.; Arrayhani, M.; Harandou, M. Outcome assessment of pregnancy-related acute kidney injury in Morocco: A national prospective study. *Saudi J. Kidney Dis. Transpl.* **2015**, *26*, 619–624. [CrossRef] [PubMed]
54. Cooke, W.R.; Hemmilä, U.K.; Craik, A.L.; Mandula, C.H. Incidence, aetiology and outcomes of obstetric-related acute kidney injury in Malawi: A prospective observational study. *BMC Nephrol.* **2018**, *19*, 1–9. [CrossRef]
55. Villie, P.; Dommergues, M.; Brocheriou, I.; Piccoli, G.B. Why kidneys fail post-partum: A tubulocentric viewpoint. *J. Nephrol.* **2018**, *31*, 645–651. [CrossRef]
56. Gui, J.; Ling, Z.; Hou, X.; Fan, Y.; Xie, K.; Shen, R. In vitro fertilization is associated with the onset and progression of preeclampsia. *Placenta* **2020**, *89*, 50–57. [CrossRef]
57. Hildebrand, A.M.; Liu, K.; Shariff, S.Z.; Rai, J.G. Characteristics and outcomes of AKI treated with dialysis during pregnancy and the postpartum period. *J. Am. Soc. Nephrol.* **2015**, *26*, 3085–3091. [CrossRef] [PubMed]
58. Ayansina, D.; Black, C.; Hall, S.J.; Mark, A. Long term effects of gestational hypertension and pre-eclampsia on kidney function: Record linkage study. *Pregnancy Hypertens.* **2016**, *6*, 344–349. [CrossRef] [PubMed]
59. Bhattacharya, S.; Ayansina, D.; Black, C.; Hall, S. Are women with gestational hypertension or preeclampsia at an increased long term risk of kidney function impairment? *Pregnancy Hypertens.* **2012**, *2*, 262–269. [CrossRef]
60. Kaze, F.F.; Njukeng, F.A.; Kengne, A.P.; Ashuntantang, G. Post-partum trend in blood pressure levels, renal function and proteinuria in women with severe preeclampsia and eclampsia in Sub-Saharan Africa: A 6-months cohort study. *BMC Pregnancy Childbirth* **2014**, *14*, 134. [CrossRef] [PubMed]

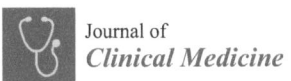

Article

Epidemiology of Antepartum Stillbirths in Austria—A Population-Based Study between 2008 and 2020

Dana Anaïs Muin [1,*], Hanns Helmer [1], Hermann Leitner [2] and Sabrina Neururer [2]

1 Department of Obstetrics and Gynecology, Division of Fetomaternal Medicine, Comprehensive Center for Pediatrics, Medical University of Vienna, Waehringer Guertel 18-20, 1090 Vienna, Austria; hanns.helmer@meduniwien.ac.at
2 Department of Clinical Epidemiology, Tyrolean Federal Institute for Integrated Care, Tirol Kliniken GmbH, Anichstraße 35, 6020 Innsbruck, Austria; hermann.leitner@tirol-kliniken.at (H.L.); s.neururer@tirol-kliniken.at (S.N.)
* Correspondence: dana.muin@meduniwien.ac.at; Tel.: +43-1-40400-28210

Abstract: (1) Background: Across Europe, the incidence of antepartum stillbirth varies greatly, partly because of heterogeneous definitions regarding gestational weeks and differences in legislation. With this study, we sought to provide a comprehensive overview on the demographics of antepartum stillbirth in Austria, defined as non-iatrogenic fetal demise $\geq 22^{+0}$ gestational weeks (/40). (2) Methods: We conducted a population-based study on epidemiological characteristics of singleton antepartum stillbirth in Austria between January 2008 and December 2020. Data were derived from the validated Austrian Birth Registry. (3) Results: From January 2008 through December 2020, the antepartum stillbirth rate $\geq 20^{+0}/40$ was 3.10, $\geq 22^{+0}/40$ 3.14, and $\geq 24^{+0}/40$ 2.83 per 1000 births in Austria. The highest incidence was recorded in the federal states of Vienna, Styria, and Lower and Upper Austria, contributing to 71.9% of all stillbirths in the country. In the last decade, significant fluctuations in incidence were noted: from 2011 to 2012, the rate significantly declined from 3.40 to 3.07‰, whilst it significantly increased from 2.76 to 3.49‰ between 2019 and 2020. The median gestational age of antepartum stillbirth in Austria was 33^{+0} (27^{+2}–37^{+4}) weeks. Stillbirth rates $\leq 26/40$ ranged from 164.98 to 334.18‰, whilst the lowest rates of 0.58–8.4‰ were observed $\geq 36/40$. The main demographic risk factors were maternal obesity and low parity. (4) Conclusions: In Austria, the antepartum stillbirth rate has remained relatively stable at 2.83–3.10 per 1000 births for the last decade, despite a significant decline in 2012 and an increase in 2020.

Keywords: stillbirth; fetal death; perinatal mortality; epidemiology; registration

Citation: Muin, D.A.; Helmer, H.; Leitner, H.; Neururer, S. Epidemiology of Antepartum Stillbirths in Austria—A Population-Based Study between 2008 and 2020. *J. Clin. Med.* **2021**, *10*, 5828. https://doi.org/10.3390/jcm10245828

Academic Editor: Rinat Gabbay-Benziv

Received: 29 October 2021
Accepted: 10 December 2021
Published: 13 December 2021

Publisher's Note: MDPI stays neutral with regard to jurisdictional claims in published maps and institutional affiliations.

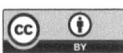

Copyright: © 2021 by the authors. Licensee MDPI, Basel, Switzerland. This article is an open access article distributed under the terms and conditions of the Creative Commons Attribution (CC BY) license (https://creativecommons.org/licenses/by/4.0/).

1. Introduction

Live birth rates and perinatal mortality statistics are considered two of the paramount parameters which shape national demographics and reflect the general population qualities and public health standards within a system. Whilst these may differ grossly between low- and high-income countries across the world, basic characteristics in live birth and stillbirth rates are approximately similar within Europe [1]. After all, minor influences in regional legislation and definition may contribute to major differences even within Europe, which make continental stillbirth rates, in particular, range from 2.6 to 9.1 per 1000 total births [2,3].

The differences in the legislation of perinatal mortality statistics primarily concern definitions of stillbirth with regard to gestational age of delivery, birth weight, and timing or way of demise. While some countries differentiate between antepartum and peripartum fetal death, others include terminations of pregnancies into their fetal mortality statistics [4]. Since the Lancet Stillbirth Series in 2011, a common consciousness emerged for the necessity to harmonize definitions, reporting standards, and legislations internationally to allow valid comparisons between nations and expand knowledge for better prevention of stillbirths worldwide [5].

In Austria, stillbirth is defined as the delivery of a baby of ≥500 g birth weight, irrespective of gestational age, with no signs of life, such as pulsation of the umbilical cord, positive heartbeats, and involuntary muscle contractions. Perinatal mortality is defined as the summary of both stillbirth and early neonatal death up to seven days of life. The Austrian perinatal mortality statistics are annually published by Statistics Austria and gather live birth and mortality data from the Austrian Birth Registry.

To date, stillbirth data as such are not precisely differentiated between the actual timing of stillbirth (i.e., antepartum versus intrapartum) and termination of pregnancy. In view of the profound differences in both the etiology and clinical implications of antepartum versus intrapartum stillbirths, we hereby aim to provide accurate and clean data from the Austrian Birth Registry to portray the demography of antepartum stillbirths in Austria since the implementation of the registry. We furthermore set out to assess regional differences in antepartum stillbirths and evaluate potential risk factors in the Austrian population.

2. Materials and Methods

2.1. Data Collection

The Austrian Birth Registry, founded in 2008, is maintained by the Institute of Clinical Epidemiology, Tyrolean Federal Institute for Integrated Care (https://www.iet.at/) and collects perinatal data from all maternity units in Austria (Supplementary Figure S1). It provides epidemiological data from all deliveries for Austria's Federal Statistical Office (https://pic.statistik.at). Data are regularly checked for accuracy and consistency and therefore assure validity.

For this study and statistical analyses, data from the Austrian Birth Registry were extracted which fulfilled the following criteria: singleton intrauterine fetal death (IUFD) above 22 weeks of gestation followed by stillbirth between 1 January 2008 and 31 December 2020 at an Austrian maternity unit. Exclusion criteria were terminations of pregnancy, and intrapartum or perinatal demise (Figure 1). For the sake of international comparison, the incidence of IUFDs above 20 weeks of gestation, excluding terminations, is provided.

2.2. Statistical Analyses

Continuous data are described as mean (M) and standard deviation (SD) or median and 25th and 75th percentiles (interquartile range, IQR). Categorical data are described as absolute (n) and relative frequencies (%). Comparison of categorical variables was conducted with the chi^2 (χ^2) test; comparison of continuous data was conducted with an independent t-test and the Wilcoxon rank test. Discrepancy between values was reported with standard error of the mean (SEM) and the value of discrepancy ± standard deviation of discrepancy with a 95% confidence interval (CI). A binary logistic regression was performed in order to assess the influence of feto-maternal characteristics on stillbirth. A two-tailed p-value below 0.05 was considered significant. Statistical tests were performed with GraphPad Prism 9 for macOS (GraphPad Software, LLC) and STATA (16.0, StataCorp LLC, College Station, TX, USA). Figures were designed with GraphPad Prism 9 and Microsoft Excel (Version 16.53; Microsoft Corporation, Redmond, WA, USA).

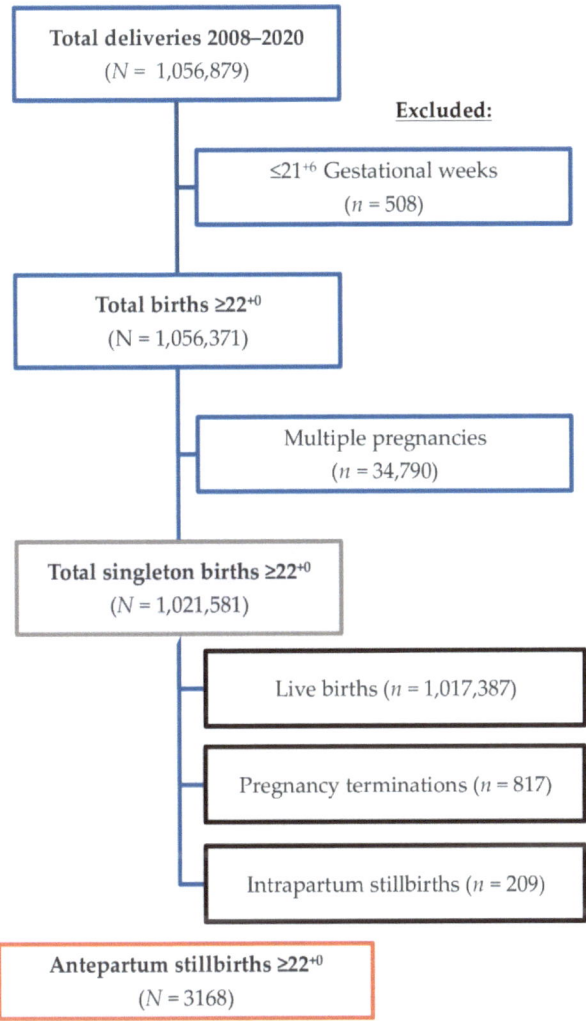

Figure 1. Flowchart on eligibility and selection of study population.

2.3. Ethical Approval and Consent

This study was approved by the Ethics Committee of the Medical University of Vienna (Registration number 1154/2019) and complied with the principles as outlined in the Declaration of Helsinki and Good Clinical Practice guidelines. Participants' written consent was not required as per the Austrian Federal Act (Protection of Personal Data Regulation, §46, Paragraph 1; 2000).

3. Results

3.1. Incidence of Antepartum Stillbirths in Austria

From January 2008 through December 2020, a total of 2888 antepartum stillbirths were registered $\geq 24^{+0}$ gestational weeks in Austria, resulting in a national stillbirth rate of 2.83 ± 0.21 per 1000 births. After lowering the threshold of fetal death to $\geq 20^{+0}$ and $\geq 22^{+0}$ gestational weeks, a total of 3208 and 3168 fetal deaths, respectively, occurred, increasing the rate to 3.14 ± 0.22 and 3.10 ± 0.21 per 1000 births, respectively (Figure 2).

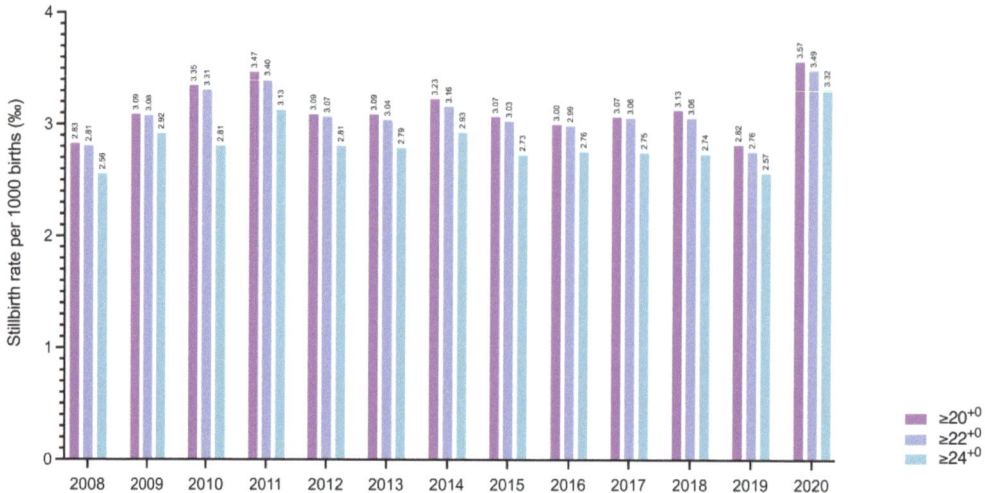

Figure 2. Interleaved contingency bar graph showing the stillbirth rate per 1000 births $\geq 20^{+0}$, $\geq 22^{+0}$, and $\geq 24^{+0}$ gestational weeks in Austria between 2008 and 2020.

In total, 275 (8.69%) antepartum singleton stillbirths were registered between 22^{+0} and 23^{+6} gestational weeks, 573 (18.12%) stillbirths occurred between 24^{+0} and 27^{+6}, and 2315 (73.19%) stillbirths occurred $\geq 28^{+0}$ gestational weeks in Austria from 2008 to 2020.

Across the country, the highest incidence of antepartum stillbirth $\geq 22^{+0}$ was registered in the capital state, Vienna, with a rate of 3.81 ± 0.33 per 1000 births, contributing to 28.0% (n = 884) of all stillbirths in Austria. The lowest rate was reported in the federal state of Burgenland, with an incidence of 2.07 ± 0.74 antepartum stillbirths per 1000 births (Figure 3). A total of 71.9% (n = 2274) of all stillbirths in Austria occurred in the states Lower Austria (n = 499; 15.78%), Upper Austria (n = 489; 15.46%), Styria (n = 402; 12.71%), and Vienna between 2008 and 2020.

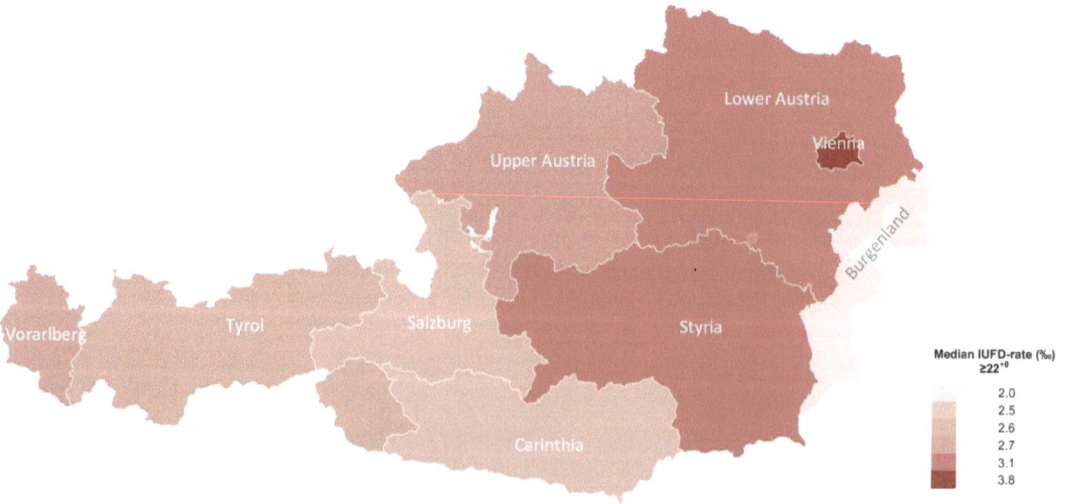

Figure 3. Map chart illustrating the rate of antepartum stillbirths per 1000 births $\geq 22^{+0}$ weeks of gestation in the nine Austrian federal states between January 2008 and December 2020.

Maternal and fetal characteristics per federal state are shown in Table 1. While the antepartum stillbirth rate was the highest in Vienna, demographics show no significant difference regarding maternal age or BMI compared to other states in Austria; however, smoking has been more commonly registered among Viennese women.

Longitudinal analysis on the trend of the incidence over time showed a significant change and increase in all states across Austria (Figure 4). The highest rate discrepancy over time was reported in Vorarlberg (SEM 0.25; 2.79 ± 0.92 (95% CI 2.23–3.34); $p < 0.0001$), followed by Styria (SEM 0.23; 3.1 ± 0.81 (95% CI 2.61–3.59); $p < 0.0001$) and Burgenland (SEM 0.20; 2.07 ± 0.74 (95% CI 1.63–2.52); $p < 0.0001$). The lowest, yet still statistically significant, time trend was observed in Vienna (SEM 0.09; 3.81 ± 0.33 (95% CI 3.62–4.01); $p < 0.0001$).

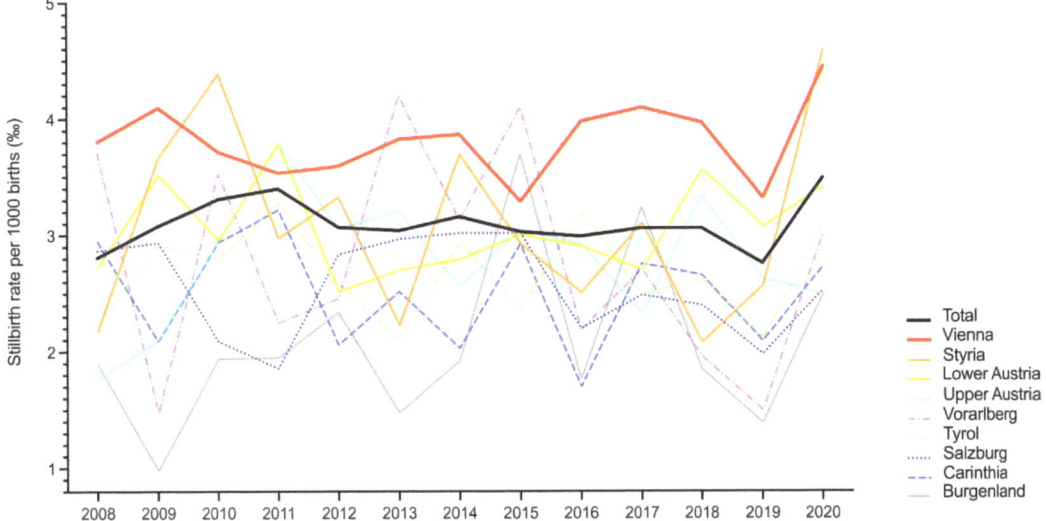

Figure 4. Trends in rates of antepartum stillbirth $\geq 22^{+0}$ gestational weeks in Austria between January 2008 and December 2020.

From 2011 to 2012, the total antepartum stillbirth rate ≥ 22 gestational weeks significantly declined from 3.40 to 3.07‰, whereas from 2019 to 2020, it significantly increased from 2.76 to 3.49‰. Thus far, the rate of 2.76‰ in the year 2019 has been the lowest rate of antepartum stillbirths $\geq 22^{+0}$ ever documented in Austria since the implementation of the Austrian Birth Registry.

Table 1. Maternal and fetal characteristics of antepartum stillbirths ≥22^{+0} gestational weeks in Austria between January 2008 and December 2020.

Antepartum Stillbirth	Total	Non-Specified	Vienna	Styria	Lower Austria	Upper Austria	Tyrol	Salzburg	Carinthia	Vorarlberg	Burgenland	p-Value [4]
Total deliveries (n)	1,021,581	32,165	231,674	130,211	163,290	175,254	88,325	66,727	57,734	48,785	27,416	.
Total antepartum stillbirths (n; ≥22^{+0})	3163	146	884	402	499	489	236	170	145	135	57	<0.001
Antepartum stillbirth rate (‰; ≥22^{+0})	3.10	.	3.82	3.09	3.06	2.79	2.67	2.55	2.51	2.77	2.08	<0.001
Median gestational age of stillbirth (IQR)	33^{+0} (27^{+2}–37^{+4})	32^{+3} (27^{+6}–37^{+0})	32^{+6} (26^{+5}–37^{+2})	31^{+6} (26^{+1}–36^{+6})	32^{+0} (26^{+5}–37^{+0})	34^{+2} (29^{+1}–38^{+1})	32^{+5} (27^{+6}–37^{+2})	33^{+5} (28^{+5}–38^{+0})	34^{+3} (27^{+3}–38^{+3})	33^{+0} (28^{+0}–37^{+5})	32^{+1} (27^{+5}–36^{+6})	0.188
Median maternal age at stillbirth (IQR)	31 (26–35)	32 (29–36)	30 (26–35)	31 (26–35)	31 (27–35)	30 (26–34)	31 (27–35)	31 (27–36)	30 (26–34)	31 (27–36)	33 (29–37)	0.244
Median BMI (IQR; kg/m^2)	23.4 (20.7–27.0)	22.9 (20.7–26.9)	23.4 (20.7–27.3)	23.4 (20.4–26.6)	23.8 (21.4–27.1)	23.5 (20.8–27.6)	22.8 (20.7–25.7)	22.8 (20.2–26.9)	23.1 (20.9–26.0)	22.4 (20.3–27.7)	23.5 (21.8–28.0)	0.241
BMI category [1] Underweight	122 (6.0%)	3 (5.3%)	38 (6.6%)	16 (6.9%)	6 (2.1%)	24 (7.2%)	17 (7.7%)	9 (6.9%)	3 (2.7%)	4 (6.0%)	2 (5.9%)	
Normal weight	1205 (59.0%)	36 (63.2%)	330 (57.1%)	138 (59.5%)	166 (59.1%)	182 (54.7%)	140 (63.6%)	76 (58.5%)	76 (67.9%)	41 (61.2%)	20 (58.8%)	
Overweight	443 (21.7%)	12 (21.1%)	126 (21.8%)	49 (21.1%)	70 (24.9%)	73 (21.9%)	45 (20.5%)	28 (21.5%)	23 (20.5%)	10 (14.9%)	7 (20.6%)	
Obese	274 (13.4%)	6 (10.5%)	84 (14.5%)	29 (12.5%)	39 (13.9%)	54 (16.2%)	18 (8.2%)	17 (13.1%)	10 (8.9%)	12 (17.9%)	5 (14.7%)	
Parity 0	1605 (50.7%)	90 (61.6%)	447 (50.6%)	191 (47.5%)	251 (50.3%)	244 (49.9%)	119 (50.4%)	94 (55.3%)	80 (55.2%)	62 (45.9%)	27 (47.4%)	0.201
1–3	1416 (44.8%)	48 (32.9%)	387 (43.8%)	193 (48.0%)	226 (45.3%)	222 (45.4%)	114 (48.3%)	71 (41.8%)	64 (44.1%)	65 (48.1%)	26 (45.6%)	
≥4	142 (4.5%)	8 (5.5%)	50 (5.7%)	18 (4.5%)	22 (4.4%)	23 (4.7%)	3 (1.3%)	5 (2.9%)	1 (0.7%)	8 (5.9%)	4 (7.0%)	
Nicotine consumption	327 (10.3%)	13 (8.9%)	131 (14.8%)	38 (9.5%)	39 (7.8%)	35 (7.2%)	22 (9.3%)	20 (11.8%)	15 (10.3%)	9 (6.7%)	5 (8.8%)	<0.001
Obstetric risk factors [2]	200 (6.3%)	2 (1.4%)	58 (6.6%)	59 (14.7%)	30 (6.0%)	16 (3.3%)	18 (7.6%)	0 (0%)	8 (5.5%)	5 (3.7%)	4 (7.0%)	<0.001
Fetal sex [3] Male	1639 (52.0%)	71 (49.0%)	479 (54.3%)	196 (48.9%)	251 (50.8%)	265 (54.4%)	129 (54.7%)	89 (53.0%)	63 (43.4%)	62 (45.9%)	34 (60.7%)	0.096
Female	1510 (48.0%)	74 (51.0%)	403 (45.7%)	205 (51.1%)	243 (49.2%)	222 (45.6%)	107 (45.3%)	79 (47.0%)	82 (56.6%)	73 (54.1%)	22 (39.3%)	
Median birth weight (g) [IQR]	1700 (860–2700)	1570 (850–2810)	1634.5 (781–2685)	1575 (770–2580)	1590 (817–2643)	1988 (1050–2850)	1565 (868–2625)	1815 (990–2776)	1912 (890–2810)	1634 (930–2740)	1380 (870–2555)	<0.001
Median birth height (cm) [IQR]	43 (35–49)	42 (35–50)	43 (34–49)	42 (34–49)	42 (34–49)	45 (36–50)	42 (35–49)	44 (38–50)	46 (36–51)	43 (36–50)	41.5 (34–48)	<0.001

Note: [1] n = 1119 missing. BMI category: underweight <18.5 kg/m^2; normal weight 18.6–24.9 kg/m^2; overweight 25.0–29.9 kg/m^2; obese ≥30.0 kg/m^2. [2] Obstetric risk factors including risk for premature delivery and/or adverse neonatal outcome. [3] n = 14 missing data. [4] χ^2 test for categorical variables, t-test for continuous variables. Abbreviations: BMI, body mass index; IQR, interquartile range.

3.2. Timing of Antepartum Stillbirths

The median gestational age of antepartum stillbirth in Austria between 2008 and 2020 was 33^{+0} (27^{+2}–37^{+4}) weeks. Stillbirths at higher gestational weeks more frequently occurred in Upper Austria (34^{+2} (29^{+1}–38^{+1}) weeks), whereas stillbirths in early gestational weeks were more commonly reported in Styria (31^{+6} (26^{+1}–36^{+6}) weeks) (Figure 5).

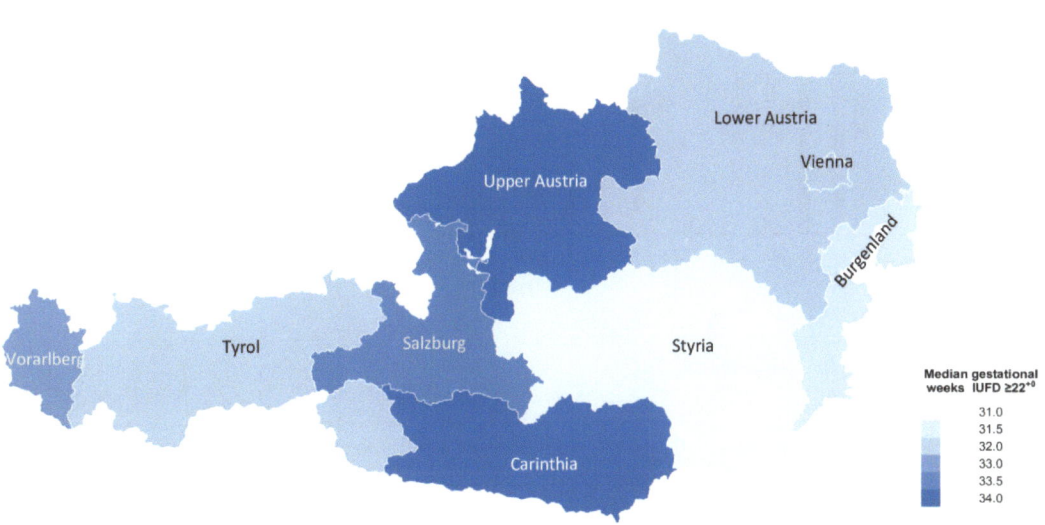

Figure 5. Map chart illustrating the median gestational age of antepartum stillbirths $\geq 22^{+0}$ gestational weeks across Austria between 2008 and 2020.

Considering the gestational age throughout the study period, the highest prevalence of fetal deaths was noted for pregnancies below 26 gestational weeks, with a rate ranging from 164.98‰ at 26^{+0} to 334.18‰ at 22^{+0}. The lowest prevalence was observed above 35 gestational weeks, with a rate ranging from 8.4‰ at 36^{+0} to 0.84‰ at 39^{+0} and 0.58‰ at term at 40^{+0} gestational weeks (Figure 6).

Over the years, there have been significant fluctuations in the stillbirth prevalence as per age of gestation (Figure 7). The highest fluctuation over time was observed at weeks 22 and 23, with a discrepancy in prevalence of SEM 25.52 (328.8 ± 92.0 (95% CI 273.2–384.4); $p < 0.0001$) and SEM 28.07 (271.9 ± 101.2 (95% CI 210.8–333.1); $p < 0.0001$), respectively. Meanwhile, in 2017, the antepartum stillbirth rate peaked at 466.7‰ for fetuses of 22^{+0}–22^{+6} gestational age, and it significantly declined to 230.8‰ in 2019, reflecting a reduction of 235.9‰ within only two years. An even greater reduction of 274.8‰ was noted for stillborn fetuses at 23^{+0}–23^{+6} gestation, with a significant decrease from 428.6‰ in 2018 to 153.8‰ in 2020. The steadiest prevalence was observed for stillbirths occurring ≥ 38 gestational weeks.

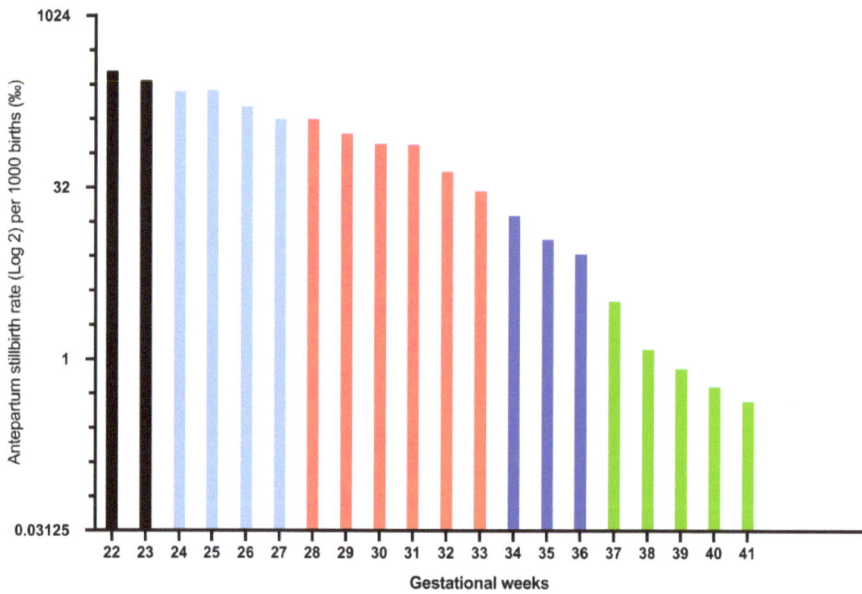

Figure 6. Bar graph illustrating the prevalence of antepartum stillbirth in Austria per gestational week (stillbirth rate per 1000 births in logarithmic scale to the base 2).

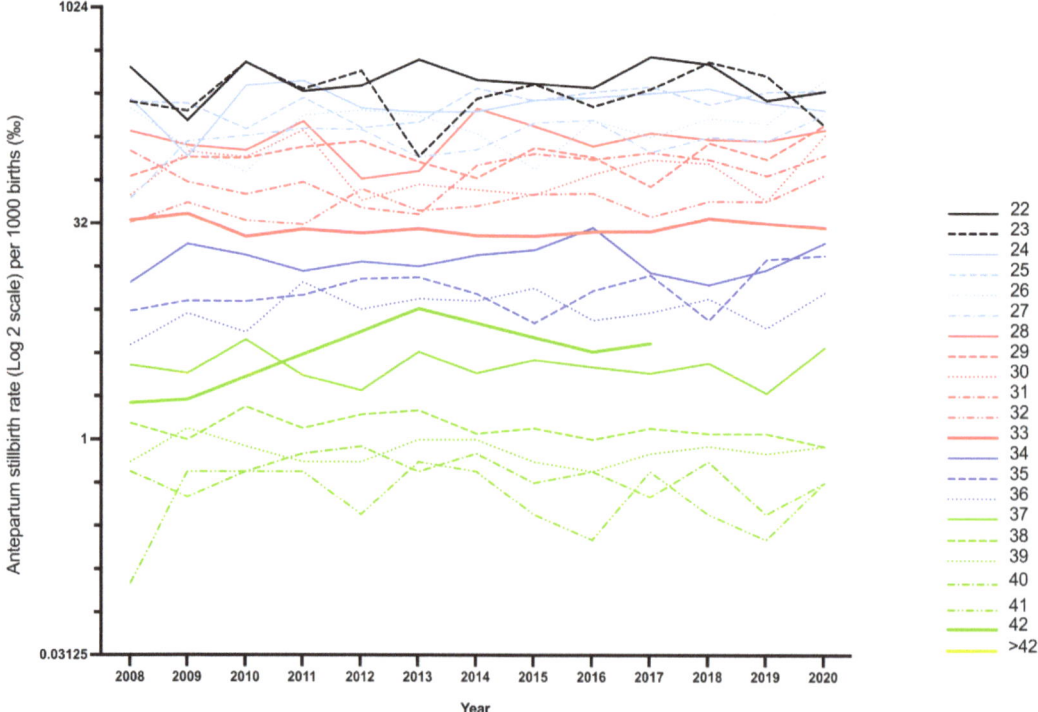

Figure 7. Time trend of stillbirth prevalence as per gestational age in Austria between January 2008 and December 2020: stillbirth rate per 1000 births in logarithmic scale to the base 2.

3.3. Risk Factors for Suffering Antepartum Stillbirth in Austria

Factors associated with antepartum stillbirth in Austria are increased maternal BMI (OR 0.98 (95% CI 0.972–0.989); $p < 0.001$), nulliparity (OR 1.32 (95% CI 1.031–1.679); $p < 0.001$), primiparity (OR 1.04 (95% CI 0.822–1.327); $p = 0.027$), and fetal growth restriction (OR 1.00 (95% CI 1.001–1.001); $p < 0.001$). Maternal age (OR 1.00 (95% CI 0.998–1.015); $p = 0.148$), nicotine consumption (OR 1.14 (95% CI 0.989–1.325); $p = 0.070$), and fetal sex (OR 1.08 (95% CI 0.986–1.188); $p = 0.096$) showed no significant association in logistic regression analyses.

4. Discussion

4.1. Main Findings and Interpretation

With this population-based study, we sought to assess the antepartum stillbirth rate in a validated cohort restricted to singleton fetuses excluding terminations of pregnancies and intrapartum or peripartum fetal demise in Austria. We generated four main findings, which are of note.

First, reflecting the medical advances in neonatal intensive care for extremely premature infants [6,7], our Austrian data confirm a significant and steep reduction in stillbirths for gestational weeks 22^{+0} to 23^{+6}, which is regarded as the period of fetal viability. Although data are missing regarding the precise cause of death in these fetuses, we may assume that the reduction in stillbirths at such a gestational age in recent years may have involved fetuses who had been rescued from intrauterine demise by early delivery and thus were subjected to iatrogenic extreme prematurity.

Second, our temporal analysis over the last 13 years showed two significant changes in the overall incidence of antepartum stillbirths in Austria: whilst the average stillbirth rate has remained relatively stable, there was a significant decline in the national antepartum stillbirth rate between January 2011 and December 2012 by 0.34‰ and a significant increase between January 2019 and December 2020 by 0.73‰. In a previous population-based study, we investigated the effect of the implementation of universal gestational diabetes screening (OGTT) in an Austrian pregnant population within the frame of the Mother and Child Booklet (Muin et al. 2021 Manuscript under revision): in consideration of singleton antepartum stillbirths $\geq 24^{+0}$ gestational weeks, we found that, whilst, following the implementation of OGTT between 24^{+0} and 28^{+0} in the year 2011, the annual stillbirth rate in the general population remained stable with 2.76 to 2.74 per 1000 births ($p = 0.845$), the stillbirth rate declined from 4.10 to 2.96 per 1000 live births ($p = 0.043$), resulting in an absolute risk reduction of 0.11% and a relative risk reduction of 27.73% in women at greater risk for stillbirths. Despite the lack of valid data on how many women had indeed received treatment for gestational diabetes, we acknowledge that untreated gestational diabetes may contribute to placental dysfunction, causing intrauterine hypoxia and, furthermore, disturbing the fetal metabolic state, resulting in acidosis, especially in later stages of pregnancy; early detection and, therefore, treatment of maternal diabetes are considered important measures in preventing fetal death in these women.

The pandemic caused by the coronavirus SARS-CoV-2 (COVID-19) in 2020 has conveyed profound direct and indirect effects on pregnant women worldwide. In a population-based study involving singleton antepartum stillbirths $\geq 24^{+0}$ gestational weeks, we confirmed that, during the pandemic in Austria, the national stillbirth rate had increased from 2.49‰ to 2.60‰ ($p = 0.601$), yielding a significant increase during the first lockdown phase ($p = 0.021$), with an adjusted odds ratio of 1.57 (95% CI 1.08–2.27; $p = 0.018$), compared to matched historical months [8]. We, therefore, assume that the significant increase by 0.73‰ from 2019 to 2020, as shown by our present data on stillbirths $\geq 22^{+0}$ weeks of gestation, may have been, partly, an effect of the pandemic, as observed elsewhere [9–17].

Our third imminent finding is the geographical distribution of antepartum stillbirths being centered in and around the capital city of Vienna, accounting for approximately 50% of all antepartum stillbirth cases in Austria. In a previous study, we illustrated the adverse perinatal outcome by increased light pollution, as naturally observed in urban areas [18].

At the same time, we acknowledge a provider bias in larger hospitals, as supported by more accurate registrations of stillbirths in maternity units, along with a higher prevalence of dealing with high-risk pregnancies. Additionally, urbanization has been consistently associated with poorer lifestyle habits and thus greater health risks, which might, therefore, also account for overall greater perinatal risks [19,20].

Our fourth finding of note is the prevalence of stillbirth as per gestational age: In acknowledgement of varying definitions and legal cut-offs for registering fetal deaths as stillbirths versus late miscarriages, the current study confirms that when counting stillbirths ≥ 28 weeks, as suggested by the WHO, only 73% of all late stillbirths would be represented in our country, i.e., 27% of losses ≥ 22 weeks would be neglected in their registration. Additionally, taking the threshold ≥ 24 weeks, as supposed by a birth weight ≥ 500 g to officially register a stillbirth as per current Austrian law, approximately 9% of late stillbirths (≥ 22 weeks) are left underrepresented in annual official statistics. This finding supports prior population-based studies showing the underestimated and unrecognized burden of late fetal losses which are not fully acknowledged by law due to limitations in local legislations [2,3,21].

4.2. Strengths and Limitations

The accuracy and validity of the dataset from the Austrian Birth Registry provide a precise overview on the epidemiological landscape in Austria. The exact differentiation between three different thresholds for antepartum stillbirth definition, as early as by gestational week 20^{+0}, may allow future accurate comparison with international data. Furthermore, we strictly defined antepartum stillbirth as singleton fetal death in utero, excluding elective termination of pregnancy, multiple pregnancies, and perinatal deaths, as epidemiology and etiology in these are known to differ greatly and may cause heterogeneity in incidence and data interpretation.

Our study is limited by its retrospective, multicenter setting with data unavoidably missing and potential data errors inherent to recall bias in participating maternity units. We also acknowledge the lack of a national classification system for defining the cause of fetal death and are, therefore, unable to provide an overview on causes of stillbirth in Austria, as yet. In consideration of the importance of assessing the cause of fetal death in each case, we are currently establishing a prospective national collaboration for acquisition of post-mortem diagnoses for future public health measures.

5. Conclusions

In Austria, the antepartum stillbirth rate per 1000 births was 3.10 for $\geq 20^{+0}$ gestational week, 3.14 for $\geq 22^{+0}$ gestational week, and 2.83 for $\geq 24^{+0}$ gestational week from 2008 to 2020. Whilst there was a significant decline from 2011 to 2012, followed by a significant increase from 2019 to 2020, the overall rate has remained relatively stable compared to other European countries. The most prevalent risk factors were high maternal BMI and low parity.

Supplementary Materials: The following are available online at https://www.mdpi.com/article/10.3390/jcm10245828/s1, Figure S1: Maternity units contributing with their perinatal data to the Austrian Stillbirth Registry (as per 1 October 2021).

Author Contributions: Conceptualization, D.A.M., H.H., H.L. and S.N.; methodology, D.A.M., H.H., H.L. and S.N.; software, S.N.; validation, H.L. and S.N.; formal analysis, H.L. and S.N.; investigation, D.A.M., H.H., H.L. and S.N.; resources, H.L. and S.N.; data curation, D.A.M., H.H., H.L. and S.N.; writing—original draft preparation, D.A.M.; writing—review and editing, D.A.M., H.H., H.L. and S.N.; visualization, D.A.M.; supervision, S.N. and H.H.; project administration, H.L. All authors have read and agreed to the published version of the manuscript.

Funding: This research received no external funding.

Institutional Review Board Statement: This study was approved by the Ethics Committee of the Medical University of Vienna (Registration number 1154/2019) and complied with the principles as outlined in the Declaration of Helsinki and Good Clinical Practice guidelines.

Informed Consent Statement: Informed consent was not required per Austrian Federal Act concerning Protection of Personal Data (DSG 2000). All patient data were de-identified prior to analyses.

Data Availability Statement: The data that support the findings of this study are available from the corresponding author, D.A.M., upon reasonable request.

Conflicts of Interest: The authors declare no conflict of interest.

References

1. Hug, L.; You, D.; Blencowe, H.; Mishra, A.; Wang, Z.; Fix, M.J.; Wakefield, J.; Moran, A.C.; Gaigbe-Togbe, V.; Suzuki, E.; et al. Global, regional, and national estimates and trends in stillbirths from 2000 to 2019: A systematic assessment. *Lancet* **2021**, *398*, 772–785. [CrossRef]
2. Smith, L.K.; Blondel, B.; Zeitlin, J. Producing valid statistics when legislation, culture and medical practices differ for births at or before the threshold of survival: Report of a European workshop. *BJOG* **2020**, *127*, 314–318. [CrossRef] [PubMed]
3. Mohangoo, A.D.; Buitendijk, S.E.; Szamotulska, K.; Chalmers, J.; Irgens, L.M.; Bolumar, F.; Nijhuis, J.G.; Zeitlin, J.; Euro-Peristat Scientific Committee. Gestational age patterns of fetal and neonatal mortality in Europe: Results from the Euro-Peristat project. *PLoS ONE* **2011**, *6*, e24727. [CrossRef]
4. Blondel, B.; Cuttini, M.; Hindori-Mohangoo, A.D.; Gissler, M.; Loghi, M.; Prunet, C.; Heino, A.; Smith, L.; van der Pal-de Bruin, K.; Macfarlane, A.; et al. How do late terminations of pregnancy affect comparisons of stillbirth rates in Europe? Analyses of aggregated routine data from the Euro-Peristat Project. *BJOG* **2018**, *125*, 226–234. [CrossRef]
5. Spong, C.Y.; Reddy, U.M.; Willinger, M. Addressing the complexity of disparities in stillbirths. *Lancet* **2011**, *377*, 1635–1636. [CrossRef]
6. Klebermass-Schrehof, K.; Wald, M.; Schwindt, J.; Grill, A.; Prusa, A.R.; Haiden, N.; Hayde, M.; Waldhoer, T.; Fuiko, R.; Berger, A. Less invasive surfactant administration in extremely preterm infants: Impact on mortality and morbidity. *Neonatology* **2013**, *103*, 252–258. [CrossRef] [PubMed]
7. Gulland, A. Fall in rate of stillbirth drives down perinatal mortality. *BMJ* **2017**, *357*, j3050. [CrossRef] [PubMed]
8. Muin, D.A.; Neururer, S.; Falcone, V.; Windsperger, K.; Helmer, H.; Leitner, H.; Kiss, H.; Farr, A. Antepartum stillbirth rates during the COVID-19 pandemic in Austria: A population-based study. *Int. J. Gynaecol. Obstet.* **2021**. [CrossRef] [PubMed]
9. Ashish, K.C.; Gurung, R.; Kinney, M.V.; Sunny, A.K.; Moinuddin, M.; Basnet, O.; Paudel, P.; Bhattarai, P.; Subedi, K.; Shrestha, M.P.; et al. Effect of the COVID-19 pandemic response on intrapartum care, stillbirth, and neonatal mortality outcomes in Nepal: A prospective observational study. *Lancet Glob. Health* **2020**, *8*, e1273–e1281.
10. Knight, M.; Bunch, K.; Vousden, N.; Morris, E.; Simpson, N.; Gale, C.; O'Brien, P.; Quigley, M.; Brocklehurst, P.; Kurinczuk, J.J. Characteristics and outcomes of pregnant women admitted to hospital with confirmed SARS-CoV-2 infection in UK: National population based cohort study. *BMJ* **2020**, *369*, m2107. [CrossRef] [PubMed]
11. Chmielewska, B.; Barratt, I.; Townsend, R.; Kalafat, E.; van der Meulen, J.; Gurol-Urganci, I.; O'Brien, P.; Morris, E.; Draycott, T.; Thangaratinam, S.; et al. Effects of the COVID-19 pandemic on maternal and perinatal outcomes: A systematic review and meta-analysis. *Lancet Glob. Health* **2021**, *9*, e759–e772. [CrossRef]
12. De Curtis, M.; Villani, L.; Polo, A. Increase of stillbirth and decrease of late preterm infants during the COVID-19 pandemic lockdown. *Arch. Dis. Child. Fetal Neonatal Ed.* **2020**, *106*, 456. [CrossRef] [PubMed]
13. Magee, L.A.; Khalil, A.; von Dadelszen, P. Covid-19: UK Obstetric Surveillance System (UKOSS) study in context. *BMJ* **2020**, *370*, m2915. [CrossRef]
14. Khalil, A.; von Dadelszen, P.; Ugwumadu, A.; Draycott, T.; Magee, L.A. Effect of COVID-19 on maternal and neonatal services. *Lancet Glob. Health* **2021**, *9*, e112. [CrossRef]
15. Khalil, A.; von Dadelszen, P.; Draycott, T.; Ugwumadu, A.; O'Brien, P.; Magee, L. Change in the Incidence of Stillbirth and Preterm Delivery During the COVID-19 Pandemic. *JAMA* **2020**, *324*, 705–706. [CrossRef] [PubMed]
16. Hedermann, G.; Hedley, P.L.; Bækvad-Hansen, M.; Hjalgrim, H.; Rostgaard, K.; Poorisrisak, P.; Breindahl, M.; Melbye, M.; Hougaard, D.M.; Christiansen, M.; et al. Danish premature birth rates during the COVID-19 lockdown. *Arch. Dis. Child. Fetal Neonatal Ed.* **2021**, *106*, 93–95. [CrossRef]
17. Philip, R.K.; Purtill, H.; Reidy, E.; Daly, M.; Imcha, M.; McGrath, D.; O'Connell, N.H.; Dunne, C.P. Unprecedented reduction in births of very low birthweight (VLBW) and extremely low birthweight (ELBW) infants during the COVID-19 lockdown in Ireland: A 'natural experiment' allowing analysis of data from the prior two decades. *BMJ Glob. Health* **2020**, *5*, e003075. [CrossRef]
18. Windsperger, K.; Kiss, H.; Oberaigner, W.; Leitner, H.; Binder, F.; Muin, D.A.; Foessleitner, P.; Husslein, P.W.; Farr, A. Exposure to night-time light pollution and risk of prolonged duration of labor: A nationwide cohort study. *Birth* **2021**. [CrossRef]
19. Jiang, T.B.; Deng, Z.W.; Zhi, Y.P.; Cheng, H.; Gao, Q. The Effect of Urbanization on Population Health: Evidence From China. *Front. Public Health* **2021**, *9*, 706982. [CrossRef]

20. Zhu, J.; Liang, J.; Mu, Y.; Li, X.; Guo, S.; Scherpbier, R.; Wang, Y.; Dai, L.; Liu, Z.; Li, M.; et al. Sociodemographic and obstetric characteristics of stillbirths in China: A census of nearly 4 million health facility births between 2012 and 2014. *Lancet Glob. Health* **2016**, *4*, e109–e118. [CrossRef]
21. Smith, L.K.; Hindori-Mohangoo, A.D.; Delnord, M.; Durox, M.; Szamotulska, K.; Macfarlane, A.; Alexander, S.; Barros, H.; Gissler, M.; Blondel, B.; et al. Quantifying the burden of stillbirths before 28 weeks of completed gestational age in high-income countries: A population-based study of 19 European countries. *Lancet* **2018**, *392*, 1639–1646. [CrossRef]

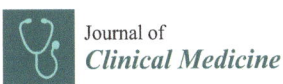

Article

Awakened Beta-Cell Function Decreases the Risk of Hypoglycemia in Pregnant Women with Type 1 Diabetes Mellitus

Josip Delmis * and Marina Ivanisevic

Clinical Department of Obstetrics and Gynecology, University Hospital Centre Zagreb, School of Medicine, University of Zagreb, 10000 Zagreb, Croatia; marina.ivanisevic@pronatal.hr
* Correspondence: josip.djelmis@zg.t-com.hr; Tel.: +385-98460485

Abstract: Diabetes in pregnancy creates many problems for both the mother and child. Pregnant women with type 1 diabetes experience more frequent hypoglycemic and hyperglycemic episodes. This study aimed to determine the risk of clinically significant biochemical hypoglycemia (CSBH) by HbA1c, fasting C-peptide, mean plasma glucose (PG), and insulin dose in pregnant women type 1 diabetes mellitus according to each trimester of the pregnancy. Methods. We conducted a prospective observational study of 84 pregnant women with type 1 diabetes in an academic hospital. To present the hypoglycemia, we divided the participants into two groups: those who did not have clinically significant biochemical hypoglycemia (CSBH−; n = 30) and those who had clinically significant biochemical hypoglycemia (CSBH+; n = 54). Results. In the first, second, and third trimesters, the duration of T1DM, fasting C-peptide, and mean glucose concentration was inversely associated with CSBH. Conclusions. Insulin overdose is the most common risk factor for hypoglycemia. In pregnant women with type 1 diabetes with elevated fasting C-peptide levels, the insulin dose should be diminished to reduce the risk of hypoglycemia.

Keywords: C-peptide; diabetes mellitus type 1; hypoglycemia; pregnancy

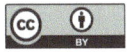

1. Introduction

Poor metabolic control in pregnant women with type 1 diabetes mellitus is associated with an increased risk of spontaneous abortion, preeclampsia, congenital malformations, asphyxia, macrosomia, and neonatal morbidity and mortality [1–3]. For a successful perinatal outcome, an intensive clinical approach is required to achieve normoglycemia before conception and pregnancy. Good metabolic control (fasting plasma glucose of 3.9–5.3 mmol/L and 1 h postprandial values between the glucose of 6.1–7.8 mmol/L or 2 h postprandial glucose of 5.6–6.7 mmol/L, and HbA1c values <6.0% (<42 mmol/mol)) exhibits potential pregnancy complications as being equal to those in the healthy pregnant population [2]. Treating women with type 1 diabetes mellitus aims to achieve normoglycemia before and during pregnancy to reduce spontaneous abortion, congenital malformations, fetal macrosomia, and neonatal complications. Tight glycemic control improves pregnancy outcomes; however, it also increases the risk of hypoglycemia [3,4] and possibly causes maternal complications, including coma, convulsion, and death [5]. Severe hypoglycemia affects up to 19–44% of pregnant women with type 1 diabetes and is 15 times higher than that observed with intensified treatment outside of pregnancy [3,6]. The risk of hypoglycemia is usually highest in early pregnancy, especially during the first trimester, due to overinsulinization [6,7].

The known risk factors for hypoglycemia are the duration of diabetes, history of previous severe hypoglycemia, hypoglycemia unawareness, change in insulin treatment, and HbA1c <6.0% (42 mmol/mol) [1,3]. A successful pregnancy outcome needs to achieve normoglycemia, with HbA1c levels between 4.0 and 6.0% (20 and 42 mmol/mol) [3,8]. Reducing the risk of hypoglycemia is a significant challenge for doctors who care for pregnant women with type 1 diabetes mellitus. The International Hypoglycemia Study Group (IHSG) considers glucose concentration levels of <3.0 mmol/L unequivocally hypoglycemic values, which are detected by self-monitoring of plasma glucose, continuous glucose monitoring (for at least 20 min), or laboratory measurement of plasma glucose [3,7]. The glycemic threshold for cognitive impairment is <2.8 mmol/L [7]. The IHSG considers a glucose concentration <3.0 mmol/L low enough to indicate severe, clinically significant hypoglycemia [8]. The same group suggested that a glucose value of 3.9 mmol/L or less should only indicate possible hypoglycemia. Severe hypoglycemia is considered a hypoglycemic episode requiring external assistance for recovery [7].

This study aimed to determine the risk of clinically significant biochemical hypoglycemia (CSBH) by HbA1c, gestational weight gain, C-peptide, mean capillary plasma glucose, and total insulin dose in pregnant women with type 1 diabetes mellitus in each trimester of pregnancy. The specific aim was to establish the effect of the C-peptide concentration on the prevalence of CSBH in pregnant women with type 1 diabetes and its association with insulin dosage.

2. Materials and Methods

2.1. Ethical Statements

The Ethics Committee of the School of Medicine, the University of Zagreb (No. 380-59-10106-19-111/26), approved the study within the scientific project PRE-HYPO No. IP-2018-01-1284. All women included in the study provided written informed consent for themselves and their newborns.

2.2. Study Participants

In the prospective observational study, we consecutively included 84 women with type 1 diabetes mellitus before completing 10 gestational weeks with a single living fetus during the study period from 1 January 2018 to 31 December 2019. Pregnant women without complications of diabetes and those with non-proliferative retinopathy and diabetic neuropathy were included in the study. All participants were admitted to the Department of Obstetrics and Gynecology at least once or repeatedly in each trimester. The daily glucose profiles of patients with type 1 diabetes were determined, and plasma glucose (9/day) was monitored for 2–3 days. Glucose was measured in capillary plasma at the following time intervals: 7, 10, 13, 16, 19, 22, 1, 4, and 7 h.

Clinically significant biochemical hypoglycemia was defined as a glucose concentration of ≤ 3.0 mmol/L detected by laboratory measurement of plasma glucose. None of the pregnant participants in this study experienced a hypoglycemic coma or needed third-party assistance during hypoglycemia or glucagon/intravenous glucose during the hypoglycemic event. No episodes of severe hypoglycemia were reported for the whole pregnancy.

We included 84 women with type 1 diabetes and singleton pregnancies who received insulin therapy for ≥ 2 years. At pregnancy confirmation, the HbA1c was $\leq 8\%$ (≤ 64 mmol/mol). All pregnant women received intensified insulin therapy with fast-acting insulin aspart and long-acting insulin detemir.

We divided the participants into two groups according to the prevalence of CSBH events: into the group of participants who did not have CSBH− ($n = 30$) and into the group with CSBH+ ($n = 54$).

The maternal and umbilical vein sera were analyzed for fasting C-peptide concentration, and the HbA1c percentage, along with glucose levels, were measured in maternal blood only.

Pregnant women with T1DM who had proliferative retinopathy, nephropathy, and chronic hypertension were excluded from the study.

2.3. Data Collection

The following parameters were recorded: maternal height (cm) and weight (kg) before pregnancy, gestational weight gain, which was the difference in weight before pregnancy (self-reported) and at time of delivery; and the pre-pregnancy body mass index (kg/m^2; BMI), calculated from the pre-pregnancy values.

Neonatal macrosomia was defined as $\geq$4000 g. Blood samples were obtained from the antecubital vein for glucose measurements when indicated, as well as HbA1c determination in each trimester throughout pregnancy in the type 1 diabetes mellitus groups. Umbilical vein blood samples were obtained immediately after birth but before the placenta was removed through puncture of the umbilical vein for glucose and C-peptide. Neonatal birth weight (g), length (cm), and the 1 min and 5 min Apgar scores were measured postnatally.

2.4. Blood Sample Analyses

The glucose levels were quantified by the hexokinase method on a Cobas C301 analyzer with reagents from the same manufacturer (Roche, Basel, Switzerland). The HbA1c levels in whole blood were measured by turbidimetric inhibition immunoassays on a Cobas C501 instrument (Roche, Basel, Switzerland). The C-peptide concentrations were determined by electrochemiluminescence immunoassays (ECLIA) with Elecsys immunoassay analyzers (Roche Diagnostics, Switzerland). The lower detection limit of C-peptide in serum is 0.003 nmol/L.

According to a homeostasis model assessment, neonatal insulin resistance was calculated using online software (https://homa-calculator.informer.com/2.2/, accessed on 15 January 2022).

2.5. Sample Size

We performed a power calculation using G*power 3.1.9.4 (https://g-power.apponic.com/, accessed on 15 January 2022). For sample size calculation, we tested the mean difference in C-peptide concentration between CSBH− and CSBH+ in the first trimester of pregnancy. For 80% power $p < 0.05$, a total sample size of 45 participants was needed.

2.6. Statistical Analyses

Statistical analyses were performed using the statistical package of SPSS version 24 (IBM, Armonk, NY, USA). Continuous variables are expressed as the mean ± SD, or median (25th–75th percentile) for a skewed distribution, and qualitative variables are presented as frequencies and percentages. Between-group differences in normally distributed continuous variables were assessed with Student's t-test. The Mann–Whitney U test was used for variables with a skewed distribution, and the χ^2 test was used for proportions. For repeated measurements of continuous data, the Wilcoxon signed-rank test was used. Data that were not normally distributed were log-transformed before Spearman's nonparametric correlation analyses. Statistical tests were two-sided.

3. Results

Impact of Clinically Significant Biochemical Hypoglycemia (CSBH) on Maternal and Neonatal Characteristics

The duration of diabetes is a significant risk factor for developing CSBH in pregnant women with type 1 diabetes, as demonstrated in Table 1.

The age, height, body weight, BMI, and weight gain did not differ between pregnant women and those without CSBH. We found the difference in prescribed total insulin doses between the groups with and without CSBH.

In all trimesters of pregnancy, the women with CSBH had lower C-peptide levels and glucose concentration in the daily profile, as demonstrated in Table 1, Figure 1a,b. The HbA1c values were significantly lower in the second trimester in the group of pregnant women with CSBH+ ($p = 0.004$).

Table 1. Maternal characteristics according to groups and trimesters of pregnancy.

	CSBH− (n = 30)	CSBH+ (n = 54)	p
Maternal characteristics in 1st trimester			
Maternal age (years)	29.8 ± 5.3	29.3 ± 6.3	0.693
Maternal height (cm)	166.3 ± 7.4	166.7 ± 6.9	0.798
Maternal pre-pregnancy weight (kg)	63.5 ± 10.9	63.8 ± 8.0	0.804
Pre-pregnancy body mass index (kg/m^2)	22.8 ± 2.9	22.9 ± 2.8	0.755
Gestational weight gain (kg)	13.3 ± 4.4	13.5 ± 4.8	0.858
Duration of type 1 diabetes mellitus (years)	10.1 ± 6.6	13.5 ± 7.1	0.032
Total insulin dose (IU/kg) 1st trimester	0.74 ± 0.15	0.82 ± 0.18	0.044
Total insulin dose (IU/kg) 2nd trimester	0.75 ± 0.18	0.84 ± 0.21	0.045
Total insulin dose (IU/kg) 3rd trimester	0.80 ± 0.13	0.89 ± 0.17	0.015
Maternal vein blood (serum and plasma) measurements in 1st trimester of pregnancy			
HbA1c % (mmol/mol)	6.8 ± 1.3 ** (51)	6.7 ± 1.0 ** (50)	0.296
Fasting C-peptide (pmol/L)	180.0 * (90.0–230.0)	50.0 (30.0–70.0)	0.005
Fasting glucose (mmol/L)	5.1 ± 1.9	5.0 ± 2.0	0.870
Mean glucose concentration (mmol/L)	5.9 ± 1.4	5.1 ± 0.9	0.004
Maternal vein blood (serum and plasma) measurements in 2nd trimester of pregnancy			
HbA1c % (mmol/mol)	5.9 ± 0.5 (41)	5.5 ± 0.6 (37)	0.004
Fasting C-peptide (pmol/L)	130 (80–220)	60 (30–90)	0.004
Fasting glucose (mmol/L)	5.0 ± 1.8	4.4 ± 1.8	0.165
Mean glucose concentration (mmol/L)	5.9 ± 1.4	5.1 ± 0.9	0.016
Maternal vein blood (serum and plasma) measurements in 3rd trimester of pregnancy			
HbA1c % (mmol/mol)	6.9 ± 0.7 ** (52)	5.8 ± 0.8 ** (40)	0.142
Fasting C-peptide (pmol/L)	210 (130–240) *	60 (30–90)	0.001
Fasting glucose (mmol/L)	5.1 ± 1.4	4.8 ± 1.8	0.508
Mean glucose concentration (mmol/L)	5.3 ± 1.0	4.6 ± 1.3	0.009

CSBH—Clinically Significant Biochemical Hypoglycemia; Wilcoxon test * $p < 0.05$; ** $p < 0.001$.

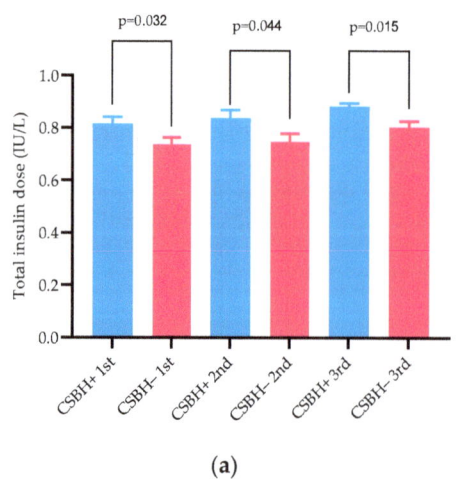
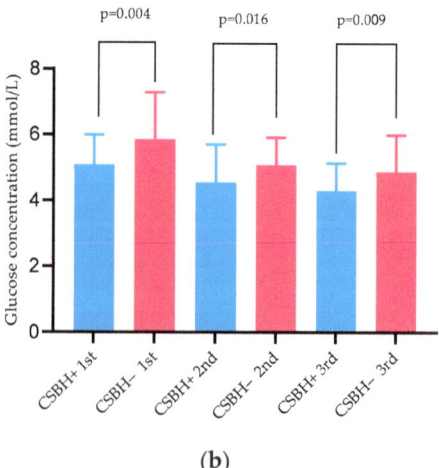

Figure 1. (**a**) Mean and standard deviation total insulin dose in two study groups in three trimesters of pregnancy (IU/kg). (**b**) Mean and standard deviation of glucose concentration in capillary plasma study groups in three trimesters of pregnancy (mmol/L).

The newborns did not differ in gestational age, birth weight and length, Apgar index at 1 and 5 min, or macrosomia prevalence. No difference was found in the glucose, C-peptide concentration, and insulin resistance HOMA 2 between the study groups (Table 2).

Table 2. Neonatal characteristics.

	CSBH− (n = 30)	CSBH+ (n = 54)	p
Gestational age at delivery (weeks)	38.5 ± 0.7	38.3 ± 1.1	0.488
Birth weight (g)	3573.0 ± 542.1	3449.3 ± 421.2	0.231
Birth length (cm)	49.6 ± 2.1	49.0 ± 1.8	0.178
Ponderal index	2.9 ± 0.2	2.9 ± 0.3	0.822
Fetal macrosomia >4000 g n Yes/No (%)	7/23 (23.3/76.7)	5/49 (9.3/90.7)	0.071
Apgar score at 1 min	9.7 ± 1.0	9.9 ± 0.4	0.217
Apgar score at 5 min	9.8 ± 0.5	9.9 ± 0.2	0.157
Umbilical vein serum measurements			
C-peptide (pmol/L)	580.0 (340.0–1100.0)	850.0 (580.0–1250.0)	0.056
Umbilical vein glucose mmo/L	4.7 ± 1.5	4.6 ± 1.4	0.428
IR HOMA 2	1.9 (0.9–2.8)	2.1 (1.4–2.9)	0.492

A significant positive correlation was obtained between CSBH+ and the duration of T1DM ($p < 0.05$). Comparing CSBH+ with C-peptide concentration, a significant negative correlation was found in all pregnancy trimesters, as shown in Table 3. A significant negative correlation was obtained between the mean value of glucose and CSBH+: Table 3.

Table 3. Nonparametric correlations between the CSBH duration of T1DM, C-peptide and mean glucose concentration according to the trimesters of pregnancy.

	CSBH+	Duration of T1DM
DurationT1DM	0.224 *	
Mean glucose concentration in 1st trimester of pregnancy	−0.375 **	−0.073
Mean glucose concentration in 2nd trimester of pregnancy	−0.256 *	−0.028
Mean glucose concentration in 3rd trimester of pregnancy	−0.387 **	−0.115
C-peptide in 1st trimester of pregnancy	−0.331 **	−0.552 **
C-peptide in 2nd trimester of pregnancy	−0.332 **	−0.564 **
C-peptide in 3rd trimester of pregnancy	−0.314 **	−0.546 **

* $p < 0.05$; ** $p < 0.01$.

The duration of T1DM is inversely correlated with C-peptide concentration: Figure 2a. The total insulin dose is inversely correlated with C-peptide: Figure 2b.

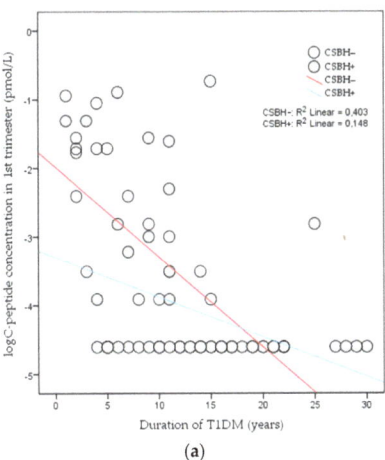
(a)

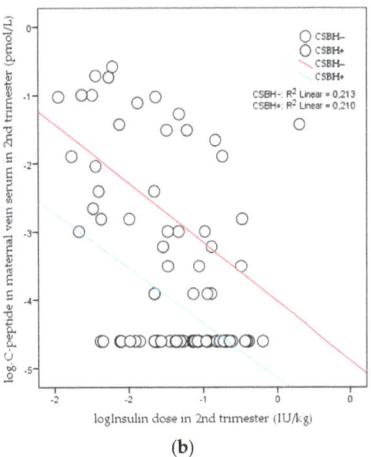
(b)

Figure 2. (a) Nonparametric linear correlation between duration of T1DM and log C-peptide concentration (CSBH+, $R^2 = -0.148$, $p = 0.005$; CSBH−, $R^2 = -0.403$, $p < 0.001$). (b) Nonparametric linear correlation between total log insulin dose and log C-peptide concentration (CSBH+: $R^2 = -0.210$, $p < 0.031$; CSBH−: $R^2 = -0.213$, $p < 0.001$).

4. Discussion

4.1. C-Peptide Concentration in Pregnant Women with Type 1 Diabetes Mellitus

The most reliable indicator of maintaining beta-cell function is the concentration of C-peptide in the blood. Measurement of the C-peptide concentration provides a validated way to quantify secreted endogenous insulin. The close association between C-peptide in the systemic circulation and endogenous insulin in the portal system is well-established [3,9–11]. Nielsen et al. showed that the C-peptide concentration gradually increases during pregnancy, independent of blood glucose concentration, in pregnant women suffering from type 1 diabetes mellitus [3,10]. Comparing C-peptide concentrations across all three trimesters, we found an increase in the CSBH− group from the first to the third trimester. This finding is consistent with our previous research showing that pregnancy increases the C-peptide concentration in healthy pregnant women and women with type 1 diabetes [11] and is compatible with the reported C-peptide increase throughout pregnancy (Nielsen et al.) [3,10]. As the C-peptide does not cross the placenta in either direction, the high C-peptide values detected during pregnancy originate from the maternal beta-cells rather than the fetus.

The increase in the C-peptide concentration in both groups of pregnant women might be mirrored by suppression of the inflammatory immune system during pregnancy, which enhances the ability of the mother to have a genetically and immunologically diverse fetus [3,12,13]. Consequently, the mother's immune system undergoes significant changes, including developing several specific pathways to protect the fetus from maternal cytotoxic attack. One mechanism reduces the expression of classical HLA class I molecules, while the other mechanisms are associated with an altered Th1 and Th2 balance [3,12]. Cellular immune function and pro-inflammatory Th1 cytokines (e.g., IL-2, TNF-α, and INF-γ) are suppressed during pregnancy. In contrast, humoral immunity and the production of anti-inflammatory Th2 cytokines (e.g., IL-4 and IL 10) are enhanced. This immune function pattern is reversed in the postpartum period [12,13]. A partial decrease in the activity of the inflammatory immune system leads to the suppression of various autoimmune diseases during pregnancy, including diabetes. In type 1 diabetes, these changes are expressed through the growth and functional modification of the Langerhans pancreatic islets. The most significant difference that the Langerhans islets undergo during pregnancy is insulin secretion enhancement or improved beta-cell proliferation [3,14].

Numerous animal model studies have shown that the beta-cell mass increases 3–4 times during pregnancy. In addition to significant maternal beta-cell hypertrophy, beta-cell proliferation during pregnancy dramatically increases [14,15]. Nielsen et al. [10] observed a rapid decrease in the postpartum C-peptide concentration. This finding also indicates the active role of the placenta in increasing the concentration of C-peptide during pregnancy. Placental growth factors and hormones that reduce maternal lymphocyte response of the fetoplacental unit [15,16] and beta-cell hyperplasia are no longer excreted after pregnancy.

The data acquired in this study are consistent with earlier studies because the concentration of C-peptide in both study groups was higher in the third trimester than in the first trimester. Tight glycemic control during pregnancy was mirrored by a significant decline in the HbA1c percentage in the third trimester, with average values below 6%. The strict glycemic control also resulted in a low rate of macrosomic infants, although the high percentage of severe hypoglycemia continued during pregnancy.

4.2. C-Peptide, Insulin Doses, and Glycemic Control

We compared the insulin dose between the first and third trimesters. We found that they were significantly reduced with a simultaneous increase in the C-peptide levels in both groups [3] (Figure 2b).

Earlier studies have shown that improved glycemic control during pregnancy leads to increased C-peptide concentrations in pregnant women with type 1 diabetes [16,17]. Although they found no association between the reduced insulin doses at the end of pregnancy and the increased C-peptide concentrations, Nielsen et al. concluded that improved glycemic control facilitates C-peptide production [10]. The authors believe that achieving and maintaining reasonable metabolic control in pregnancy plays a role in beta-cell regeneration. However, our study showed that the C-peptide concentrations affect the insulin dose. A higher C-peptide concentration decreases the total insulin dose, and a lower C-peptide level increases the total insulin dose. We obtained these results thanks to accurate data on the need for daily insulin doses and the determination of glucose and C-peptide concentrations in the same hospital laboratory. So far, only Ilic et al. [18] found a decrease in insulin dose with increased C-peptide concentration in the first trimester of pregnancy.

However, the results of this study did not show a significant correlation between the HbA1c percentage and fasting glucose with the serum C-peptide concentrations. Although this result may seem unexpected, the reason may be that pregnant women in both groups had well-controlled glycemia.

Preservation of beta-cell function decreases the number of hypoglycemic events during pregnancy. It improves metabolic control and reduces the risk of long-term diabetic complications and the adverse effects of intensive therapy, primarily hypoglycemia [3,18,19].

The umbilical vein glucose and C-peptide concentrations differed between the study groups. In a previous study, Delmis et al. showed a significant positive association between the glucose and insulin levels in the umbilical vein [20], that is, increased glucose concentrations increased the synthesis and release of fetal insulin and vice versa. In this study, the concentration of C-peptide in the umbilical vein was correlated with the umbilical vein glucose level.

This research has its advantages and limitations. To the best of our knowledge, this is the first study to investigate the effect of C-peptide on the prevalence of severe hypoglycemia and the insulin dose in pregnant women with type 1 diabetes mellitus. A strength of this report is that this is a prospective study with evidence of fasting glucose and C-peptide values in capillary plasma and 8-point glucose profiles determined in the same hospital laboratory with accurate fast-acting and long-acting insulin dose data. Another advantage is the determination of glucose in the maternal capillary plasma and the glucose and C peptides in the umbilical vein immediately after delivery while the placenta was still in situ. The potential limitation of this study is that no C-peptide values were determined postprandially.

5. Conclusions

Although insulin overdose is the most common risk factor for hypoglycemia, there are more subtle endogenous actors in diabetic pregnancy, which impact hypoglycemia occurrence. An increase in fasting C-peptide in the CSBH group occurred in the third trimester of pregnancy compared to the first. The lower prevalence of clinically significant biochemical hypoglycemia and the decrease in the required dose of insulin during pregnancy were associated with increased endogenous insulin secretion. The duration of pregnancy serves as a mediator between CSBH and C-peptide. Our suggestion would be to introduce fasting and postprandial C peptide as additional valuable laboratory parameters in the conventional clinical approach as a complementary tool for insulin dose titration throughout diabetic pregnancy.

Author Contributions: Conceptualization, M.I. and J.D.; methodology, M.I.; software, J.D.; validation, M.I., J.D.; formal analysis, M.I.; investigation, M.I.; resources, J.D.; writing—original draft preparation, J.D.; writing—review and editing, J.D. All authors have read and agreed to the published version of the manuscript.

Funding: This research was funded by the CROATIAN SCIENCE FOUNDATION, grant number project PRE-HYPO No. IP-2018-01-1284. https://mef.unizg.hr/znanost/istrazivanje/web-stranice-projekata/projekt-hrzz-pre-hypo/ (accessed on 1 February 2019).

Institutional Review Board Statement: The study was conducted in accordance with the Declaration of Helsinki, and approved by the Ethics Committee of School of Medicine, the University of Zagreb (No. 380-59-10106-19-111/26).

Informed Consent Statement: Informed consent was obtained from all subjects involved in the study.

Data Availability Statement: Data can be found on URL https://figshare.com/s/971031f799498beb2 274, accessed on 15 January 2022.

Conflicts of Interest: The authors declare no conflict of interest.

References

1. Persson, M.; Norman, M.; Hanson, U. Obstetric and perinatal outcomes in type 1 diabetic pregnancies: A large, population-based study. *Diabetes Care* **2009**, *32*, 2005–2009. [CrossRef] [PubMed]
2. American Diabetes Association. 14. Management of Diabetes in Pregnancy: Standards of Medical Care in Diabetes. *Diabetes Care* **2021**, *44* (Suppl. 1), S200–S210. [CrossRef] [PubMed]
3. Delmis, J.; Ivanisevic, M.; Horvaticek, M. N-3 PUFA and Pregnancy Preserve C-Peptide in Women with Type 1 Diabetes Mellitus. *Pharmaceutics* **2021**, *4*, 2082. [CrossRef] [PubMed]
4. Ringholm, L.; Pedersen-Bjergaard, U.; Thorsteinsson, B.; Damm, P.; Mathiesen, E.R. Hypoglycaemia during pregnancy in women with type 1 diabetes. *Diabet Med.* **2012**, *29*, 558–566. [CrossRef] [PubMed]
5. Leinonen, P.; Hiilesmaa, V.; Kaaja, R.; Teramo, K.A. Maternal Mortality in Type 1 Diabetes. *Diabetes Care* **2001**, *24*, 1501–1502. [CrossRef] [PubMed]
6. Evers, I.M.; ter Braak, E.W.; de Valk, H.W.; van Der Schoot, B.; Hanssen, N.; Visser, G.H.A. Risk indicators predictive for severe hypoglycemia during first trimester of type 1 diabetic pregnancy. *Diabetes Care* **2002**, *25*, 554–559. [CrossRef] [PubMed]
7. IHSG. Glucose Concentrations of Less Than 3.0 mmol/L Should Be Reported in Clinical Trials: A Joint Position Statement of the American Diabetes Association and the European Association for the Study of Diabetes. *Diabetes Care* **2017**, *40*, 155–157. [CrossRef] [PubMed]
8. Kinsley, B. Achieving better outcomes in pregnancies complicated by type 1 and type 2 diabetes mellitus. *Clin. Ther.* **2007**, *29* (Suppl. D), S153–S160. [CrossRef] [PubMed]
9. Palmer, J.P.; Fleming, G.A.; Greenbaum, C.J.; Herold, K.C.; Jansa, L.D.; Kolb, H.; Lachin, J.M.; Polonsky, K.S.; Pozzilli, P.; Skyler, J.S.; et al. ADA Workshop Report: C-Peptide Is the Appropriate Outcome Measure for Type 1 Diabetes Clinical Trials to Preserve β-Cell Function. *Diabetes* **2004**, *53*, 250–264. [CrossRef] [PubMed]
10. Nielsen, L.R.; Rehfeld, J.F.; Pedersen-Bjergaard, U.; Damm, P.; Mathiesen, E.R. Pregnancy-induced rise in serum C-peptide concentrations in women with type 1 diabetes. *Diabetes Care* **2009**, *32*, 1052–1057. [CrossRef] [PubMed]
11. Horvaticek, M.; Djelmis, J.; Ivanisevic, M.; Oreskovic, S.; Herman, M. Effect of eicosapentaenoic acid and docosahexaenoic acid supplementation on C-peptide preservation in pregnant women with type-1 diabetes: A randomized placebo-controlled clinical trial. *Eur. J. Clin. Nutr.* **2017**, *71*, 968–972. [CrossRef] [PubMed]
12. Wilder, R.L. Hormones, pregnancy, and autoimmune diseases. *Ann. N.Y. Acad. Sci.* **1998**, *840*, 45–50. [CrossRef]
13. Poole, J.A.; Claman, H.N. Immunology of Pregnancy: Implications for the Mother. *Clin. Rev. Allergy Immunol.* **2004**, *26*, 161–170. [CrossRef]
14. Sorenson, R.; Brelje, T. Adaptation of Islets of Langerhans to Pregnancy: β-Cell Growth, Enhanced Insulin Secretion and the Role of Lactogenic Hormones. *Horm. Metab. Res.* **1997**, *29*, 301–307. [CrossRef] [PubMed]
15. Parsons, J.A.; Brelje, T.C.; Sorenson, R.I. Adaptation of Islets of Langerhans to Pregnancy: Increased Islet Cell Proliferation and Insulin Secretion Correlates with the Onset of Placental Lactogen Secretion. *Endocrinology* **1992**, *130*, 1459–1466. [PubMed]
16. Rieck, S.; Kaestner, K.H. Expansion of b-cell mass in response to pregnancy. *Trends Endocrinol. Metab.* **2013**, *21*, 151–158. [CrossRef] [PubMed]
17. Madsbad, S.; Krarup, T.; Reguer, L.; Faber, O.K.; Binder, C. Effect of strict blood glucose control on residual b-cell Function in insulin-dependent diabetics. *Diabetologia* **1981**, *20*, 530–534. [CrossRef] [PubMed]
18. Ilic, S.; Jovanovic, L.; Wolitzer, A.O. Is the paradoxical first trimester drop in insulin requirement due to an increase in C-peptide concentration in pregnant Type 1 diabetic women? *Diabetologia* **2000**, *43*, 1329–1336. [PubMed]
19. Gumpel, R.C. Intensive therapy preserves insulin secretion. *Ann. Intern. Med.* **1998**, *129*, 913–914. [CrossRef]
20. Djelmis, J.; Ivanišević, M.; Desoye, G.; van Poppel, M.; Berberovic, E.; Soldo, D.; Oreskovic, S. Higher Cord Blood Levels of Fatty Acids in Pregnant Women with Type 1 Diabetes Mellitus. *J. Clin. Endocrinol. Metab.* **2018**, *103*, 2620–2629. [CrossRef] [PubMed]

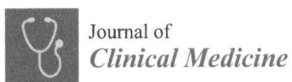

Article

Validation and Psychometric Properties of the Spanish Version of the Fear of Childbirth Questionnaire (CFQ-e)

Héctor González-de la Torre [1,2,*], Adela Domínguez-Gil [3], Cintia Padrón-Brito [3], Carla Rosillo-Otero [3], Miriam Berenguer-Pérez [4] and José Verdú-Soriano [4,*]

1. Research Unit, Insular Maternal and Child University Hospital Complex of Gran Canaria, Canary Health Service, 35016 Las Palmas de Gran Canaria, Spain
2. Department of Nursing, Nursing School La Palma, University of La Laguna, 38200 San Cristóbal de La Laguna, Spain
3. Obstetrics and Gynaecology Department, Insular Maternal and Child University Hospital Complex of Gran Canaria, Canary Health Service, 35016 Las Palmas de Gran Canaria, Spain; adeadg96@gmail.com (A.D.-G.); cintiapb992@gmail.com (C.P.-B.); carlarosillo@gmail.com (C.R.-O.)
4. Department of Community Nursing, Preventive Medicine, Public Health and History of Science, Faculty of Health Sciences, University of Alicante, 03690 Alicante, Spain; miriam.berenguer@ua.es
* Correspondence: hgontor@gobiernodecanarias.org (H.G.-d.l.T.); pepe.verdu@ua.es (J.V.-S.)

Abstract: The fear of childbirth is a topical concern, yet the issue has barely been studied in Spain, and only one fear of childbirth measurement instrument has been validated in the country. The aim of this study was to translate, adapt and validate the Fear of Childbirth Questionnaire (CFQ) for use in Spain, as well as to describe and evaluate the psychometric properties of the Spanish version of this instrument. In a first phase, a methodological study was carried out (translation–backtranslation and cross-cultural adaptation), and pilot study was carried out in the target population. In addition, content validation of the instrument was obtained (CFQ-e) from 10 experts. In the second phase, a cross-sectional study was carried out at several centres in Gran Canaria Island to obtain a validation sample. The evaluation of the psychometric properties of the CFQ-e, including construct validity through exploratory factor analysis and confirmatory factor analysis, the calculation of reliability via factor consistency using the ORION coefficients as well as alpha and omega coefficients were carried out. The CFQ-e showed evidence of content validity, adequate construct validity and reliability. The CFQ-e is composed of 37 items distributed in four subscales or dimensions: "fear of medical interventions"; "fear of harm and dying"; "fear of pain" and "fears relating to sexual aspects and embarrassment". The CFQ-e constitutes a valid and reliable tool to measure the fear of childbirth in the Spanish pregnant population.

Keywords: fear of childbirth; pregnancy; surveys and questionnaires; validation studies as topic

1. Introduction

The fear of childbirth (FOC) is a state of intense anxiety that leads some pregnant women to a fear of childbirth that interferes with their daily lives [1–3].

This fear can become pathological, in which case, it is called tokophobia and can negatively affect the development of the pregnancy and childbirth, as well as favour the development of post-traumatic stress disorders, postpartum depression and anxiety [4–7].

There seems to be a consensus that both FOC and tokophobia rates are increasing in pregnant women [3,8]. The global prevalence of FOC is, however, difficult to estimate [3,9,10]. A global FOC prevalence of 14% has been suggested [9], but this figure is disputed; reported rates vary widely from one study to another, and the problem is often under-detected [11,12].

There are various possible explanations for this. On the one hand, different definitions of the fear of childbirth and tokophobia have been proposed. This makes it very difficult to establish a clear divide between both conditions, distorting the calculations of real and accurate prevalence rates [3,8,13]. On the other hand, FOC is known to be linked to certain factors. For example, FOC prevalence differs according to the woman's previous number of childbirths, showing higher rates in nulliparous women compared to multiparous women [14,15]. Some authors therefore argue that both groups of women should be studied separately regarding FOC [16,17].

Nevertheless, a decisive factor in the detection, diagnosis and evaluation of FOC is the availability of various measurement instruments [18,19]. The use of different scales or instruments conditions the calculation of cut-off points and the determination of mild, moderate or severe fear. It also obstructs the comparative analyses of different studies that address this issue [8,10,20].

Although many tools and measuring instruments exist to assess the fear of childbirth, the most widely known and applied is the Wijma Delivery Expectancy/Experience Questionnaire (W-DEQ) [10,18,19]. Developed in Sweden in 1998, the W-DEQ is a two-part questionnaire (W-DEQ-A and W-DEQ-B) [21]. Part A measures FOC based on women's expectations, and Part B measures FOC based on prior experience [21].

The W-DEQ has been validated in several languages and settings and has been extensively used in FOC studies [10,18,20]. It is worth noting that the W-DEQ was initially conceived as a unidimensional tool [18], despite the causes of FOC being multifactorial [10,22,23].

Other multidimensional tools have thus been developed to measure FOC. One example is the Slade–Pais Expectations of Childbirth Scale (SPECS) [24], or more recently, the Fear of Childbirth Questionnaire (CFQ) [17,22,25].

The CFQ's creators designed the instrument so that it could both measure FOC symptom severity and be used as a screening tool for clinically significant symptoms. To do this, the CFQ includes a wide range of fears related to childbirth that can be perceived by women, reflected in 40 items and organised into 9 dimensions or subscales [17,22,25]. This feature is important, as it allows one to detect and determine the domains in which health professionals should further educate and/or intervene when addressing a pregnant woman with FOC. Additionally, the CFQ includes another scale that measures the interference of FOC in the different spheres of the pregnant woman's life [17].

An increased risk of elective caesarean section has been linked to severe cases of FOC [26,27]. The CFQ design therefore took into account the fact that it was useful for measuring the fear of both vaginal delivery and caesarean section.

The CFQ was validated in a sample of 643 pregnant women from different English-speaking countries (Canada, the United States and the United Kingdom). A Cronbach's alpha of 0.94 was obtained for the general 40-item scale and 0.85 for the interference scale [17,25].

The fear of childbirth is widely studied in certain countries, such as Scandinavian countries [20]. In Finland, for example, FOC measurement and treatment is regulated during pregnancy [5], and in Sweden, midwives offer routine counselling [28]. In Spain, the existence of FOC has been recognised [29], but the problem has barely been studied, partly due to a lack of validated measurement tools [19]. The W-DEQ-A [30] and W-DEQ-B [31] have only very recently been validated in Spain.

Given the growing interest in this topic and the lack of measurement instruments in Spain, the aim was to translate, adapt and validate the Fear of Childbirth Questionnaire (CFQ) for use in Spanish settings, as well as to describe and evaluate the psychometric properties of the Spanish version of this instrument.

2. Materials and Methods

The present study took place over two phases:

First Phase: The translation and cross-cultural adaptation of the CFQ and content validation by experts.

Second Phase: A cross-sectional observational study to evaluate the psychometric properties of the Spanish version of the CFQ (CFQ-e).

2.1. Phase 1

2.1.1. Starting Instrument

The original version of the CFQ consists of 40 items based on a positive Likert scale ranging from 0 points to 4 points. The total score can therefore range from 0 to 160 points (the higher the score, the greater the fear). These items are grouped into 9 subscales, which represent different dimensions or constructs of the fear of childbirth [17,25].

The subscales considered were as follows: fear of loss of sexual pleasure/attractiveness (6 items); fear of pain from a vaginal birth (5 items); fear of medical interventions (7 items); fear of embarrassment (5 items); fear of harm to baby (3 items); fear of caesarean birth (3 items); fear of mum or baby dying (3 items); fear of insufficient pain medication (3 items); fear of body damage from a vaginal birth (5 items). To obtain each subscale's score, the scores of the items in each subscale are added up, and the sum was divided by the number of items within each subscale. This made it possible to compare the different subscale scores [17,22,25].

In addition, the CFQ includes another scale that measures the degree of FOC interference in the different spheres of the pregnant woman's life. This scale consists of 7 Likert-type items, with 0 points meaning no interference and 4 points signifying extreme interference (between 0 and 28 points/the higher the score, the greater the interference) [17].

2.1.2. Translation and Cross-Cultural Adaptation

In order to translate and culturally adapt the questionnaire, the stages proposed by Sousa et al. were followed [32]. The author of the original questionnaire was first contacted to ask for her approval, and her authorisation to adapt it was obtained.

The process unfolded from April to June 2020. Two freelance translators performed two translations from English to Spanish. The first translator was a midwife who had completed her professional studies in England, was a native Spanish speaker, but had been bilingual English/Spanish since childhood. The second was Spanish and a professional translator. The first translator was knowledgeable in the subject, while the second was not. Both translations were analysed and discussed by the research team to obtain an initial unified version (preliminary version 1 of the CFQ-e).

This preliminary version 1 was sent to two independent bilingual translators—who were different from the initial translators—and they performed two backtranslations. The first was a native English translator, who was bilingual and had been residing in Spain for many years. The second was a native Spanish speaker, an obstetrician, who was also bilingual English/Spanish, having spent all her childhood in an English-speaking country (Australia). This second translator was knowledgeable in the subject, while the first was not.

The research team compared the two backtranslations with the original version of the questionnaire, discussing possible discrepancies until a consensus was reached. They were also sent to the original author via email for evaluation. No item was considered necessary to modify, and the similarity of the two backtranslations with the original version of the CFQ was confirmed. This phase thus led to preliminary version 2 of the CFQ-e.

Finally, this version was evaluated and compared with the original CFQ by an external bilingual researcher, an expert in Health Science research methodology and highly experienced in the adaptation and validation of questionnaires.

2.1.3. Pretest

A pilot of the preliminary CFQ-e version 2 was administered to the population under study by means of convenience sampling in order to estimate the instrument's feasibility and viability, as well as its cultural adequacy in the Spanish population. In this phase, the aim was to identify ambiguous items, possible errors and misunderstandings of the items, as well as to assess the burden of administering the questionnaire. Sampling was considered completed when none of the participants expressed any comprehension problems with the questionnaire.

2.1.4. Content Validation

To evaluate the total content validity (CVI-T), the expert test described by Polit and Hungler was performed [33]. The content validity of each item (CVI-I) and the content validity index per expert (CVI-E), as well as the total content validity (CVI-T = sum of the CVI of each expert/total number of experts) were also calculated based on the expert scores. To ensure the validity of the items in the content validity index calculation, the likely random agreement (Pa) was corrected using the formula Pa = $[N!/(A!(NA)!)] \times 0.5N$, where N = expert number and A = n° according to good relevance and the statistical calculation of the modified Kappa ($K^* = (CVI-I - Pa)/(1 - Pa)$) for each instrument item [33,34].

2.2. Phase 2

2.2.1. Design

A cross-sectional observational study was proposed to obtain a validation sample for the CFQ-e questionnaire.

2.2.2. Population to Study

The population to be studied was pregnant women living in Gran Canaria Island. The inclusion criteria were as follows: pregnant women aged 18 years or above, with a gestational age equal to or over 16 weeks and with pregnancies with a live foetus. The exclusion criteria were the following: scheduled/elective caesarean section, in active stage of labour and having a language barrier (difficulty reading or understanding the Spanish language).

Withdrawal criteria included incorrectly or incompletely completing the questionnaire (unanswered items or multiple answers where inappropriate) or wishing to leave the study after having given informed consent.

2.2.3. Sampling and Data Collection

Non-probabilistic convenience sampling was applied. Participants were recruited among women whose pregnancy was being followed up at primary care centres and specialised care centres, or pregnant women who went to consultations and the emergency service of the Insular Maternal and Child University Hospital Complex of Gran Canaria. Each centre's responsible obstetrician or midwife collaborated in the recruitment process. Data were collected from 1 August to 15 November 2020.

It is usually considered that at least 10 subjects need to be studied for each questionnaire item in order to obtain a sufficient number of subjects for an exploratory factor analysis (EFA) [35,36]. Given that the original questionnaire consisted of 40 items, the intention was to reach a minimum sample size of 400 pregnant women.

2.2.4. Variables and Collection Instrument

The questionnaire consisted of two parts. The first part was created "ad hoc" to collect some sociodemographic variables (age, education level and marital status) and obstetric variables (gestational age, previous offspring, type of previous childbirths, how the current pregnancy was achieved, single or twin gestation and the existence of any risk factors). All these variables were gathered by the midwives or obstetricians from the clinical history records.

The second part collected answers to the first version of the CFQ-e. It maintained the same number of items as the original CFQ (40 items) and the interference scale (7 items).

2.2.5. Data Analysis

A descriptive analysis of the variables was conducted using the IBM© SPSS Statistics v.28.0 statistical program, expressing the qualitative variables in percentages and frequencies, and in the case of quantitative variables, in means, standard deviation and minimum-maximum values.

2.2.6. Construct Validation

To evaluate construct validity, a factor analysis was performed using the FACTOR program v.11.05.01 [37–39]. To estimate whether the common variance justified a factor analysis, the Kaiser–Meyer–Olkin index (KMO) was used, with values above 0.75 being considered adequate, as well as Bartlett's statistic, with values $p \leq 0.05$ being considered statistically significant [35,36]. The following indices were used to evaluate the adequacy of the Factorial Solution: Root Mean Square Error of Approximation (RMSEA), Non-Normed Fit Index (NNFI), Comparative Fit Index (CFI), Goodness of Fit Index (GFI) and the Adjusted Goodness of Fit Index (AGFI). RMSEA values less than 0.05 were considered a good fit and values between 0.05 and 0.08 a reasonable fit [35]. NNFI and CFI values of 0.95 or higher were accepted as indicators of good fit, with values for GFI and AGFI over 0.90 generally indicating acceptable model fit [35,38].

To examine the questionnaire's factorial structure, a random sample was initially selected using the Solomon method [35,40], based on 279 participants out of the 557 included in the total sample. An EFA was carried out with the Pearson correlation matrix (according to the result of the Mardia test for symmetry and kurtosis) and the extraction of factors by unweighted least squares and PROMIN rotation [35,41,42]. A parallel analysis was used to establish the number of factors to retain. The consistency (reliability) of the retained factors was calculated. Using bootstrapping, 95% confidence intervals (95%CI) were calculated for the model measurements. Initially, the EFA was performed for a nine-factor model to verify its similarity with the original model proposed for the CFQ, and, subsequently, for a four-factor model, according to the solution suggested in the first EFA, via parallel analysis.

Subsequently, a confirmatory factor analysis (CFA) was performed using the data of the remaining 278 participants, taking as a reference the factor loadings matrix obtained from the first sample's EFA. The loading matrix was semi-specified, with non-zero values attributed to coefficients above 0.30 for each factor and zero to the rest. In cases in which an item's factor loading was above 0.30 in more than one factor, a value other than 0 was assigned in the one with the highest loading and 0 in the rest.

2.2.7. Internal Consistency

Factor consistency was evaluated using the ORION coefficients (Overall Reliability of fully Informative prior Oblique N-EAP scores) [35,43]. Moreover, the questionnaire's reliability was calculated based on the alpha coefficient and the omega coefficient using the IBM Corp. Released 2021. IBM SPSS Statistics for Windows, Version 28.0. Armonk, NY, USA: IBM Corp.

2.2.8. Ethical Considerations

The study protocol was evaluated and approved by the Research Ethics Committee/Medicines Research Ethics Committee University Hospital of Gran Canaria Dr. Negrín (CEI/CEIm HUGCDN, CEIm HUGCDN Code: 2020-264-1). The project was explained to each participant, and their written informed consent was obtained. An anonymised matrix was used to statistically analyse the data. Confidentiality and anonymity were ensured during all of the stages of the study.

3. Results

3.1. Phase 1

3.1.1. Translation and Cross-Cultural Adaptation

The research team's review of the translated versions revealed no major discrepancies between the two initial translations. No items were controversial, and preliminary version 1 CFQ-e was obtained.

The research team compared the original questionnaire with the two backtranslations obtained from CFQ-e preliminary version 1. No significant differences were found between the two versions. The original author also evaluated them and considered that both backtranslations were faithful and conveyed the meaning of the original questionnaire. The author did show, however, a slight preference for backtranslation number 2.

The external researcher agreed that CFQ-e preliminary version 2 was similar to the CFQ original version.

3.1.2. Pretest

A total of 20 pregnant women presenting similar inclusion and exclusion criteria to those considered in phase 2 answered and completed CFQ-e preliminary version 2 in writing, expressing their opinion and providing suggestions. This pilot study was conducted in one of the health centres participating in the study and in the emergency department of the Insular Maternal and Child University Hospital Complex of Gran Canaria.

Overall, no problems were encountered regarding the participants' understanding of the questionnaire, except for item number 19 ("having an episiotomy"), since the pretest revealed that several women did not understand the term "episiotomy". This meant that the item had to be modified with an additional clarification note, as follows: Item 19—have an episiotomy performed (have a cut made in your vagina). This item was considered to be the one that differed the most from the original CFQ reference item. Regarding the efforts required to fill out the questionnaire, a number of pregnant women found that it was rather long to complete.

After the pretest, the first Spanish version of the CFQ (CFQ-e) was obtained. Similarly to the original CFQ, it included 40 items (Table S1: First version of the CFQ-e).

3.1.3. Content Validation

The expert panel was composed of ten professionals: six women and four men (two obstetricians, five midwives and three nurses). The expert assessment provided a CVI-Total of 0.77. The CVI-E values ranged from 0.52 (one expert) to 1 (two experts) (Table S2: Profile and CVI-E of the experts). According to the experts, twenty-one out of the forty items included in the CFQ-e showed an excellent CVI-I, and another ten items obtained good CVI-I. Nine items presented a CVI-I with "fair" (items 14, 21, 24 and 32) or "poor" (items 5, 12, 13, 22 and 38) values (Table S3: CVI-I scores for each CFQ-e item).

3.2. Phase 2

3.2.1. Sociodemographic Characteristics

A total of 608 women from 22 health centres, 3 specialised care centres, obstetric consultations and the emergency service of the XXXX completed the questionnaires, but 51 questionnaires were inadequately completed and had to be withdrawn. The final sample was therefore composed of a total of 557 women ($n = 557$).

The participants' mean age was 31.30 years (SD = 5.49/Minimum = 18-Maximum = 48). The mean gestational age was 29.63 weeks (SD = 7.42/Minimum = 16.00-Maximum = 42.00). Table 1 shows the frequencies and percentages for the rest of the sociodemographic and obstetric variables considered.

The final mean score obtained for fear of childbirth in the sample was 66.15 points (SD = 26.77/Minimum = 1.00-Maximum = 143.00). The final mean score obtained for the interference scale in the sample was 4.95 points (SD = 5.06/Minimum = 0-Maximum = 28). Table 2 shows the floor percentage, ceiling percentage, mean and standard deviation for each item, as well as the average scores for the nine subscales considered in the original CFQ. These same values can be found for the interference scale in Table S4.

Table 1. Sociodemographic and obstetric variables of the sample ($n = 557$).

Variables	Frequency (%) $n = 557$	M (SD)
Age (years)		31.30 (5.49)
Gestational Age (weeks)		29.63 (7.42)
Level of studies		
No studies	2 (0.4)	
Primary education	127 (22.8)	
Secondary education	229 (41.1)	
University studies	199 (35.7)	
Marital status		
Has a partner	536 (96.2)	
No Partner	21 (3.8)	
Type of Pregnancy		
Single pregnancy	550 (98.7)	
Twin pregnancy	7 (1.3)	
How the current pregnancy was achieved		
Spontaneous	529 (95.0)	
Assisted reproduction technique	28 (5.0)	
Previous offspring [a]		
Nulliparous	365 (65.5)	
Primiparous	146 (26.2)	
Multiparous	46 (8.3)	
Existence of at least one risk factor [b]		
Yes	99 (17.8)	
No	458 (82.2)	
Gestational hypertension risk factor		
Yes	24 (4.3)	
No	533 (95.7)	
Preeclampsia risk factor		
Yes	4 (0.7)	
No	553 (99.3)	
Pregestational Diabetes risk factor		
Yes	4 (0.7)	
No	553 (99.3)	
Gestational Diabetes risk factor		
Yes	60 (10.8)	
No	497 (89.2)	
Intrauterine Growth Restriction risk factor		
Yes	9 (1.6)	
No	548 (98.4)	
Coagulopathies risk factor		
Yes	7 (1.3)	
No	550 (98.7)	
Anterior Eutocic delivery		
Yes	173 (31.1)	
No	384 (68.9)	
Anterior Dystopian delivery (Forceps)		
Yes	20 (3.6)	
No	537 (96.4)	
Previous caesarean section		
Yes	31 (5.6)	
No	526 (94.4)	

M = Mean/SD = standard deviation; [a] = nulliparous: woman with no vaginal births/primiparous: woman who had given birth vaginally only once/multiparous: woman who had had two or more vaginal births; [b] = existence of at least one of the risk factors considered in the study.

Table 2. Floor and ceiling scores and means and standard deviations for each of the items in the CFQ-e (n = 557).

Subscales and Items of the CFQ [a]	Floor Not at All [b] n (%)	Ceiling Extremely [b] n (%)	M (SD)
Subscale Fear of loss of sexual pleasure/attractiveness			1.07 (0.86)
12—That your vagina stretches by having a vaginal birth	272 (48.8%)	9 (1.6%)	0.86 (1.02)
13—Enjoy less sexual intercourse by stretching the vagina because of vaginal birth	212 (38.1%)	19 (3.4%)	1.17 (1.15)
15—That your body is less attractive after childbirth	254 (45.6%)	18 (3.2%)	0.90 (1.05)
24—Make your vagina look less attractive after a vaginal birth	301 (54.0%)	9 (1.6%)	0.73 (0.94)
26—Enjoy less sexual intercourse because you feel pain or discomfort after childbirth	127 (22.8%)	25 (4.5%)	1.47 (1.15)
27—That your partner enjoys less of sexual intercourse after childbirth by stretching your vagina after childbirth	175 (31.4%)	20 (3.6%)	1.30 (1.15)
Subscale Fear of pain from a vaginal birth			1.33 (0.95)
30—Feeling pain during childbirth	117 (21.0%)	59 (10.6%)	1.77 (1.28)
31—Have a vaginal birth	333 (59.8%)	9 (1.6%)	0.71 (1.02)
34—Feel pain while pushing the baby	139 (25.0%)	20 (3.6%)	1.35 (1.09)
35—Feeling pain during a vaginal birth	133 (23.9%)	27 (4.8%)	1.41 (1.12)
37—Feeling pain during contractions	120 (21.5%)	22 (3.9%)	1.45 (1.08)
Subscale Fear of medical interventions			1.45 (0.79)
1—That you are harmed by incompetent medical assistance	44 (7.9%)	104 (18.7%)	2.25 (1.22)
4—Receive general anaesthesia	162 (29.1%)	38 (6.8%)	1.44 (1.24)
5—To be given injections	295 (53.0%)	15 (2.7%)	0.85 (1.09)
22—That you get the epidural	252 (45.2%)	27 (4.8%)	0.99 (1.15)
25—That you have scars after the caesarean section	288 (51.7%)	14 (2.5%)	0.82 (1.03)
38—To be probed (a tube that is inserted into the urethra to collect urine)	136 (24.4%)	57 (10.2%)	1.70 (1.31)
39—Feeling pain during a C-section	63 (11.3%)	88 (15.8%)	2.15 (1.24)
Subscale Fear of embarrassment			0.72 (0.69)
7—That other people see you naked during childbirth	428 (76.8%)	2 (0.4%)	0.34 (0.70)
14—Losing control of your emotions in front of other people (being rude, screaming) during childbirth	241 (43.3%)	14 (2.5%)	0.94 (1.04)
21—That other people see you urinating during childbirth	328 (58.9%)	7 (1.3%)	0.63 (0.90)
23—Feeling observed by strangers during childbirth	355 (63.7%)	8 (1.4%)	0.58 (0.91)
32—That other people see you defecate during childbirth	216 (38.8%)	26 (4.7%)	1.12 (1.17)
Subscale Fear of harm to baby			3.25 (0.97)
6—That damage or harm the baby as a result of childbirth	19 (3.4%)	307 (55.1%)	3.18 (1.11)
9—That the baby suffers some damage during childbirth	9 (1.6%)	329 (59.1%)	3.33 (0.96)
10—That harm the baby in a medical intervention during childbirth (e.g., vacuum, anaesthesia, forceps...)	13 (2.3%)	307 (55.1%)	3.24 (1.02)
Subscale Fear of caesarean birth			1.72 (1.10)
33—Not being able to have a vaginal birth despite being what you prefer	132 (23.7%)	44 (7.9%)	1.58 (1.23)
36—Having a caesarean section	116 (20.8%)	73 (13.1%)	1.86 (1.31)
40—Not being able to have the type of birth you would like (for example, vaginal or caesarean section)	119 (21.4%)	63 (11.3%)	1.73 (1.28)
Subscale Fear of mom or baby dying			3.06 (1.06)
3—Dying during childbirth	98 (17.6%)	233 (41.8%)	2.46 (1.57)
16—That the baby suffocates during childbirth	15 (2.7%)	324 (58.2%)	3.24 (1.08)
20—That the baby dies during childbirth	18 (3.2%)	415 (74.5%)	3.49 (1.04)
Subscale Fear of insufficient pain medication			1.66 (1.01)
11—That you do not have a caesarean section when it is what you want	242 (43.4%)	32 (5.7%)	1.21 (1.29)
18—Not getting the pain medication you need	67 (12.0%)	57 (10.2%)	1.92 (1.18)
29—That you do not put the epidural during childbirth in the case of wanting it or needing it	102 (18.3%)	65 (11.7%)	1.87 (1.29)
Subscale Fear of body damage from a vaginal birth			2.01 (0.90)
2—Suffer a tear or rectal damage as a result of childbirth	33 (5.9%)	85 (15.3%)	2.31 (1.12)
8—Suffering a vaginal tear during childbirth	37 (6.6%)	72 (12.9%)	2.12 (1.14)
17—Need a forceps or suction cup	38 (6.8%)	133 (23.9%)	2.48 (1.21)
19—Have an episiotomy performed (have a cut made in your vagina)	82 (14.7%)	76 (13.6%)	1.96 (1.26)
28—Need stitches after childbirth	181 (32.5%)	23 (4.1%)	1.22 (1.12)

M = Mean/SD = standard deviation; [a] For each of the nine-subscale listed, sum the items in the subscale. To create mean score (to be able to compare across subscales), divide the subscale score by the number of items in the subscale. [b] Only the highest (ceiling) and lowest scores (floor) per question are shown.

3.2.2. Preliminary Factor Analysis

Initially, a preliminary EFA was performed for a nine-factor model, according to the model proposed in the original questionnaire. Although it presented very good adequacy, with a Kaiser–Meyer–Olkin measure (KMO) = 0.918 (95%CI: 0.867–0.911) and a significant Bartlett statistic (p = 0.00001), and it showed excellent goodness of fit indices (Root Mean

Square Error of Approximation (RMSEA) = 0.000 (95%CI: could not be computed), Non-Normed Fit Index (NNFI) = 1.020 (95%CI: 1.015–1.026) and Comparative Fit Index (CFI) = 0.999 (95%CI: 0.999–0.999), the parallel analysis recommended a four-factor solution. Because of this, an EFA was carried out for a four-factor model.

The EFA for this four-factor model presented very good adequacy, with KMO = 0.918 (95%CI: 0.867–0.911) and Bartlett's statistic p = 0.00001, with the goodness of fit indices being RMSEA = 0.021 (95%CI: 0.015–0.015), NNFI = 0.996 (95%CI: 0.997–0.998) and CFI = 0.997 (95%CI: 0.997–0.999). In this model, all items had a factor loading above 0.30 in the assigned factor, except item numbers 8 and 14, which did not obtain sufficiently satisfactory loading for any factor (less than 0.30 in both cases) (Table S5: Factor loadings obtained in the EFA of the model of 4 factors and 40 items).

The CFA subsequently performed on the second sample (278 participants) to confirm the model showed excellent adjustment (RMSEA = 0.022 (95%CI: 0.001–0.022), NNFI = 0.996 (95%CI: 0.995–1.000) and CFI = 0.997 (95%CI: 0.996–1.000) but suggested problems in the case of some items. Thus, two items (items 11 and 14) had loadings below 0.30. Moreover, a change of factor assignment with respect to the EFA was proposed for another, with the factor loading of "Item 19-have an episiotomy performed (have a cut made in your vagina)" being the lowest of all those that exceeded the established limit of 0.30 (0.311) (Table S6: Factor loadings obtained in the CFA of the four-factor forty-item model). The analysis of the estimated congruences for each item [44] indicated comparatively lower values for these three items compared to the rest, especially in the case of item 19 (Congruence Index = 0.208/95%CI: −0.165–0.531) (Table S7).

Based on the results obtained in this preliminary factor analysis, a CFQ-e four-factor model with thirty-seven items was tested via a new factor analysis, eliminating items number 11, 14 and 19 of the first version of the questionnaire and maintaining the rest of the conditions that were specified in the Materials and Methods section.

3.2.3. Exploratory Factor Analysis (EFA) of the Four-Factor and Thirty-Seven-Item Model

The EFA for this model also presented very good adequacy, with KMO = 0.913 (95%CI: 0.864–0.908) and a significant Bartlett statistic (p = 0.00001), with Normed item-MSA indices above 0.85 in all items. The four-factor solution provided a total explained variance of 58.75% according to the parallel analysis. The goodness of fit indices for the model were RMSEA = 0.025 (95%CI: 0.013–0.024)—i.e., below the 0.05 limit to be considered a good fit—NNFI = 0.995 (95%CI: 0.994–0.999), CFI = 0.996 (95%CI: 0.995–0.999) and above 0.95, also indicating an excellent fit.

Table 3 presents the factor loadings (after rotation) of the four-factor and thirty-seven-item model. According to the analysis, in this model, Factor 1 groups all the "fear of caesarean birth" and "fear of medical interventions" subscale items (except items 1 and 25) in addition to item 28; Factor 2 includes all the items relating to "fear of harm to baby", "fear of mum or baby dying" and "fear of body damage from a vaginal birth" subscales, plus item 1; Factor 3 includes all the items from the "fear of pain from a vaginal birth" and "fear of insufficient pain medication" subscales, and finally Factor 4, includes the items from the subscales "fear of loss of pleasure/sexual attractiveness" and "fear of embarrassment", plus item 25.

In this initial model, F1 is called "fear of medical interventions" (9 items), F2 is "fear of harm and dying" (10 items), F3 refers to "fear of pain" (7 items) and Factor 4 is called "fear relating to sexual aspects and embarrassment" (11 items).

The results obtained can generally be observed to maintain the structure of the original questionnaire, although some subscales were grouped until they reached a reduction in four dimensions or subscales. With this structure, all items had a factor loading above 0.30 in the assigned factor, with the lowest value corresponding to item number 8 (0.307). The items could have been assigned differently to the factors, since some items (items number 18, 23 and 25) had a loading above 0.3 in several factors. These items could therefore be assigned to the factor presenting the highest factor loading to perform the subsequent CFA.

Table 3. Factorial loads (after rotation) of the 4-factor, 37-item model obtained on the first sample (n = 279).

	F1	F2	F3	F4
Item 1	0.097	0.503	0.037	0.101
Item 2	−0.037	0.427	0.276	0.136
Item 3	−0.004	0.659	−0.081	0.089
Item 4	0.442	0.191	−0.136	0.172
Item 5	0.418	0.060	−0.085	0.180
Item 6	0.099	0.872	−0.010	−0.154
Item 7	0.149	−0.177	0.036	0.483
Item 8	−0.037	0.307	0.225	0.259
Item 9	−0.018	0.880	−0.076	0.044
Item 10	0.087	0.886	−0.048	−0.075
Item 12	−0.126	0.139	0.162	0.514
Item 13	−0.158	−0.228	0.014	0.686
Item 15	−0.014	−0.116	−0.026	0.775
Item 16	−0.039	0.882	−0.038	−0.050
Item 17	0.193	0.463	0.109	0.049
Item 18	−0.104	0.362	0.499	0.064
Item 20	0.013	0.817	−0.017	−0.077
Item 21	0.164	−0.142	0.029	0.509
Item 22	0.524	0.074	−0.109	0.131
Item 23	0.323	−0.191	0.043	0.456
Item 24	−0.005	−0.069	0.052	0.812
Item 25	0.314	−0.135	−0.089	0.538
Item 26	−0.002	0.215	−0.076	0.685
Item 27	0.020	0.205	−0.165	0.718
Item 28	0.357	0.001	0.258	0.212
Item 29	−0.075	0.219	0.618	0.004
Item 30	−0.027	0.038	0.800	−0.019
Item 31	−0.087	−0.002	0.471	0.283
Item 32	0.171	−0.100	0.104	0.512
Item 33	0.772	−0.013	−0.061	−0.005
Item 34	0.027	−0.075	0.987	−0.099
Item 35	0.068	−0.075	0.934	−0.050
Item 36	0.882	−0.046	0.042	−0.098
Item 37	0.087	−0.070	0.775	−0.036
Item 38	0.477	0.089	0.289	−0.103
Item 39	0.566	0.224	0.266	−0.172
Item 40	0.634	0.101	0.046	0.015

3.2.4. Confirmatory Factor Analysis (CFA) for the Four-Factor and Thirty-Seven-Item Model

The factorial model obtained from four factors with the first sample (n = 279) was confirmed via CFA using the second sample with the remaining 278 participants. To do this, a CFA was performed using a semi-specified matrix of factor loading coefficients. This procedure compares the congruence or similarity with a model for which the factor loadings are 0 in specified items and other than 0 in the rest. Accordingly, the factor loadings matrix to be confirmed were factor loadings other than 0 in the items obtained from the EFA of the four-factor and thirty-seven-item model in the first sample.

The second sample (n = 278) presented very good adequacy, with a KMO = 0.914 (95%CI: 0.864–0.908) and a significant Bartlett statistic ($p = 0.00001$), and with an explained variance by the four factors of 59.84% according to the parallel analysis. The model's goodness of fit indices were RMSEA = 0.028 (95%CI: 0.018–0.030) (below the 0.05 limit to be considered a good fit), NNFI = 0.994 (95%CI: 0.992–0.998) and CFI = 0.995 (95%CI: 0.993–0.998), above 0.95, thus confirming the model's excellent fit. The Goodness of Fit Index (GFI) was 0.984 (95%CI: 0.981–0.988), and the Adjusted Goodness of Fit Index (AGFI) = 0.980 (95%CI: 0.976–0.984).

Table 4 presents the model's factor loadings (after rotation) obtained after the CFA. All items had loadings above 0.30. The analysis confirmed the assignment of most items to the factors proposed by the EFA, although three items had loadings above 0.30 in two factors (items number 18, 25 and 28). Depending on the loadings, the CFA led to a change in factor assignment for items 18 and 25.

Table 4. Factorial loads (after rotation) of the model obtained from 4-factor, 37-item model in the second sample (n = 278) (loadings lower than absolute 0.300 omitted).

	F1 Fear of Medical Interventions	F2 Fear of Harm and Dying	F3 Fear of Pain	F4 Fears Relating to Sexual Aspects and Embarrassment
Item 1—That you are harmed by incompetent medical assistance		0.565		
Item 2—Suffer a tear or rectal damage as a result of childbirth		0.443		
Item 3—Dying during childbirth		0.764		
Item 4—Receive general anaesthesia	0.493			
Item 5—Get injections	0.551			
Item 6—That harm or harm the baby as a result of childbirth		0.894		
Item 7—That other people see you naked during childbirth				0.568
Item 8—Suffering a vaginal tear during childbirth		0.355		
Item 9—That the baby suffers some damage during childbirth		0.940		
Item 10—That harm the baby in a medical intervention during childbirth (e.g., vacuum, anaesthesia, forceps...)		0.890		
Item 12—That your vagina stretches from having a vaginal birth				0.619
Item 13—Enjoy less sexual intercourse by stretching the vagina because of vaginal birth				0.852
Item 15—Make your body less attractive after childbirth				0.688
Item 16—That the baby suffocates during childbirth		0.929		
Item 17—Need a forceps or suction cup		0.474		
Item 18—Not getting the pain medication you need		0.470	0.386	
Item 20—That the baby dies during childbirth		0.715		
Item 21—Other people see you urinating during childbirth				0.565
Item 22—Have your epidural administered	0.703			
Item 23—Feeling observed by strangers during childbirth				0.646
Item 24—Make your vagina look less attractive after a vaginal birth				0.898
Item 25—That you have scars after the caesarean section	0.388			0.376
Item 26—Enjoying sex less because of feeling pain or discomfort after childbirth				0.696
Item 27—That your partner enjoys less of sexual intercourse after childbirth by stretching your vagina after childbirth				0.771
Item 28—Needing stitches after childbirth	0.435			0.309
Item 29—That you do not get the epidural during childbirth in the case of wanting or needing it			0.457	
Item 30—Feeling pain during childbirth			0.846	
Item 31—Having a vaginal birth			0.487	
Item 32—That other people see you defecate during childbirth				0.709
Item 33—Not being able to have a vaginal birth despite being what you prefer	0.758			
Item 34—Feel pain while pushing the baby			0.955	
Item 35—Feeling pain during a vaginal birth			0.962	
Item 36—Have a C-section	0.915			
Item 37—Feeling pain during contractions			0.845	
Item 38—To be probed (a tube that is inserted into the urethra to collect urine	0.534			
Item 39—Feeling pain during a C-section	0.541			
Item 40—Not being able to have the type of birth you would like (for example vaginal or caesarean section)	0.632			

"Item 18—not receiving adequate pain relief" had loadings for factors F2 (0.470) and F3 (0.386). Although the highest loading was for F2, it was considered more appropriate and in line with the theoretical framework to maintain this item in factor F3 ("fear of pain").

Regarding "item 28—needing stitches after childbirth", despite receiving loadings for two factors (F1 and F4), the F4 loading was minimal (0.309), so the factor change was not considered and F1 was maintained, as suggested by the EFA.

The only item that was considered problematic in this model was "item 25—scars after a C-section", since it had very similar loadings for Factors F1 (0.388) and F4 (0.376). In this case, a change of factor was chosen, assigning it to F1 (fear of medical interventions).

Table S8 illustrates the root mean square discrepancy (RMSD) between the rotated loading matrix and the target matrix for each variable under study between the data of the second sample and the semi-specified four-factor model. The global RSMDs estimated for each factor were 0.086 (95%CI: 0.065–0.100) for F1, 0.108 (95%CI: 0.077–0.128) for F2, 0.104 (95%CI: 0.078–0.115) for F3 and 0.120 (95%CI: 0.085–0.137), with an overall model discrepancy coefficient of 0.105 (95%CI: 0.103–0.104). Table 5 shows the correlations between the model factors, presenting all significant factor correlations.

Table 5. Correlations (and 95% confidence intervals) between the factors of the obtained model.

Factors	Correlation Values	Bias-Corrected Bootstrap 95% Confidence Intervals
1——2	0.479 *	(0.403–0.579)
1——3	0.537 *	(0.480–0.646)
1——4	0.533 *	(0.464–0.680)
2——3	0.380 *	(0.288–0.472)
2——4	0.399 *	(0.315–0.485)
3——4	0.588 *	(0.539–0.674)

* Significantly different from zero at population.

3.2.5. CFQ-e Final Instrument

The analysis gave rise to a final version of the CFQ-e, consisting of 37 items (items number 11, 14 and 19 in the original CFQ questionnaire were eliminated), distributed in 4 dimensions or subscales called: "fear of medical interventions" (10 items), "fear of harm and dying" (10 items), "fear of pain" (7 items) and "fear relating to sexual aspects and embarrassment" (10 items). In this way, the total score can range between 0 and 148 points (a higher score corresponds to greater fear). The interference scale remains unchanged. The final version of the CFQ-e can be found in Table S9.

3.2.6. Internal Consistency

The values obtained for the ORION coefficients for the final version of the CFQ-e were 0.900 (95%CI: 0.800–0.916) for F1, 0.954 (95%CI: 0.938–0.962) for F2, 0.940 (95%CI: 0.924–0.955) for F3 and 0.930 (95%CI: 0.914–0.941) for F4. All values were above 0.80, thus showing adequate consistency [43,45].

A total alpha of 0.947 was obtained for the final version of the CFQ-e and 0.898 for the interference scale. The total omega coefficient was 0.945 for the CFQ-e and 0.898 for the interference scale. All alpha and omega coefficient values calculated for the subscales in this study can be seen in Table S10.

4. Discussion

Despite extensive interest in FOC and the large amount of research published on the subject, FOC has barely been studied in Spain [30,46]. The absence of validated FOC measurement tools in Spain has undoubtedly contributed to this situation.

Some authors have pointed out the need for measuring instruments that assess the different dimensions that could be related to the fear of childbirth [8]. The FCQ's multidimensionality is regarded by its creators as one of its greatest strengths compared to the W-DEQ [17,25], which was hitherto considered the "gold standard" of FOC measurement [10,18,30].

The unidimensional nature of the W-DEQ has been much discussed, as many studies suggest that this measuring instrument should in fact be considered multidimensional [47–49]. Despite this, no consensus has been reached regarding the number of factors or dimensions included or their composition [50]. In fact, the authors who performed the Spanish validation (W-DEQ-A-Sp) suggested that this version had four factors or dimensions [30].

Unlike W-DEQ, the CFQ was conceived as a multidimensional tool from the outset. For this reason—and because another research group was already validating the W-DEQ in Spain—we chose the CFQ as the tool to validate, regarding it as a potentially effective way to study FOC in the Spanish population.

The performed factor analysis indicates that the Spanish version of the CFQ-e is composed of thirty-seven items and four factors/subscales, achieving an appropriate model adjustment. The model's goodness of fit indices were greater than that of the original version of the CFQ, with RMSEA = 0.028 (95%CI: 0.018–0.030) and CFI = 0.995 (95%CI: 0.993–0.998) compared to RMSEA = 0.064 (90% CI: 0.062–0.066) and CFI = 0.977, reported by Fairbrother [25].

We cannot yet compare these results with other validation studies in other language populations since, to the best of our knowledge, this is the first CFQ validation study in a non-English-speaking setting. Further validation studies are required in other contexts to provide more information in this regard and to confirm or discard this model.

Regarding the sample size, we followed the classic factorial analysis recommendation of having at least 10 subjects for each item. We do accept, however, that such a recommendation is highly controversial [36]. Conversely, when using Pearson correlation matrices, as in this case, the recommendation is to use a minimum sample of 200 subjects [35,36]. We therefore consider that the sample size achieved was sufficient to ensure the results' internal validity. The KMO and Barlett statistic values obtained supported this assumption.

While the EFA was initially conducted for nine subscales and showed excellent goodness of fit indices, the parallel analysis suggested four factors. A parallel analysis method was chosen, since this system allows one to perform the most rigorous identification of a questionnaire's numbers of dimensions [36,51]. In addition, it was also used by Fairbrother et al. and Ortega-Cejas et al. to validate the W-DEQ-Sp [25,30,31].

The number of items that should be included in each factor is an object of discussion. The common procedure is to select a minimum of three items with high saturations (factor loadings above 0.60) by factor [36,52]. This practice, however, has been described as counterproductive, as it can affect the stability of the results [36]. It seems clear that the greater the number of items, and the more accurately they measure a factor, the more stable the factor solution [35,36]. The distribution of the items and factor loadings obtained for the four-factor model proposed for CFQ-e is robust in this regard.

The analysis revealed problems with three items. Item numbers "11—that you do not have a caesarean section when it is what you want" and "14—losing control of your emotions in front of other people (being rude, screaming) during childbirth" had loadings below 0.30 in the preliminary factor analysis. These items obtained kappa values of 0.66 (good) and 0.50 (fair), respectively, in the content validation process. The latter suggests that the experts had assessed, a priori, the existence of cultural aspects that could affect the adequacy of these items in Spanish settings.

In Fairbrother's factor analysis, the item "11—that you do not have a caesarean section when it is what you want" was the item with the lowest factor loading in the EFA (0.297), discarding items with similar and even higher loadings during the creation and validation of the CFQ [25]. These results indicate that this item is problematic in both versions, perhaps because there may be a contradiction between women who desire a caesarean section and those who wish to avoid it at all costs, which is reflected in the item's construct.

Fairbrother's study did not identify any problems with the item "14—losing control of your emotions in front of other people (being rude, screaming) during childbirth", with loadings above 0.35 (0.446), although this item had the lowest loading in its dimension [25].

The results of our study indicate that the item is complex, at least in the case of our sample, since it had much lower loadings, as well as the highest loading (0.208) in a subscale factor which was not very consistent with the theoretical framework (F4–fear of harm and dying). Although a possible explanation may be that Spanish women are not afraid of losing control of their emotions during labour, this item's average score in our sample was 0.94, i.e., higher than that obtained for other items of the original subscale. The relationship between the loss of self-control during labour and fear in the Spanish population should thus be explored more in depth.

"Item 19–Have an episiotomy performed (have a cut made in your vagina)" deserves special attention. In the pilot study, it was found that several women did not understand this term, so it had to be substantially modified with respect to that of the original questionnaire. Although the item obtained a discrete factor loading (0.311), the estimated congruence value was extremely low (Congruence Index = 0.208). While this index has given rise to different interpretations, most authors agree that values above 0.85 can be considered adequate, indicating a similarity of the items with the model [44]. Values below 0.68 are considered "terrible" [44]. Based on the latter, item 19 was removed from the final CFQ-e model, although we recommend assessing this aspect in future studies on the CFQ-e. In Spain, episiotomy rates are even higher than the recommended number [53–55], suggesting that Spanish women are still insufficiently aware of certain childbirth interventions, and this could influence FOC.

The obtained alpha coefficients, with a total value of 0.947, and values above 0.85 for the four factor-subscales indicated the adequate reliability of the final version of the CFQ-e for practical use [56], the values being almost identical to those reported by Fairbrother and her team [17,25].

In recent years, the widespread use of the alpha coefficient as the only index to evaluate the reliability of a measuring instrument has been criticised [57,58]. This has led some authors to recommend the use of other estimators such as the omega coefficient [59,60]. Indeed, this latter index, unlike the alpha coefficient, works directly with the factor loadings, making the calculations more stable and reducing the dependence on the number of instrument items to be evaluated [58,61]. Values above 0.80 are considered adequate [59,61].

This aspect was not taken into account by the authors of the CFQ, who did not report the omega coefficients. They were, however, considered by those responsible for validating the W-DEQ-A-Sp, who mentioned a total omega coefficient of 0.936 and values between 0.80 and 0.90 for the four identified factors [30].

In our study, the omega coefficients were calculated both for the original nine-subscale model proposed by the original CFQ and for the final model of the proposed four-subscale and thirty-seven-item CFQ-e. The analysis indicated that despite an almost complete absence of variation in the total omega coefficient in our sample, the subscale values obtained were more suitable for the four-factor model of the CFQ-e. Indeed, the values were above 0.85 for all the subscales, while in the original model, the omega values were below 0.80 in three subscales.

Based on these results, we can affirm that the decision to remove the items mentioned above did not affect the reliability of the CFQ-e. Considering that, as identified in the pilot study, some women found that the questionnaire was long to complete, this decision improves the instrument's applicability in practice.

Fairbrother et al., in their assessment of the CFQ's convergent validity, reported a correlation value between CFQ and W-DEQ-A of 0.58 ($p < 0.001$) [25]. Since both the validation process of the W-DEQ-A-Sp and this study were conducted during the same period, it was not possible to explore the convergent validity between both tools. This step has thus been left for future studies.

Another unresolved question is the CFQ-e cut-off points between moderate fear and extreme fear, compared to the 83 and 104 points, respectively, proposed for the CFQ [17]. Further studies in the rest of Spain should explore and confirm the cut-off points, taking into account the fact that the scores must be adjusted (total score between 0 and 148 points for the CFQ-e, unlike the CFQ, whose total score can range between 0 and 160 points). Another line to explore is converting the scores to a standard scale, for example, with values 0–100, which would facilitate comparisons with other studies.

The study presented a number of limitations. We chose non-probabilistic convenience sampling, i.e., a type of sampling which presents certain shortcomings. We do not believe, however, that this affected the sample's representativeness. Indeed, pregnant women were recruited from a large number of health centres. Moreover, numerous professionals, both obstetricians and midwives, also participated in the process. In addition, the sociodemographic and clinical characteristics of the Canarian's pregnant population can be considered to be similar to the rest of Spain's pregnant women, so the CFQ-e properties can be generalised.

A notable limitation is that women were recruited exclusively from public health services. Therefore, no data were obtained for women who had chosen to follow-up their pregnancies exclusively in private centres or services.

The present study was conducted in 2020, the year in which the SARS-CoV-2 global pandemic unfolded, also affecting pregnant women around the world [62]. This situation had an impact both on the data collection and women's emotions, so it should be considered as a possible external confounding factor. In this respect, several studies have highlighted the influence of the pandemic on pregnant women's mental health [63–65], so we can consider that the pandemic did influence the results obtained in this study.

5. Conclusions

The present work is the second validation study of a FOC evaluation instrument in Spain and the first validation of the CFQ in a non-English-speaking setting. The Spanish version of the CFQ (CFQ-e) consists of thirty-seven items distributed into four subscales or dimensions: "fear of medical interventions", "fear of harm and dying", "fear of pain" and "fears relating to sexual aspects and embarrassment". The psychometric characteristics of the CFQ-e indicate that this instrument is useful, valid and reliable to measure fear of childbirth. In addition, it allows one to assess different dimensions associated with FOC in the Spanish population.

Further studies are needed to evaluate the prevalence of FOC in Spanish settings, as well as to explore the convergent validity of CFQ-e with other FOC measurement instruments.

Supplementary Materials: The following supporting information can be downloaded at: https://www.mdpi.com/article/10.3390/jcm11071843/s1, Table S1: First version of the CFQ-e; Table S2: Profile and CVI-E of the experts; Table S3: CVI-I scores for each CFQ-e item; Table S4: Floor and ceiling scores, means and standard deviation for each item in the interference scale; Table S5: Factor loadings obtained in the EFA of the model of 4 factors/40 items; Table S6: Factor loadings obtained in the CFA of the four-factor, 40-item model; Table S7: Table of data congruence indices with the semi-specified four-factor, 40-item model based on the results of the first sample's EFA; Table S8: root mean square discrepancy between rotated loading matrix and target matrix; Table S9: Final version of the CFQ-e (English and Spanish version); Table S10: CFQ-e reliability scores.

Author Contributions: Conceptualisation, H.G.-d.l.T., C.R.-O., A.D.-G. and C.P.-B.; methodology, H.G.-d.l.T., A.D.-G., C.P.-B., C.R.-O. and J.V.-S.; software, H.G.-d.l.T., M.B.-P. and J.V.-S.; formal analysis, H.G.-d.l.T., M.B.-P. and J.V.-S.; investigation, H.G.-d.l.T., A.D.-G., C.P.-B. and C.R.-O.; writing—original draft preparation, H.G.-d.l.T.; writing—review and editing, H.G.-d.l.T., M.B.-P. and J.V.-S. All authors have read and agreed to the published version of the manuscript.

Funding: This research received no external funding.

Institutional Review Board Statement: The study was conducted according to the guidelines of the Declaration of Helsinki and approved by the Ethics Committee of Universityy Hospital of Gran Canaria Dr. Negrín (CEI/CEIm HUGCDN, CEIm HUGCDN Code: 2020-264-1) (protocol code 2020-264-1 Date 4 June 2020).

Informed Consent Statement: Informed consent was obtained from all subjects involved in the study.

Data Availability Statement: The data used in this research are confidential and are protected in a coded and anonymised database kept by the research group in accordance with Spanish regulations. Because of the sensitive nature of the questions asked in this study, respondents were assured that the raw data would be kept confidential and would not be shared. However, the raw data from the CFQ-e survey (response to each item) and without the rest of the sociodemographic–obstetric variables could be shared with those researchers who contact the corresponding authors with a reasonable and logical request.

Acknowledgments: Thanks to all the women who participated in this study, the 10 experts who participated in the content validation process, the midwife Julia Jeppesen and the obstetrician Ismael Ortega who participated in the translation process of the questionnaire, the Multi-Professional Educational Unit of Obstetrics and Gynaecology of las Palmas de Gran Canaria and to all the midwives and obstetricians who collaborated in the data collection.

Conflicts of Interest: The authors declare no conflict of interest.

References

1. Wijma, K. Why focus on 'fear of childbirth'? *J. Psychosom. Obstet. Gynecol.* **2003**, *24*, 141–143. [CrossRef]
2. O'Connell, M.; Leahy-Warren, P.; Khashan, A.S.; Kenny, L.C. Tocophobia—The new hysteria? *Obstet. Gynaecol. Reprod. Med.* **2015**, *25*, 175–177. [CrossRef]
3. Jomeen, J.; Martin, C.R.; Jones, C.; Marshall, C.; Ayers, S.; Burt, K.; Frodsham, L.; Horsch, A.; Midwinter, D.; O'Connell, M.; et al. Tokophobia and fear of birth: A workshop consensus statement on current issues and recommendations for future research. *J. Reprod. Infant Psychol.* **2021**, *39*, 2–15. [CrossRef] [PubMed]
4. Ayers, S. Fear of childbirth, postnatal post-traumatic stress disorder and midwifery care. *Midwifery* **2014**, *30*, 145–148. [CrossRef]
5. Raisanen, S.; Lehto, S.; Nielsen, H.; Gissler, M.; Kramer, M.; Heinonen, S.; Lehto, S. Fear of childbirth in nulliparous and multiparous women: A population-based analysis of all singleton births in Finland in 1997–2010. *BJOG Int. J. Obstet. Gynaecol.* **2014**, *121*, 965–970. [CrossRef] [PubMed]
6. Rondung, E.; Thomtén, J.; Sundin, Ö. Psychological perspectives on fear of childbirth. *J. Anxiety Disord.* **2016**, *44*, 80–91. [CrossRef]
7. Demšar, K.; Svetina, M.; Verdenik, I.; Tul, N.; Blickstein, I.; Velikonja, V.G. Tokophobia (fear of childbirth): Prevalence and risk factors. *J. Périnat. Med.* **2017**, *46*, 151–154. [CrossRef] [PubMed]
8. Nilsson, C.; Hessman, E.; Sjöblom, H.; Dencker, A.; Jangsten, E.; Mollberg, M.; Patel, H.; Sparud-Lundin, C.; Wigert, H.; Begley, C. Definitions, measurements and prevalence of fear of childbirth: A systematic review. *BMC Pregnancy Childbirth* **2018**, *18*. [CrossRef]
9. O'Connell, M.A.; Leahy-Warren, P.; Khashan, A.S.; Kenny, L.C.; O'Neill, S.M. Worldwide prevalence of tocophobia in pregnant women: Systematic review and meta-analysis. *Acta Obstet. Et Gynecol. Scand.* **2017**, *96*, 907–920. [CrossRef] [PubMed]
10. O'Connell, M.A.; Khashan, A.S.; Leahy-Warren, P.; Stewart, F.; O'Neill, S.M. Interventions for fear of childbirth including tocophobia. *Cochrane Database Syst. Rev.* **2021**, *2021*, CD013321. [CrossRef]
11. Richens, Y.; Hindley, C.; Lavender, T. A national online survey of UK maternity unit service provision for women with fear of birth. *Br. J. Midwifery* **2015**, *23*, 574–579. [CrossRef]
12. Nath, S.; Busuulwa, P.; Ryan, E.G.; Challacombe, F.L.; Howard, L.M. The characteristics and prevalence of phobias in pregnancy. *Midwifery* **2019**, *82*, 102590. [CrossRef] [PubMed]
13. O'Connell, M.; Martin, C.; Jomeen, J. Reconsidering fear of birth: Language matters. *Midwifery* **2021**, *102*, 103079. [CrossRef] [PubMed]
14. O'Connell, M.A.; Leahy-Warren, P.; Kenny, L.C.; O'Neill, S.M.; Khashan, A.S. The prevalence and risk factors of fear of childbirth among pregnant women: A cross-sectional study in Ireland. *Acta Obstet. Et Gynecol. Scand.* **2019**, *98*, 1014–1023. [CrossRef] [PubMed]
15. Jokić-Begić, N.; Žigić, L.; Radoš, S.N. Anxiety and anxiety sensitivity as predictors of fear of childbirth: Different patterns for nulliparous and parous women. *J. Psychosom. Obstet. Gynecol.* **2013**, *35*, 22–28. [CrossRef]
16. Weaver, J.; Browne, J.; Aras-Payne, A.; Magill-Cuerden, J. A comprehensive systematic review of the impact of planned interventions offered to pregnant women who have requested a caesarean section as a result of tokophobia (fear of childbirth). *JBI Libr. Syst. Rev.* **2012**, *10*, 1–20. [CrossRef]
17. Fairbrother, N.; Thordarson, D.S.; Stoll, K. Fine tuning fear of childbirth: The relationship between Childbirth Fear Questionnaire subscales and demographic and reproductive variables. *J. Reprod. Infant Psychol.* **2017**, *36*, 15–29. [CrossRef] [PubMed]
18. Richens, Y.; Smith, D.M.; Lavender, D.T. Fear of birth in clinical practice: A structured review of current measurement tools. *Sex. Reprod. Health* **2018**, *16*, 98–112. [CrossRef] [PubMed]
19. Ortega-Cejas, C.M.; Roldán-Merino, J.; Biurrun-Garrido, A.; Isabel Castrillo-Pérez, M.I.; Vicente-Hernández, M.M.; Lluch-Canut, T.; Cabrera-Jaime, S. Fear of Childbirth: Literature review of measuring intruments. *Matronas Prof.* **2019**, *20*, e36–e42.
20. Striebich, S.; Mattern, E.; Ayerle, G.M. Support for pregnant women identified with fear of childbirth (FOC)/tokophobia— A systematic review of approaches and interventions. *Midwifery* **2018**, *61*, 97–115. [CrossRef]
21. Wijma, K.; Wijma, B.; Zar, M. Psychometric aspects of the W-DEQ; a new questionnaire for the measurement of fear of childbirth. *J. Psychosom. Obstet. Gynecol.* **1998**, *19*, 84–97. [CrossRef] [PubMed]

22. Stoll, K.; Fairbrother, N.; Thordarson, D.S. Childbirth Fear: Relation to Birth and Care Provider Preferences. *J. Midwifery Women's Health* **2018**, *63*, 58–67. [CrossRef] [PubMed]
23. Slade, P.; Balling, K.; Sheen, K.; Houghton, G. Establishing a valid construct of fear of childbirth: Findings from in-depth interviews with women and midwives. *BMC Pregnancy Childbirth* **2019**, *19*, 96. [CrossRef] [PubMed]
24. Slade, P.; Pais, T.; Fairlie, F.; Simpson, A.; Sheen, K. The development of the Slade-Pais Expectations of Childbirth Scale (SPECS). *J. Reprod. Infant Psychol.* **2016**, *34*, 495–510. [CrossRef]
25. Fairbrother, N.; Collardeau, F.; Albert, A.; Stoll, K. The Childbirth Fear Questionnaire: A New Measure of Fear of Childbirth. Research Square. *Int. J. Environ. Res. Public Health* **2022**, *19*, 2223. [CrossRef]
26. Ryding, E.L.; Lukasse, M.; Van Parys, A.-S.; Wangel, A.-M.; Karro, H.; Kristjansdottir, H.; Schroll, A.-M.; Schei, B.; Bidens Group. Fear of childbirth and risk of cesarean delivery: A cohort study in six European countries. *Birth* **2015**, *42*, 48–55. [CrossRef]
27. Olieman, R.M.; Siemonsma, F.; Bartens, M.A.; Garthus-Niegel, S.; Scheele, F.; Honig, A. The effect of an elective cesarean section on maternal request on peripartum anxiety and depression in women with childbirth fear: A systematic review. *BMC Pregnancy Childbirth* **2017**, *17*, 195. [CrossRef]
28. Larsson, B.; Karlström, A.; Rubertsson, C.; Hildingsson, I. Counseling for childbirth fear-a national survey. *Sex. Reprod. Health* **2016**, *8*, 82–87. [CrossRef]
29. Mena-Tudela, D.; Iglesias-Casás, S.; González-Chordá, V.M.; Cervera-Gasch, Á.; Andreu-Pejó, L.; Valero-Chillerón, M.J. Obstetric Violence in Spain (Part I): Women's Perception and Interterritorial Differences. *Int. J. Environ. Res. Public Health* **2020**, *17*, 7726. [CrossRef]
30. Ortega-Cejas, C.M.; Roldán-Merino, J.; Lluch-Canut, T.; Castrillo-Pérez, M.I.; Vicente-Hernández, M.M.; Jimenez-Barragan, M.; Biurrun-Garrido, A.; Farres-Tarafa, M.; Casas, I.; Cabrera-Jaime, S. Reliability and validity study of the Spanish adaptation of the "Wijma Delivery Expectancy/Experience Questionnaire" (W-DEQ-A). *PLoS ONE* **2021**, *16*, e0248595. [CrossRef]
31. Roldán-Merino, J.; Ortega-Cejas, C.M.; Lluch-Canut, T.; Farres-Tarafa, M.; Biurrun-Garrido, A.; Casas, I.; Castrillo-Pérez, M.I.; Vicente-Hernández, M.M.; Jimenez-Barragan, M.; Martínez-Mondejar, R.; et al. Validity and reliability of the Spanish version of the "Wijma Delivery Expectancy/Experience Questionnaire" (W-DEQ-B). *PLoS ONE* **2021**, *16*, e0249942. [CrossRef]
32. Sousa, V.D.; Rojjanasrirat, W. Translation, adaptation and validation of instruments or scales for use in cross-cultural health care research: A clear and user-friendly guideline. *J. Eval. Clin. Pr.* **2010**, *17*, 268–274. [CrossRef] [PubMed]
33. Polit, D.F.; Beck, C.T. The content validity index: Are you sure you know what's being reported? critique and recommendations. *Res. Nurs. Health* **2006**, *29*, 489–497. [CrossRef] [PubMed]
34. Beckstead, J.W. Content validity is naught. *Int. J. Nurs. Stud.* **2009**, *46*, 1274–1283. [CrossRef] [PubMed]
35. Ferrando, P.J.; Lorenzo-Seva, U.; Hernández-Dorado, A.; Muñiz, J. Decálogo para el Análisis Factorial de los Ítems de un Test. *Psicothema* **2022**, *34*, 7–17. [PubMed]
36. Lloret-Segura, S.; Ferreres-Traver, A.; Hernandez, A.; Tomás, I. Exploratory Item Factor Analysis: A practical guide revised and updated. *An. De Psicol.* **2014**, *30*, 1151–1169. [CrossRef]
37. Lorenzo-Seva, U.; Ferrando, P.J. FACTOR: A computer program to fit the exploratory factor analysis model. *Behav. Res. Methods* **2006**, *38*, 88–91. [CrossRef]
38. Lorenzo-Seva, U.; Ferrando, P.J. FACTOR 9.2: A comprehensive program for fitting exploratory and semiconfirmatory factor analysis and IRT models. *Appl. Psychol. Meas.* **2013**, *37*, 497–498. [CrossRef]
39. Ferrando, P.J.; Lorenzo-Seva, U. Program FACTOR at 10: Origins, development and future directions. *Psicothema* **2017**, *29*, 236–240. [CrossRef] [PubMed]
40. Lorenzo-Seva, U. SOLOMON: A method for splitting a sample into equivalent subsamples in factor analysis. *Behav. Res. Methods* **2021**. [CrossRef]
41. Lorenzo-Seva, U. Promin: A Method for Oblique Factor Rotation. *Multivar. Behav. Res.* **1999**, *34*, 347–365. [CrossRef]
42. Lorenzo-Seva, U.; Ferrando, P.J. Robust Promin: A method for diagonally weighted factor rotation. *Liberabit* **2019**, *25*, 99–106. [CrossRef]
43. Ferrando, P.J.; Lorenzo-Seva, U. A note on improving EAP trait estimation in oblique factor-analytic and item response theory models. *Psicologica* **2016**, *37*, 235–247.
44. Lorenzo-Seva, U.; Berge, J.M.F.T. Tucker's Congruence Coefficient as a Meaningful Index of Factor Similarity. *Methodology* **2006**, *2*, 57–64. [CrossRef]
45. Ferrando, P.J.; Lorenzo-Seva, U. Assessing the Quality and Appropriateness of Factor Solutions and Factor Score Estimates in Exploratory Item Factor Analysis. *Educ. Psychol. Meas.* **2018**, *78*, 762–780. [CrossRef]
46. Dai, Z.; Zhang, N.; Rong, L.; Ouyang, Y.-Q. Worldwide research on fear of childbirth: A bibliometric analysis. *PLoS ONE* **2020**, *15*, e0236567. [CrossRef]
47. Andaroon, N.; Kordi, M.; Ghasemi, M.; Mazlom, R. The Validity and Reliability of the Wijma Delivery Expectancy/Experience Questionnaire (Version A) in Primiparous Women in Mashhad, Iran. *Iran J. Med. Sci.* **2020**, *45*, 110–117. [CrossRef]
48. Takegata, M.; Haruna, M.; Matsuzaki, M.; Shiraishi, M.; Murayama, R.; Okano, T.; Severinsson, E. Translation and validation of the Japanese version of the Wijma Delivery Expectancy/Experience Questionnaire version A. *Nurs. Health Sci.* **2013**, *15*, 326–332. [CrossRef]
49. Fenaroli, V.; Saita, E. Fear of childbirth: A contribution to the validation of the Italian version of the Wijma Delivery Expectancy/Experience Questionnaire (WDEQ). *TPM-Test. Psychom. Methodol. Appl. Psychol.* **2013**, *20*, 131–154.

50. Pallant, J.F.; Haines, H.M.; Green, P.; Toohill, J.; Gamble, J.; Creedy, D.K.; Fenwick, J. Assessment of the dimensionality of the Wijma delivery expectancy/experience questionnaire using factor analysis and Rasch analysis. *BMC Pregnancy Childbirth* **2016**, *16*, 361. [CrossRef]
51. Ruscio, J.; Roche, B. Determining the number of factors to retain in an exploratory factor analysis using comparison data of known factorial structure. *Psychol. Assess.* **2012**, *24*, 282–292. [CrossRef] [PubMed]
52. Maccallum, R.C.; Widaman, K.; Preacher, K.J.; Hong, S. Sample Size in Factor Analysis: The Role of Model Error. *Multivar. Behav. Res.* **2001**, *36*, 611–637. [CrossRef]
53. Mena-Tudela, D.; Iglesias-Casás, S.; González-Chordá, V.M.; Cervera-Gasch, Á.; Andreu-Pejó, L.; Valero-Chilleron, M.J. Obstetric Violence in Spain (Part II): Interventionism and Medicalization during Birth. *Int. J. Environ. Res. Public Health* **2020**, *18*, 199. [CrossRef] [PubMed]
54. Espada-Trespalacios, X.; Ojeda, F.; Rodrigo, N.N.; Rodriguez-Biosca, A.; Coll, P.R.; Martin-Arribas, A.; Escuriet, R. Induction of labour as compared with spontaneous labour in low-risk women: A multicenter study in Catalonia. *Sex. Reprod. Health* **2021**, *29*, 100648. [CrossRef]
55. Barca, J.; Bravo, C.; Pintado-Recarte, M.; Cueto-Hernández, I.; Ruiz-Labarta, J.; Cuñarro, Y.; Buján, J.; Alvarez-Mon, M.; Ortega, M.; De León-Luis, J. Risk Factors in Third and Fourth Degree Perineal Tears in Women in a Tertiary Centre: An Observational Ambispective Cohort Study. *J. Pers. Med.* **2021**, *11*, 685. [CrossRef] [PubMed]
56. Tavakol, M.; Dennick, R. Making sense of Cronbach's alpha. *Int. J. Med. Educ.* **2011**, *2*, 53–55. [CrossRef] [PubMed]
57. Watkins, M.W. The reliability of multidimensional neuropsychological measures: From alpha to omega. *Clin. Neuropsychol.* **2017**, *31*, 1113–1126. [CrossRef] [PubMed]
58. Deng, L.; Chan, W. Testing the Difference Between Reliability Coefficients Alpha and Omega. *Educ. Psychol. Meas.* **2016**, *77*, 185–203. [CrossRef] [PubMed]
59. Viladrich, C.; Angulo-Brunet, A.; Doval, E. A journey around alpha and omega to estimate internal consistency reliability. *An. Psicol.* **2017**, *33*, 755–782. [CrossRef]
60. Taylor, J.M. Coefficient Omega. *J. Nurs. Educ.* **2021**, *60*, 429–430. [CrossRef] [PubMed]
61. McDonald, R.P. *Test Theory: A Unified Treatment*, 1st ed.; Lawrence Erlbaum Associates, Inc.: Mahwah, NJ, USA, 1999.
62. Wang, C.-L.; Liu, Y.-Y.; Wu, C.-H.; Wang, C.-Y.; Long, C.-Y. Impact of COVID-19 on Pregnancy. *Int. J. Med. Sci.* **2021**, *18*, 763–767. [CrossRef] [PubMed]
63. Yan, H.; Ding, Y.; Guo, W. Mental Health of Pregnant and Postpartum Women During the Coronavirus Disease 2019 Pandemic: A Systematic Review and Meta-Analysis. *Front. Psychol.* **2020**, *11*, 617001. [CrossRef] [PubMed]
64. Hessami, K.; Romanelli, C.; Chiurazzi, M.; Cozzolino, M. COVID-19 pandemic and maternal mental health: A systematic review and meta-analysis. *J. Matern. Neonatal Med.* **2020**, 1–8. [CrossRef]
65. Ayora, A.F.; Salas-Medina, P.; Collado-Boira, E.; Ropero-Padilla, C.; Rodriguez-Arrastia, M.; Bernat-Adell, M.D. Pregnancy during the COVID-19 pandemic: A cross-sectional observational descriptive study. *Nurs. Open* **2021**, *8*, 3016–3023. [CrossRef] [PubMed]

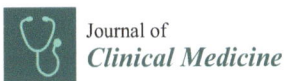

Article

Better Estimation of Spontaneous Preterm Birth Prediction Performance through Improved Gestational Age Dating

Julja Burchard [1,*], George R. Saade [2], Kim A. Boggess [3], Glenn R. Markenson [4], Jay D. Iams [5], Dean V. Coonrod [6], Leonardo M. Pereira [7], Matthew K. Hoffman [8], Ashoka D. Polpitiya [1], Ryan Treacy [1], Angela C. Fox [1], Todd L. Randolph [1], Tracey C. Fleischer [1], Max T. Dufford [1], Thomas J. Garite [1], Gregory C. Critchfield [1], J. Jay Boniface [1] and Paul E. Kearney [1]

[1] Sera Prognostics, Incorporated, Salt Lake City, UT 84109, USA; ashoka@seraprognostics.com (A.D.P.); rtreacy@seraprognostics.com (R.T.); afox@seraprognostics.com (A.C.F.); trandolph@seraprognostics.com (T.L.R.); tfleischer@seraprognostics.com (T.C.F.); mdufford@seraprognostics.com (M.T.D.); tgarite@seraprognostics.com (T.J.G.); gcritchfield@seraprognostics.com (G.C.C.); jboniface@seraprognostics.com (J.J.B.); pkearney@seraprognostics.com (P.E.K.)

[2] Department of Obstetrics & Gynecology, The University of Texas Medical Branch, Galveston, TX 77555, USA; gsaade@utmb.edu

[3] Department of Obstetrics and Gynecology, Division of Maternal-Fetal Medicine, University of North Carolina, Chapel Hill, NC 27599, USA; kim_boggess@med.unc.edu

[4] Maternal Fetal Medicine, Boston University School of Medicine, Boston, MA 02118, USA; glenn.markenson@bmc.org

[5] Department of Obstetrics & Gynecology, The Ohio State University, Columbus, OH 43210, USA; jdiamsmd@outlook.com

[6] Department of Obstetrics and Gynecology, Valleywise Health, Phoenix, AZ 85008, USA; dean_coonrod@dmgaz.org

[7] Division of Maternal-Fetal Medicine, Oregon Health & Science University, Portland, OR 97239, USA; pereiral@ohsu.edu

[8] Department of Obstetrics & Gynecology, Christiana Care Health System, Newark, DE 19718, USA; mhoffman@christianacare.org

* Correspondence: jburchard@seraprognostics.com; Tel.: +1-801-990-0597

Abstract: The clinical management of pregnancy and spontaneous preterm birth (sPTB) relies on estimates of gestational age (GA). Our objective was to evaluate the effect of GA dating uncertainty on the observed performance of a validated proteomic biomarker risk predictor, and then to test the generalizability of that effect in a broader range of GA at blood draw. In a secondary analysis of a prospective clinical trial (PAPR; NCT01371019), we compared two GA dating categories: both ultrasound and dating by last menstrual period (LMP) (all subjects) and excluding dating by LMP (excluding LMP). The risk predictor's performance was observed at the validated risk predictor threshold both in weeks $19^{1/7}$–$20^{6/7}$ and extended to weeks $18^{0/7}$–$20^{6/7}$. Strict blinding and independent statistical analyses were employed. The validated biomarker risk predictor showed greater observed sensitivity of 88% at 75% specificity (increases of 17% and 1%) in more reliably dated (excluding-LMP) subjects, relative to all subjects. Excluding dating by LMP significantly improved the sensitivity in weeks $19^{1/7}$–$20^{6/7}$. In the broader blood draw window, the previously validated risk predictor threshold significantly stratified higher and lower risk of sPTB, and the risk predictor again showed significantly greater observed sensitivity in excluding-LMP subjects. These findings have implications for testing the performance of models aimed at predicting PTB.

Keywords: gestational age; gestational age dating; preterm birth; spontaneous preterm birth; proteomic biomarker risk predictor

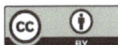

1. Introduction

Preterm birth (PTB), including both spontaneous (sPTB) and indicated delivery earlier than 37 weeks of gestational age (GA), is the leading global cause of perinatal morbidity and mortality [1]. Each year, PTB occurs in more than 10% of U.S. births [2,3]. For decades, these estimates have remained essentially unchanged, despite evolving medical technologies and clinical practices. The economic impact of PTB on the U.S. healthcare system is immense, estimated to exceed USD 25 billion annually [4]. Thus, effectively addressing PTB persists as a critical need.

PTB is an adverse outcome defined by a single endpoint: delivery before an established time period as measured by an estimate of GA [5]. Consequently, uncertainty in GA dating, defined as the variability observed between the estimated and actual GA, affects the observed performance of a predictor of PTB. Further, the clinical management of pregnancy relies on GA, which is set by establishing the estimated due date (EDD) following professional society recommendations and guidelines [6,7]. Conventionally, in the United States, the EDD is set at 280 days following the first day of the last menstrual period (LMP). However, LMP dating assumes a regular, 28-day menstrual cycle with ovulation on day 14 and set timing for implantation, though studies have shown that approximately half of all women do not recall their precise LMP date [7–10]. Even when the LMP is known, it is surprisingly uncertain in determining the EDD, with a 95% confidence interval of ±29 days [11,12]. Today, ultrasound measurements during the first trimester of pregnancy are considered the most certain method for establishing (or confirming) GA [7–9,13–16]. Ultrasound measurements through week 21 of pregnancy are regarded as standard in the obstetric estimation of EDD and can be used to confirm or replace an LMP-established EDD. Pregnancies dated by LMP without confirmation or revision based on ultrasound examination before week 22 of gestation are considered to show sub-optimal dating [7,17].

The successful application of any PTB-preventive strategy is enabled by the early and accurate identification of higher-risk pregnancies. Here, we consider the performance of a risk factor or predictor in terms of how well it identifies pregnancies destined for sPTB. A history of prior PTB and short cervical length in the current pregnancy are clinically accepted risk factors for sPTB but combine to detect less than 20% of singleton sPTBs [18,19]. A range of additional factors including body mass index (BMI), smoking, substance use and socioeconomic circumstances are commonly considered on a case-by-case basis in evaluating PTB risk but are not sufficiently prognostic for clinical use; instead, they are seen to provide opportunities for preconception and post-partum care. Untapped potential exists to develop tools, including molecular biomarkers, that sensitively identify PTB risk early in pregnancy, providing opportunities for risk-ameliorating interventions in addition to current options for acute care. Increasing true-positive and true-negative rates for prognostic tests improves the targeting of interventions and the allocation of resources, respectively.

Saade et al. [20] broadly validated a proteomic biomarker risk predictor for the assessment of sPTB risk in serum collected from asymptomatic singleton pregnancies in the United States at weeks $19^{1/7}$–$20^{6/7}$ of gestation [21]. This risk predictor is based on the ratio of insulin-like-growth-factor-binding protein 4 (IBP4) and sex-hormone-binding globulin (SHBG). Clinical validation of the test was performed in an independent and representative set of women from the prospective Proteomic Assessment of Preterm Risk (PAPR) study (NCT01371019) [20], a large, multicenter, observational study that enrolled a diverse population across 14 U.S. sites, emphasizing academic medical centers. The PAPR analysis established a predictive biomarker threshold score that significantly stratifies premature from later GAs at birth and corresponds to a 15% risk, i.e., a twofold increase compared with the average risk across U.S. singleton pregnancies [6]. Subsequently, this threshold was validated in subjects from an independent, prospective cohort (Multicenter Assessment of a Spontaneous Preterm Birth Risk Predictor (TREETOP; NCT02787213) [22,23]. The prediction of health outcomes related to prematurity by these biomarkers also was confirmed in TREETOP [22].

The PAPR trial was concluded prior to the publication of current American College of Obstetricians and Gynecologists (ACOG) guidelines for GA dating [7]. The objectives of our current study were: (1) to estimate biomarker risk predictor performance more accurately by restricting the analysis of the PAPR cohort to women who have more certain GA dating as per current practice guidelines; and (2) to test the generalizability of the effect of dating certainty upon observed performance amongst these women, by comparing performance in the previously established blood draw window of $19^{1/7}$–$20^{6/7}$ weeks' GA with that for a broader GA window, $18^{0/7}$–$20^{6/7}$ weeks.

2. Materials and Methods

The current study was a secondary analysis of the prospective PAPR clinical trial (NCT01371019), using only subjects held out for validation and not employed in the discovery or verification of biomarker prediction [20]. The PAPR study enrolled 5501 pregnant women between $17^{0/7}$ and $28^{6/7}$ weeks' GA across 11 sites in the United States for the purpose of discovering and validating a biomarker prediction of spontaneous preterm delivery (sPTB). The PAPR study was approved by the Institutional Review Boards/Ethics Committees of all participating study sites. Informed consent was obtained from all subjects involved in the study. The PAPR study was conducted before the ACOG Committee Opinion 700 (CO 700), which provides guidance on GA dating, was issued [7].

In the current analysis, we compared the performance of the proteomic biomarker risk predictor as published for women dated using any available method [20] against test performance observed in the subset of women whose pregnancies were dated with more certainty. For the purposes of our current analysis, GA calculated directly from a first- or second-trimester ultrasound was considered more certain, while GA calculated using LMP was considered less certain, consistent with current practice standards [7]. To evaluate the generalizability of the effects of GA dating on observed test performance, we also compared risk predictor performance among more certainly dated subjects. These included subjects in both the previously established blood draw window of $19^{1/7}$–$20^{6/7}$ weeks' GA and in a broader GA window of $18^{0/7}$–$20^{6/7}$ weeks, inclusive of subjects not previously assessed by these measures. The primary outcome measured was the predictive performance of the test, the endpoints for which included a regression test for sPTB case classifications, sensitivity, specificity, area under the receiver operating curve (AUC), positive predictive value (PPV) and negative predictive value (NPV), evaluated at the validated biomarker threshold score [20,23].

2.1. Study Population

The evaluated study population was the PAPR validation cohort [20], for which data were prospectively collected under a strict blinding protocol. The sample size was sufficient to power the study to >80%, assuming an AUC of 0.75 and an alpha of 0.05, and to power a regression test of classification at the validated threshold with 75% sensitivity and 74% specificity. BMI in the PAPR population was derived from height and prepregnancy self-reported weight and reported in two categories: (1) "All BMI", representing the full range of BMI scores; and (2) "Stratified BMI", which only included BMI scores in the range of >22–≤ 37 kg/m^2. Deliveries were classified as term births ($\geq 37^{0/7}$ weeks GA) or sPTBs.

2.2. Gestational Age Dating and Estimated Delivery Date

The PAPR clinical trial protocol specified an algorithm for the assessment of GA and EDD. In recognition of the importance of dating certainty, the protocol specified that ultrasound was the preferred method of dating and, when possible, the earliest available ultrasound should be used for GA determination. LMP was to be used on its own only in the absence of other dating methods. When both ultrasound and LMP were available, subjects were dated using LMP if the LMP date was <7 days different from a 1st-trimester ultrasound date, <10 days different from an early 2nd-trimester ultrasound date ($14^{0/7}$–$20^{0/7}$), <14 days different from a late 2nd-trimester ultrasound date ($20^{1/7}$–$27^{6/7}$), or <21 days different from a 3rd-trimester ultrasound date. Among 4285 PAPR subjects who had a record of GA dating method, 37.3% were dated by a 1st-trimester ultrasound, 11.0% by an early 2nd-trimester ultrasound, 2.1% by a late 2nd-trimester ultrasound and 49.5% by LMP. We classified subjects with a record of direct use of LMP to establish the EDD as "LMP" and all others as "excluding LMP." This was a conservative assumption, in that subjects without a record of a GA dating method were included in the excluding-LMP group. The population of subjects dated by any method (all subjects) was compared to the excluding-LMP subset population.

2.3. Sample Analysis

Samples were analyzed in a Clinical Laboratory Improvement Amendments, College of American Pathologists and New York State Department of Health certified laboratory according to a previously described standard operating protocol [20,21]. Briefly, serum samples were depleted of the 14 most abundant proteins, reduced, alkylated, and digested with trypsin. Samples then were spiked with stable isotope standard peptides for proteins of interest, desalted, and analyzed using reverse phase liquid chromatography, followed by multiple reaction monitoring mass spectrometry. Relative levels of IBP4 and SHBG were expressed as response ratios of the peak area for the endogenous peptide divided by the peak area of the stable isotopic standard peptide. The IBP4/SHBG proteomic biomarker was calculated as: ln(IBP4 response ratio/SHBG response ratio). Measurements within 10% of the standard analytic error (standard deviation of replicates) of the test were considered equivalent.

2.4. Statistical Analysis

All analyses of AUC, sensitivity, and specificity tested predefined hypotheses using a prespecified statistical analysis plan. The blinded assessment of hypotheses was conducted by a third-party statistician. In post hoc analyses, NPV and PPV were calculated from sensitivity, specificity, and an sPTB prevalence of 7.3%, as specified [20]. NPV and PPV confidence intervals were calculated as appropriate for a case–control study [24]. Means not contained within comparator 95% confidence intervals indicated significant differences in predictor performance metrics. Analyses were performed in R 3.5 or higher, using the packages data.table [25], pROC [26], and binom [27].

2.5. Estimation of the Effects of Certainty of Gestational Age Dating on Prediction of Prematurity

We simulated the effects of dating uncertainty on observed predictor performance using the 2019 distribution in the United States of GA at birth [28] and a simplification of intervals in guidelines for the use of ultrasound dates provided in ACOG CO 700 [7].

The United States' national distribution of GA at birth for singleton pregnancies was retrieved from the CDC for 2019, the most recent full year of data not known to be affected by the COVID-19 pandemic [28]. Spline interpolation was used to convert CDC GAs at birth from weeks to days.

ACOG guidelines' intervals for the confirmation of LMP by ultrasound were used as the half-widths of 95% confidence intervals of ultrasound dates: 7 days for 1st-trimester dating and 10 days for 2nd-trimester dating. The two-standard-deviation interval for LMP dating has been reported to be 29 days for known LMP and 53 days for uncertain LMP [11]. Based on known similar centers [7,8] and independent spreads of LMP and ultrasound dating and the above standard deviations with the assumption of normally distributed values, we estimated that about half of LMP dates would be confirmed by a 2nd-trimester ultrasound, with a two-standard-deviation interval of 14 days for the confirmed LMP dates.

We defined a perfect predictor that assigned high risk probabilities to all births below 37 weeks of GA and low risk probabilities to all births at or above 37 weeks of GA. Random sets of 0.1% of births were selected 20 times. Each set was assigned GA dating types at prevalences observed in PAPR: half LMP confirmed by ultrasound, half pure ultrasound. Random normally distributed noise was added to the GAs at birth to simulate uncertainty in

GA dating, calculated with a mean of zero and standard deviations derived from guidelines as established [7]. Lastly, the predictor perfectly matched to the original GAs was tested for the AUC of the prediction of PTB amongst the adjusted GAs.

3. Results

Table 1 summarizes the characteristics of the subjects in the study, with comparisons between the all-subject population and the excluding-LMP population for the GA windows of weeks $18^{0/7}$–$20^{6/7}$ and $19^{1/7}$–$20^{6/7}$. No significant differences were observed between the two populations across a range of demographic and clinical parameters.

Table 1. Demographic comparison of all-subject and excluding-LMP (not dated by first day of last menstrual period) populations in gestational age weeks $19^{1/7}$–$20^{6/7}$ and $18^{0/7}$–$20^{6/7}$.

Demographic/ Clinical Variable	Value	Weeks $19^{1/7}$–$20^{6/7}$			Weeks $18^{0/7}$–$20^{6/7}$		
		All-Subjects	Excluding LMP	p-Value	All Subjects	Excluding LMP	p-Value
Maternal age	Median (IQR)	24.5 (21.0–30.0)	23 (21.0–28.0)	0.72	24.5 (22.0–31.0)	23.0 (21.5–28.0)	0.7
Maternal BMI	Median (IQR)	26.5 (22.3–31.3)	28.5 (23.8–34.6)	0.7	28.0 (23.5–32.0)	29.4 (24.4–34.6)	0.7
Gravida	Primigravida	13	7	1	24	11	0.83
	Multigravida	41	22		60	33	
Race	Black	13	5	0.76	17	8	0.95
	White	38	23		61	33	
	Other	3	1		6	3	
Ethnicity	Hispanic	22	12	0.97	36	20	0.9
	Non-Hispanic	32	17		48	24	
Prior PTB	No	34	19	0.9	50	29	0.76
	Yes	20	10		34	15	
GABD	Median (IQR)	139 (135–144)	139 (135–144)	0.96	135 (130.5–142.5)	135 (130–143)	0.98
GAB	Median (IQR)	273 (256–281)	273 (258–277)	0.98	273 (256–281)	273 (257–277)	0.96
Neonatal gender	Female	22	21	0.34	39	17	0.46
	Male	32	8		45	27	
Outcome	Cases	18	10	0.95	28	15	0.97
	Controls	36	19		56	29	
	Total	54	29		84	44	

Continuous data: 2-sided Wilcoxon test. Medians and IQRs are shown. Categorical data: 2-sided Fisher's Exact test. Counts are shown. IQR, interquartile ratio; excluding LMP, not dated by first day of last menstrual period. GAB, gestational age at birth; GABD, gestational age at blood draw; LMP, last menstrual period; PTB, preterm birth.

Figure 1 shows the expected performance of a simulated perfect PTB predictor on subjects with GAs determined by LMP or excluding-LMP dating, interpreted as per ACOG CO 700 guidance. Performance was significantly lower with LMP than with excluding-LMP dating (mean LMP AUC: 0.79; mean excluding-LMP AUC: 0.89; p-value < 0.001).

Applying the ACOG estimates of reliability of dating to the present study, we estimated that in weeks $19^{1/7}$–$20^{6/7}$, three births labeled as sPTB in the all-subject population and one in the excluding-LMP group were likely to have been term births, while less than one term birth in each was likely to be a misclassified PTB. In weeks $18^{0/7}$–$20^{6/7}$, we estimated that at least one additional sPTB and one additional term birth were likely to have been misclassified.

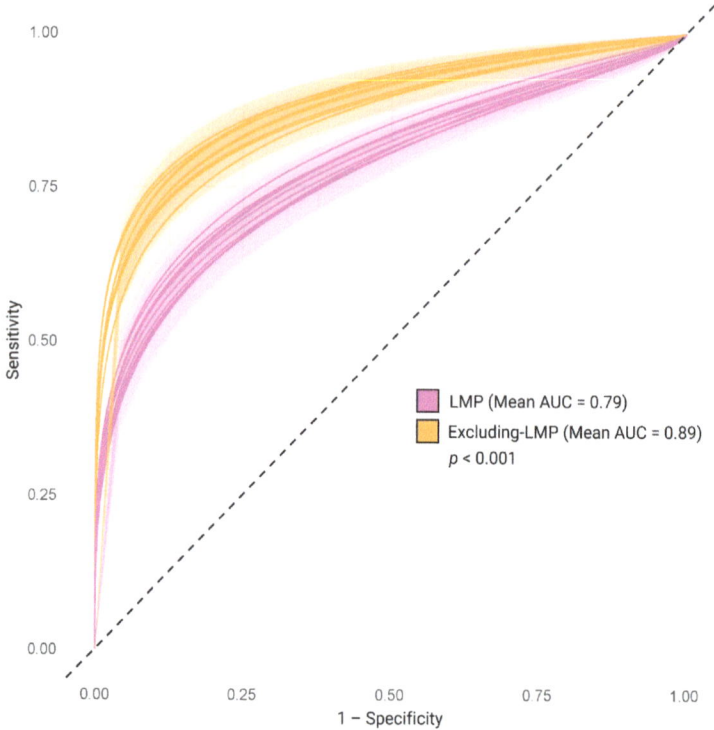

Figure 1. Performance of a hypothetical perfect preterm birth risk predictor using first date of last menstrual period (LMP) or excluding-LMP gestational age dating. Darker curves represent individual simulations, while the shaded area represents the 95% confidence interval of sensitivity at each value of 1 − specificity. AUC, area under the receiver operating curve.

Risk Predictor Performance

The AUC of the proteomic biomarker sPTB risk predictor was significant in the validated draw window, weeks $19^{1/7}$–$20^{6/7}$, for both all subjects (0.75) and excluding-LMP subjects (0.80) in the BMI-stratified population. Similarly, the correlation between the sPTB risk predictor and GA at birth was significant in both populations, with Pearson correlation coefficients −0.6 and −0.5 in the all-subject and excluding-LMP, BMI-stratified populations, respectively. At the validated threshold and the range of GA at blood draw reported in Saade et al. [28], the sPTB risk predictor showed previously reported performance within the all-subject BMI-stratified population, extended here with additional descriptive statistics: 75% sensitivity, 74% specificity, 18% PPV, and 97% NPV. At the same threshold in the excluding-LMP, BMI-stratified population, the sPTB risk predictor showed higher performance, with 88% sensitivity, 75% specificity, 22% PPV, and 99% NPV. The only significant difference in performance between the all-subject population and the excluding-LMP population was in sensitivity, although point estimates were generally numerically higher in the excluding-LMP population, while confidence intervals overlapped.

To test whether these observations extended to additional subjects whose samples were collected in a broader GA blood draw window, we compared the performance of the risk predictor in excluding-LMP subjects with blood drawn in weeks $19^{1/7}$–$20^{6/7}$ versus that in weeks $18^{0/7}$–$20^{6/7}$. As a baseline observation, we found that the validated threshold significantly stratified higher- from lower-risk subjects in weeks $18^{0/7}$–$20^{6/7}$. Additionally, there was no significant difference in sPTB risk predictor performance in the excluding-LMP population in weeks $18^{0/7}$–$20^{6/7}$ compared to $19^{1/7}$–$20^{6/7}$. Sensitivity, specificity, PPV, and NPV at the validated threshold did not differ, nor did AUC and correlation to GA at birth. As well, values did not differ significantly by BMI stratification. However, sensitivity was significantly improved in weeks $18^{0/7}$–$20^{6/7}$ in the excluding-LMP population as compared to the all-subject population. Specificity, NPV, PPV, AUC, and correlation to GA at birth showed numerical increases in point estimates in the excluding-LMP population relative to the all-subject population, with overlapping confidence intervals. Figure 2 shows the separation in risk predictor scores between sPTBs and term births (controls) for the excluding-LMP population across GA at blood draw, relative to (A) the proteomic biomarker risk predictor score and (B) the validated threshold.

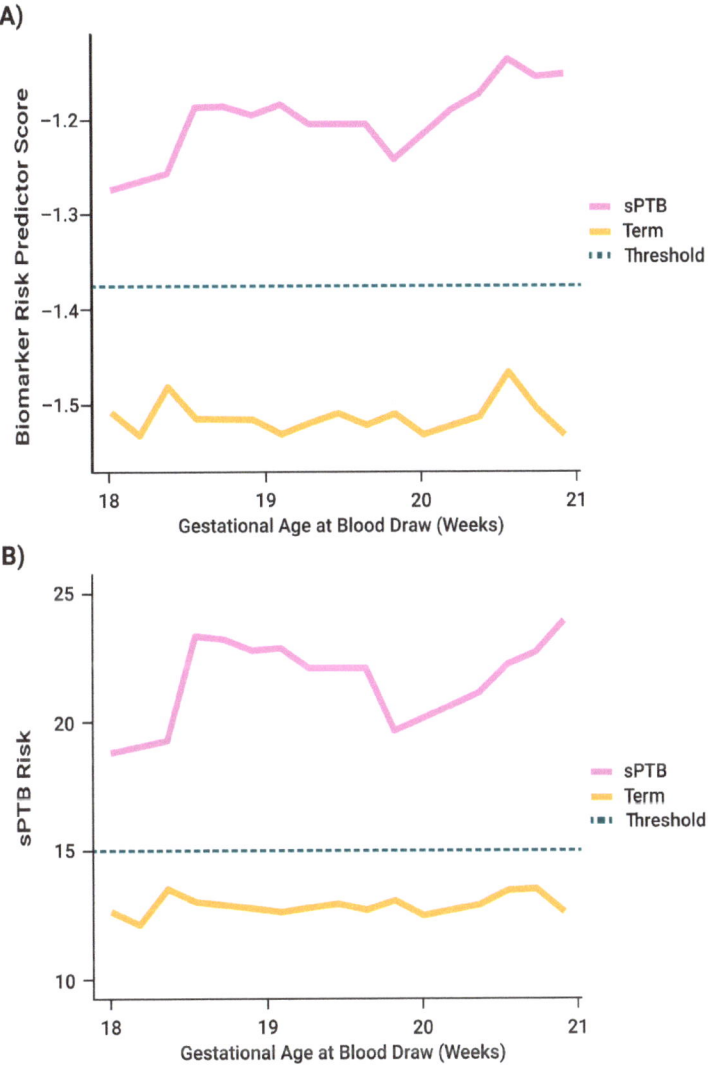

Figure 2. Separation between spontaneous preterm birth (sPTB) cases and term births (controls) across gestational age (GA) at blood draw, in the excluding-LMP (not dated by first day of last menstrual period) population. (**A**) Using the proteomic predictor score. Dashed line corresponds to the validated risk predictor threshold (−1.37), representing 15% sPTB risk, or twice the average sPTB risk across all U.S. singleton pregnancies. (**B**) Using the percent sPTB risk. Dashed line indicates 15% sPTB risk.

4. Discussion

In the current analysis, we demonstrated an improvement in observed biomarker risk predictor performance in representative subjects who had more certain GA dating. The fact that subjects with more certain dating did not differ from all subjects by any demographic or clinical factor suggests that the improvement we observed in performance is only due to more certain dating and applies to all pregnancies, no matter how they are dated. We note that the sPTB risk predictor assessed in the current analysis was developed on a broad and diverse United States pregnant population and is applicable across demographic groups, including those based on race or ethnicity. Performance improvement also was confirmed in additional subjects by extending the analysis from the current intended-use window of $19^{1/7}$–$20^{6/7}$ weeks to a broader window of $18^{0/7}$–$20^{6/7}$ weeks.

Based on the lower reliability of their GA dating, we estimated that three term births in weeks $19^{1/7}$–$20^{6/7}$ were misclassified as preterm when all dating methods were included, while only one was estimated to have been misclassified with more reliable dating. Thus, the significantly increased sensitivity that we observed at the validated risk predictor threshold is indeed the most likely result of restricting analysis to subjects with better dating. Our data suggest that lower-scoring cases contributing to the original, lower estimate of sensitivity largely had received less certain dating and that at least some are expected to represent term births misclassified as PTBs due to dating uncertainty.

ACOG guidance regarding GA dating was revised after PAPR study data were collected, providing new specifications for the uncertainty of available GA dating methods [7]. These specifications motivated the current analysis. ACOG guidance quantifies the increased certainty of GA dating with earlier GA at ultrasound. More certain dating in turn provides greater certainty for GA-related outcomes such as PTB and thus provides more accurate quantitation of risk predictor performance.

The impact of GA dating uncertainty on the assessment of the prediction of GA-dependent events such as PTB can be quantified. In our simulations, a perfect PTB predictor showed a decrease in the AUC of 21% when GA was determined by LMP dating confirmed by ultrasound and about half that decrease when GA was determined by ultrasound dating. This simulation demonstrates the inaccuracy of assessing predictor performance in a population for which the outcome (sPTB as determined by GA date) is not known reliably. While ultrasound dating is commonly accepted as a more certain dating method than LMP, our results demonstrate the novel suggestion that confirming LMP by ultrasound does not improve its certainty to the level achieved by using actual ultrasound dates. The impact of GA dating certainty can also be quantified in ways that impact daily obstetric practice. Based on the approximately nine-fold higher prevalence of term than PTBs, less certain GA dating notably increases the number of term births misclassified as preterm, while a smaller number of PTBs will be misclassified as term births. Estimated GAs that provide higher numbers of false positive and false negative calls for PTB result in more opportunities for the incorrect application of treatments such as antenatal corticosteroid administration.

Uncertainty in GA dating may be particularly impactful upon medical decisions for preterm and late-term or post-date deliveries. Maternal and neonatal care recommendations may differ strongly with threatened labor or delivery at an estimated GA of $21^{6/7}$ vs. $22^{6/7}$ weeks. Similarly, recommendations for intervention as opposed to expectant management may differ for post-term pregnancy at $41^{0/7}$ vs. $42^{0/7}$ weeks. Such challenging scenarios motivate the development of prognostics or diagnostics that can improve the certainty of GA dating beyond the current state and thus improve the performance of GA as a classifier of risk of periviable or post-term birth. These findings have wider-ranging implications beyond PTB prediction and may affect the timing of antenatal testing and induction, reductions in cesarean section, and the prevention of stillbirth. The results of the present analysis suggest that use of pure ultrasound dating with a validated proteomic biomarker risk predictor may allow the most accurate assessment of the prediction of PTB. As well, combinations of biomarkers selected for the estimation of GA at the time of sampling rather than risk prediction, in combination with ultrasound, may be of interest for the more confident estimation of GA and EDD.

Future work might include an examination of the observed performance of pregnancy predictors on additional cohorts with two or more GA dating techniques assessed on all subjects, enabling within-subject comparison of the effects of dating uncertainty on performance assessment.

The limitations of the current study include the modest size of the study and the availability of only one GA dating method per subject. In addition, the exact GA of the dating ultrasound was not available in the PAPR study. For this reason, we established biomarker performance amongst a more precisely dated population by excluding LMP-only dating. Future studies are planned to extend these analyses in clinical trials where the gestational age of the dating ultrasound is available and within-patient comparison of gestational age dating methods can be carried out. Finally, ours was a retrospective analysis, which can be enhanced by focused prospective studies.

A major strength of the study was that it applied the current best practices, including the implementation of ACOG guidance and evidence cited therein and a blinded analysis by a third-party statistician. The analysis was conducted on a well-characterized, previously studied population. Finally, the current study introduced a methodology for assessing risk predictor performance more accurately through the consideration of GA dating uncertainty.

5. Conclusions

The improved estimation of the performance of an sPTB risk predictor in subjects whose GA at delivery is more certain suggests that the risk predictor provides accurate predictions that are confirmed by better dating. Improvements in risk prediction can lead to better risk stratification, and this work suggests that more well-designed controlled studies on interventions to reduce risk are warranted and have the potential to have significant impacts.

Author Contributions: Conceptualization, J.B., T.J.G., G.C.C., J.J.B., and P.E.K.; data curation, A.D.P., A.C.F., T.C.F., and M.T.D.; formal analysis, J.B., A.D.P., R.T., M.T.D., and P.E.K.; investigation, J.B., G.R.S., K.A.B., G.R.M., J.D.I., D.V.C., L.M.P., M.K.H., R.T., M.T.D., A.C.F., and T.C.F.; methodology, J.B., T.L.R., T.C.F., M.T.D., T.J.G., G.C.C., J.J.B., and P.E.K.; project administration, J.B., J.J.B., and P.E.K.; resources, G.C.C., G.R.S., K.A.B., G.R.M., J.D.I., D.V.C., L.M.P., and M.K.H.; supervision, P.E.K.; validation, J.B., J.J.B., and P.E.K.; visualization, J.B., R.T., and M.T.D.; writing—original draft, J.B. and P.E.K.; writing—review and editing, J.B., G.R.S., K.A.B., G.R.M., J.D.I., D.V.C., L.M.P., M.K.H., A.D.P., R.T., A.C.F., T.L.R., T.C.F., M.T.D., T.J.G., G.C.C., J.J.B., and P.E.K. All authors have read and agreed to the published version of the manuscript.

Funding: This study was funded by Sera Prognostics, Inc. Sera Prognostics employees and consultants played a role in the study design, data collection and analysis, manuscript preparation, and the decision to submit.

Institutional Review Board Statement: The PAPR study (NCT01371019) was conducted according to the guidelines of the Declaration of Helsinki and approved by the Institutional Review Boards/Ethics Committees of all 11 participating study sites. The following is a list of approvals: Intermountain Healthcare Institutional Review Board (1022138, 22 December 2010), Office of Human Research Ethics, University of North Carolina (11-1641, 13 September 2011), Institutional Review Board for Human Research, Office of Research Integrity, Medical University of South Carolina (Pro00012552, 11 October 2011), Maricopa Integrated Health System Institutional Review Board (2011-078, 18 October 2011), Western IRB (used by Ohio State University (20112063, 13 December 2011), Baystate Medical Center Institutional Review Board (BH-12-020, 23 December 2011), Research Integrity Office, Oregon Health & Science University (IRB00008131, 7-February-2012), San Diego Perinatal Center (20112063, 10 February 2012), University of Texas Medical Branch Institutional Review Board (12-046, 29 March 2012), Regional Obstetrical Consultants (20112063, 20 November 2012), and Christiana Care Institutional Review Board (32234, 28 December 2012). All necessary patient/participant consent was obtained, and the appropriate institutional forms have been archived.

Informed Consent Statement: Informed consent was obtained from all subjects involved in the study.

Data Availability Statement: Data supporting the results presented here are available on request from the corresponding author. Data will not be made publicly available or in any format that may violate a subject's right to privacy. For example, dating information or identifiers that could allow data integration, thereby enabling potential identification of study subjects, are protected.

Acknowledgments: We wish to acknowledge the study coordinators and research personnel at the study sites, the participants in the TREETOP study, and the Sera Prognostics, Inc. clinical laboratory and clinical operations teams. Babak Shahbaba conducted fixed sequence hypotheses testing, and Jennifer Logan, contributed to the writing of this article and project administration.

Conflicts of Interest: The authors of this manuscript have the following competing interests: J.B., R.T., A.C.F., T.C.F., M.T.D., T.J.G., G.C.C., J.J.B., and P.E.K. are employees and stockholders of Sera Prognostics, Inc. A.D.P. and T.L.R. are consultants to Sera Prognostics, Inc. All other authors report no conflict of interest.

References

1. Liu, L.; Oza, S.; Hogan, D.; Chu, Y.; Perin, J.; Zhu, J.; Lawn, J.E.; Cousens, S.; Mathers, C.; Black, R.E. Global, regional, and national causes of under-5 mortality in 2000-15: An updated systematic analysis with implications for the Sustainable Development Goals. *Lancet* **2016**, *388*, 3027–3035. [CrossRef]
2. Chawanpaiboon, S.; Vogel, J.P.; Moller, A.B.; Lumbiganon, P.; Petzold, M.; Hogan, D.; Landoulsi, S.; Jampathong, N.; Kongwattanakul, K.; Laopaiboon, M.; et al. Global, regional, and national estimates of levels of preterm birth in 2014: A systematic review and modelling analysis. *Lancet Glob. Health* **2019**, *7*, e37–e46. [CrossRef]
3. Osterman, M.J.K.; Hamilton, B.E.; Martin, J.A.; Driscoll, A.K.; Valenzuela, C.P. Births: Final Data for 2020. Available online: https://www.cdc.gov/nchs/nvss/births.htm (accessed on 9 February 2022).
4. Waitzman, N.J.; Jalali, A.; Grosse, S.D. Preterm birth lifetime costs in the United States in 2016: An update. *Semin. Perinatol.* **2021**, *45*, 151390. [CrossRef] [PubMed]
5. Alexander, G.R.; Institute of Medicine (US) Committee on Understanding Premature Birth and Assuring Healthy Outcomes; Behrman, R.E.; Butler, A.S. Prematurity at Birth: Determinants, Consequences, and Geographic Variation (Appendix B). In *Preterm Birth: Causes, Consequences, and Prevention*; National Academies Press (US): Washington, DC, USA, 2007.
6. American College of Obstetricians and Gynecologists, Gynecologists' Committee on Practice, Bulletins-Obstetrics. Prediction and Prevention of Spontaneous Preterm Birth: ACOG Practice Bulletin, Number 234. *Obs. Gynecol* **2021**, *138*, e65–e90. [CrossRef] [PubMed]
7. American College of Obstetricians and Gynecologists. Committee Opinion No 700: Methods for Estimating the Due Date. *Obs. Gynecol.* **2017**, *129*, e150–e154. [CrossRef] [PubMed]
8. Barr, W.B.; Pecci, C.C. Last menstrual period versus ultrasound for pregnancy dating. *Int. J. Gynaecol. Obs.* **2004**, *87*, 38–39. [CrossRef] [PubMed]
9. Savitz, D.A.; Terry, J.W., Jr.; Dole, N.; Thorp, J.M., Jr.; Siega-Riz, A.M.; Herring, A.H. Comparison of pregnancy dating by last menstrual period, ultrasound scanning, and their combination. *Am. J. Obs. Gynecol.* **2002**, *187*, 1660–1666. [CrossRef]
10. Wegienka, G.; Baird, D.D. A comparison of recalled date of last menstrual period with prospectively recorded dates. *J. Womens Health* **2005**, *14*, 248–252. [CrossRef]
11. Andersen, H.F.; Barclay, M.L. Prediction of delivery date in a computerized prenatal record system. *Proc. Annu. Symp. Comput. Appl. Med. Care* **1980**, *1*, 307–310.
12. Darwish, N.A.; Thabet, S.M.; Aboul Nasr, A.L.; El Sharkawy, S.; El Tamamy, M.N. Modified Naegele's Rule for determination of the expected date of delivery irrespective of the cycle length. *Med. J. Cairo Univ.* **1994**, *62*, 39–47.
13. Caughey, A.B.; Nicholson, J.M.; Washington, A.E. First- vs second-trimester ultrasound: The effect on pregnancy dating and perinatal outcomes. *Am. J. Obs. Gynecol.* **2008**, *198*, 703.e1–703.e5. [CrossRef] [PubMed]
14. Kalish, R.B.; Thaler, H.T.; Chasen, S.T.; Gupta, M.; Berman, S.J.; Rosenwaks, Z.; Chervenak, F.A. First- and second-trimester ultrasound assessment of gestational age. *Am. J. Obs. Gynecol.* **2004**, *191*, 975–978. [CrossRef] [PubMed]
15. Verburg, B.O.; Steegers, E.A.; De Ridder, M.; Snijders, R.J.; Smith, E.; Hofman, A.; Moll, H.A.; Jaddoe, V.W.; Witteman, J.C. New charts for ultrasound dating of pregnancy and assessment of fetal growth: Longitudinal data from a population-based cohort study. *Ultrasound Obs. Gynecol.* **2008**, *31*, 388–396. [CrossRef] [PubMed]
16. Taipale, P.; Hiilesmaa, V. Predicting delivery date by ultrasound and last menstrual period in early gestation. *Obs. Gynecol.* **2001**, *97*, 189–194. [CrossRef]
17. Bennett, K.A.; Crane, J.M.; O'Shea, P.; Lacelle, J.; Hutchens, D.; Copel, J.A. First trimester ultrasound screening is effective in reducing postterm labor induction rates: A randomized controlled trial. *Am. J. Obs. Gynecol.* **2004**, *190*, 1077–1081. [CrossRef] [PubMed]

18. Hassan, S.S.; Romero, R.; Vidyadhari, D.; Fusey, S.; Baxter, J.K.; Khandelwal, M.; Vijayaraghavan, J.; Trivedi, Y.; Soma-Pillay, P.; Sambarey, P.; et al. Vaginal progesterone reduces the rate of preterm birth in women with a sonographic short cervix: A multicenter, randomized, double-blind, placebo-controlled trial. *Ultrasound Obs. Gynecol.* **2011**, *38*, 18–31. [CrossRef]
19. Petrini, J.R.; Callaghan, W.M.; Klebanoff, M.; Green, N.S.; Lackritz, E.M.; Howse, J.L.; Schwarz, R.H.; Damus, K. Estimated effect of 17 alpha-hydroxyprogesterone caproate on preterm birth in the United States. *Obs. Gynecol.* **2005**, *105*, 267–272. [CrossRef]
20. Saade, G.R.; Boggess, K.A.; Sullivan, S.A.; Markenson, G.R.; Iams, J.D.; Coonrod, D.V.; Pereira, L.M.; Esplin, M.S.; Cousins, L.M.; Lam, G.K.; et al. Development and validation of a spontaneous preterm delivery predictor in asymptomatic women. *Am. J. Obs. Gynecol.* **2016**, *214*, 633.e1–633.e24. [CrossRef]
21. Bradford, C.; Severinsen, R.; Pugmire, T.; Rasmussen, M.; Stoddard, K.; Uemura, Y.; Wheelwright, S.; Mentinova, M.; Chelsky, D.; Hunsucker, S.W.; et al. Analytical validation of protein biomarkers for risk of spontaneous preterm birth. *Clin. Mass Spectrom.* **2017**, *3*, 25–38. [CrossRef]
22. Markenson, G.R.; Saade, G.R.; Laurent, L.C.; Heyborne, K.D.; Coonrod, D.V.; Schoen, C.N.; Baxter, J.K.; Haas, D.M.; Longo, S.; Grobman, W.A.; et al. Performance of a proteomic preterm delivery predictor in a large independent prospective cohort. *Am. J. Obs. Gynecol. MFM* **2020**, *2*, 100140. [CrossRef]
23. Burchard, J.; Polpitiya, A.D.; Fox, A.C.; Randolph, T.L.; Fleischer, T.C.; Dufford, M.T.; Garite, T.J.; Critchfield, G.C.; Boniface, J.J.; Saade, G.R.; et al. Clinical Validation of a Proteomic Biomarker Threshold for Increased Risk of Spontaneous Preterm Birth and Associated Clinical Outcomes: A Replication Study. *J. Clin. Med.* **2021**, *10*, 5088. [CrossRef] [PubMed]
24. Steinberg, D.M.; Fine, J.; Chappell, R. Sample size for positive and negative predictive value in diagnostic research using case–control designs. *Biostatistics* **2008**, *10*, 94–105. [CrossRef] [PubMed]
25. Dowle, M.; Srinivasan, A. Data.Table: Extension of 'Data.Frame', Version 1.14.2. Available online: https://cran.r-project.org/web/packages/data.table/index.html (accessed on 20 December 2021).
26. Robin, X.; Turck, N.; Hainard, A.; Tiberti, N.; Lisacek, F.; Sanchez, J.C.; Müller, M. pROC: An open-source package for R and S+ to analyze and compare ROC curves. *BMC Bioinform.* **2011**, *12*, 77. [CrossRef] [PubMed]
27. Dorai-Raj, S. Binom: Binomial Confidence Intervals for Several Parameterizations. Available online: https://CRAN.R-project.org/package=binom (accessed on 1 December 2021).
28. National Center for Health Statistics, U.S. Centers for Disease Control and Prevention. Birth Data Files. Available online: https://www.cdc.gov/nchs/data_access/vitalstatsonline.htm#Births (accessed on 1 March 2022).

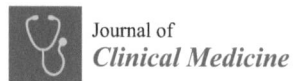

Systematic Review

Efficacy of Continuous Glucose Monitoring on Glycaemic Control in Pregnant Women with Gestational Diabetes Mellitus—A Systematic Review

Agata Majewska *, Paweł Jan Stanirowski, Mirosław Wielgoś and Dorota Bomba-Opoń

1st Department of Obstetrics and Gynaecology, Medical University of Warsaw, 02-015 Warsaw, Poland; stanirowski@gmail.com (P.J.S.); miroslaw.wielgos@wum.edu.pl (M.W.); dorota.bomba-opon@wum.edu.pl (D.B.-O.)
* Correspondence: majewska.agata@gmail.com

Abstract: Gestational diabetes mellitus (GDM) is one of the most common complications of pregnancy, affecting up to 14% of pregnant women. The population of patients with risk factors of GDM is increasing; thus, it is essential to improve management of this condition. One of the key factors affecting perinatal outcomes in GDM is glycaemic control. Until recently, glucose monitoring was only available with self-monitoring of blood glucose (SMBG). However, nowadays, there is a new method, continuous glucose monitoring (CGM), which has been shown to be safe in pregnancy. Since proper glycaemia assessment has been shown to affect perinatal outcomes, we decided to perform a systematic review to analyse the role of CGM in glycaemic control in GDM. We conducted a web search of the MEDLINE, EMBASE, Cochrane Library, Scopus, and Web of Science databases according to the PRISMA guidelines. The web search was performed by two independent researchers and resulted in 14 articles included in the systematic review. The study protocol was registered in the PROSPERO database with registration number CRD42021289883. The main outcome of the systematic review was determining that, when compared, CGM played an important role in better glycaemic control than SMBG. Furthermore, glycaemic control with CGM improved qualification for insulin therapy. However, most of the articles did not reveal CGM's role in improving neonatal outcomes. Therefore, more studies are needed to analyse the role of CGM in affecting perinatal outcomes in GDM.

Keywords: gestational diabetes mellitus; continuous glucose monitoring; self-monitoring of blood glucose; hyperglycaemia; hypoglycaemia

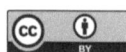

1. Introduction

Gestational diabetes mellitus (GDM) is the most common complication of pregnancy, with an incidence rate of up to 14% of all pregnant women [1]. Over a long period of time, it was defined as any degree of glucose intolerance with the onset or first recognition during pregnancy [2,3]. However, now it is debated whether this definition is appropriate due to its limitations, including imprecise information about diagnostic thresholds for GDM [4]. The population of patients with risk factors for GDM is continuously increasing, thus, it is essential to improve the management of GDM [5]. It is believed that glycaemic control plays a major role in the proper treatment of GDM [6,7]. Until recently glycaemic control in GDM was mainly based on the self-monitoring of blood glucose (SMBG) [8]. However, the main inconveniences of this method are multiple finger-pricking for a single glycaemia measurement and intermittent checking of glucose levels, which might lead to poor patient compliance [9]. Recently, a new method for glycaemic control was introduced, namely, continuous glucose monitoring (CGM) [10]. The method uses a subcutaneous sensor to collect the glycaemia results. The main benefit of CGM is that, after insertion, the system analyses the actual glycaemia constantly without any additional invasive procedure [11]. An important advantage of CGM is the evaluation of time the patient spends in normoglycaemia. It is called time-in-range, and it is defined as the percentage of time in which glycaemia is in reference range [12]. It is believed that time-in-range is a more accurate outcome to assess the patient's compliance.

There are ongoing debates about what type of glycaemia measurement method is the most effective for pregnant women diagnosed with GDM. It is hypothesized that CGM is superior to SMBG, but due to the high price of the device and a lack of reimbursement for GDM in many countries, it is not used as the method of choice [7,8].

The aim of this systematic review is to assess the efficacy of continuous glucose monitoring on glycaemic control in pregnant women with GDM. In addition, this review will focus on the need for pharmacological treatment and perinatal outcomes in the population of patients using CGM.

2. Materials and Methods

2.1. Search Strategy and Selection Criteria

We conducted a systematic web search in the MEDLINE, EMBASE, Cochrane Central Register of Controlled Trials (CENTRAL), Scopus, and Web of Science databases according to the Preferred Reporting Items for Systematic Reviews and Meta-Analyses (PRISMA) guidelines. The systematic review has been registered in the International Prospective Register of Systematic Reviews (PROSPERO) registry (CRD42021289883). The keywords utilized for the research were: continuous glucose monitoring, flash glucose monitoring, and gestational diabetes mellitus. The time frame of the research was from database inception date to November 2021. The inclusion criteria were: randomized controlled trials and observational studies, and human studies in English. The exclusion criteria were types of studies other than the inclusion criteria, animal studies, and studies in different languages than English (Table 1).

Table 1. Inclusion and exclusion criteria for the systematic review.

Inclusion Criteria	Exclusion Criteria
Randomized controlled trials and observational studies	Case reports, review articles, editorial comments
Human studies	Animal studies
Studies in English	Studies in different languages than English

Following the initial screening, publications were analysed further by title and abstract to exclude studies that did not meet the inclusion criteria. After initial selection, the remaining full articles were screened to assess the final number of eligible publications included to the systematic review. Two of the authors independently evaluated all retrieved studies against the eligibility criteria and, in cases of differing opinion, the publication was discussed with the third author.

Due to heterogeneity in terms of continuous glucose monitoring devices, study duration, and number of patients among the included articles, no meta-analysis was performed.

2.2. Data Analysis

Data were extracted independently by two researchers. The following data were extracted: type of article, year of publication, type of continuous glucose monitoring, number of patients included in the study, fasting, postprandial and nocturnal glycaemia, time in range, qualification for insulin therapy, incidence of severe nocturnal hypoglycaemia, glycosylated haemoglobin concentration (HbA1c), gestational weight gain, newborn birth weight, and other neonatal outcomes.

2.3. Outcomes

The main outcome was glycaemic control (fasting, postprandial and nocturnal glycaemia). Several secondary outcomes were also investigated, including: qualification to insulin therapy, incidence of severe nocturnal hypoglycaemia, HbA1c, gestational weight gain, newborn birth weight, and other neonatal outcomes.

3. Results

A total of 435 articles were identified through a systematic review of the literature (Figure 1).

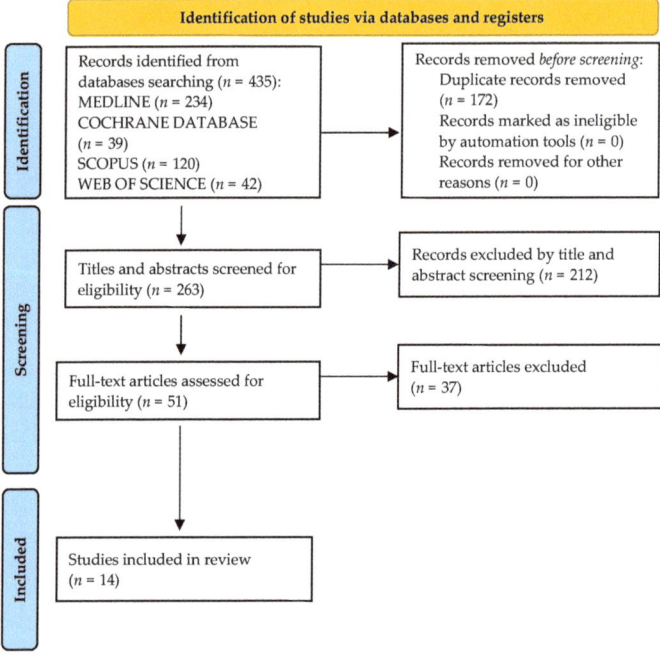

Figure 1. PRISMA flow diagram.

After initial screening, 172 duplicates were excluded and 263 titles and abstracts were screened further for eligibility criteria, leaving a total of 51 full-text publications. Review of the full-text articles resulted in 37 studies being excluded from further assessment. A total of 14 remaining publications were included in the final analysis of this systematic review (Table 2).

Table 2. Characteristics of studies included in the systematic review.

Study ID	Study Design	Study Population	Type of CGM	Duration of CGM Usage	Outcome	Results
Paramasivam S et al. [6]	RCT *	57 GDM patients	iPro™ 2 Medtronic	6 days	Incidence of hypoglycaemia, insulin therapy, maternal and neonatal outcomes	Higher detection of hypoglycaemia in CGM group; no difference in other outcomes
Afandi B et al. [7]	Prospective observational study	25 GDM patients	iPro™ 2 Medtronic	5 days	Incidence of hyper- and hypoglycaemia, HbA1c level, qualification to insulin therapy	Lower incidence of hyperglycaemia and higher detection of hypoglycaemia in CGM group

Table 2. Cont.

Study ID	Study Design	Study Population	Type of CGM	Duration of CGM Usage	Outcome	Results
Márquez-Pardo S et al. [8]	Prospective observational study	77 GDM patients	iPro™ 2 Medtronic	6 days	Incidence of hyperglycaemia, qualification to insulin therapy	Higher detection of hyperglycaemia, more qualification to insulin therapy in CGM group
Chen R et al. [9]	Prospective observational study	57 GDM patients	Medtronic MiniMed	72 h	Incidence of postprandial hyperglycaemia and nocturnal hypoglycaemia; HbA1c level	Higher detection of nocturnal hypoglycaemia and postprandial hyperglycaemia in CGM group, no difference in HbA1c level between the groups
Lane AF et al. [11]	RCT	40 GDM patients	Medtronic MiniMed/iPro™ 2 Medtronic	28 days	Incidence of hyper- and hypoglycaemia, time in range, HbA1c level, maternal and neonatal outcomes	No difference between the groups
Yu F et al. [12]	Prospective cohort study	340 GDM patients	Medtronic MiniMed	72 h a week for 5 weeks	Glycaemia control, insulin therapy, maternal and neonatal outcomes	Shorter durations of hyper- and hypoglycaemia, more patients qualified to insulin therapy in CGM group; less incidence of LGA *, neonatal hypoglycaemia and hyperbilirubinemia in CGM group
Cypryk K et al. [13]	Prospective observational study	12 GDM patients, 7 patients non-GDM	Medtronic MiniMed	72 h	Glycaemia control	No difference between the groups
Zhang X et al. [14]	RCT	110 GDM patients	ISGMS * (Abbott Diabetes Care)	14 days	Incidence of hypoglycaemia, gestational weight gain, health behaviour patterns	Lower gestational weight gain, better health behaviour patterns and lower incidence of hypoglycaemia in CGM group
Buhling KJ et al. [15]	Prospective observational study	63 GDM, 17 IGT, 24 non-GDM, 9 non-pregnant patients	Medtronic MiniMed	72 h	Glycaemia control, neonatal outcomes	Higher detection of hyperglycaemia in CGM group, no difference in other outcomes between the groups
Zaharieva D et al. [16]	Prospective Observational Study	90 GDM patients	iPRO Medtronic	7 days	Incidence of hyperglycaemia	Higher detection of hyperglycaemia in CGM group
Alfadhli E et al. [17]	RCT	130 GDM patients	Guardian® RT-CGMS MiniMed	3–7 days	Fasting and postprandial glycaemia, HbA1c level, insulin therapy, maternal and neonatal outcomes	No difference between the groups

Table 2. Cont.

Study ID	Study Design	Study Population	Type of CGM	Duration of CGM Usage	Outcome	Results
Kestila K et al. [18]	RCT	73 GDM patients	Medtronic MiniMed	Mean 47.4 h	Insulin therapy, maternal and neonatal outcomes	Higher number of patients qualified for insulin therapy in CGM group; no difference in maternal and neonatal outcomes between the groups
Yogev Y et al. [19]	Prospective observational study	6 PGDM, 2 GDM patients,	Medtronic MiniMed	72 h	Glycaemia, HbA1c level, insulin therapy, maternal and neonatal outcomes	Higher detection of nocturnal hypoglycaemia and postprandial hyperglycaemia, better modification of insulin therapy in CGM group; no difference in other outcomes between the groups
Wei Q et al. [20]	RCT	106 GDM patients	Medtronic MiniMed	48–72 h	Glycaemia, HbA1c level, insulin therapy, maternal and neonatal outcomes	Higher number of patients qualified to insulin therapy, better detection of nocturnal hypoglycaemia and postprandial hyperglycaemia, less gestational weight gain in CGM group; No difference in other outcomes between the groups

* RCT = Randomised controlled trial; LGA = large for gestational age; ISGMS: instantaneous scanning glucose monitoring system.

3.1. Glycaemic Control

3.1.1. Hyperglycaemia

In five studies, it was found that CGM is better at detecting episodes of hyperglycaemia as compared to SMBG [7,9,12,15,16]. In two studies, it was found that CGM detected more hyperglycaemic events than SMBG [9,15]. However, Afandi et al. demonstrated that the incidence rate of hyperglycaemia in all patients included in the study reached 5.65% using CGM versus 14.2% using SMBG ($p < 0.05$) [7]. The incidence of hyperglycaemia above 180 mg/dL in the CGM and SMBG groups was estimated to be <1.0% and 2% of all readings, respectively ($p < 0.05$). In another prospective study, hyperglycaemic events were analysed further, and the result was that, in the CGM group, the duration of time spent in hyperglycaemia was shorter than in the SMBG group [12]. One study found that CGM is a better detector of nocturnal hyperglycaemia than SMBG [16]. On the other hand, three studies described no statistical difference between the SMBG and CGM groups in detecting glycaemia above the reference range [11,13,17].

3.1.2. Hypoglycaemia

We found eight articles about incidences of hypoglycaemia [6,7,9,11–15]. In most studies, the outcome was that CGM detects a higher number of hypoglycaemia episodes than SMBG [6,7,9,15]. It played an especially significant role in pregnant women qualified for insulin therapy [9,19]. Chen et al. underlined CGM's role in especially detecting nocturnal hypoglycaemia in patients requiring pharmacological treatment [9].

There was only one study, by Zhang et al., that calculated a significantly lower number of patients with hypoglycaemic events in the CGM group (overall, 3 patients with hypoglyceamic episodes (5.45%) in CGM versus 12 patients (21.82%) in SMBG group; $\chi^2 = 6.253$, $p = 0.012$) [13]. Yu at el analysed hypoglycaemia further and showed significant a difference in the duration of time spent in hypoglycaemia, with lower results in the CGM group [12].

3.2. Insulin Therapy

Five studies analysed how qualification to insulin therapy differs between the CGM and SMBG groups [6,8,18–20]. In three of them, it was noted that CGM is a better predictor for the initiation of antihyperglycaemic treatment [8,18,20]. Kestilä et al. found that using SMBG only leads to underestimation of the actual number of patients requiring insulin therapy [18]. In another study, it was also confirmed that CGM detects a higher number of patients who should be qualified for pharmacological treatment [8].

Two studies analysed whether CGM has an impact on insulin dosage. Paramasivan et al. conducted a randomised, controlled trial and revealed that the total insulin requirement was higher in the CGM group throughout pregnancy; however, there was no significant difference in the insulin dosage between the groups (CGM vs. control: 16.2 ± 6.4 vs. 11.8 ± 13.6 units, $p = 0.314$) [6]. An interesting outcome was demonstrated in the study by Yogev et al.; namely, the CGM group demanded 33% less long and intermediate-acting insulin, while, simultaneously, having higher (mean 20%) postprandial morning and afternoon insulin doses than the SMBG group [19].

3.3. HBA1c

HBA1c levels were analysed in six studies [5,8,10,16,18,19]. A randomized, controlled trial assessing HbA1c results in patients with GDM treated with insulin revealed significantly lower HbA1c concentration in the CGM group (CGM group: $5.2 \pm 0.4\%$ vs. SMBG group: $5.6 \pm 0.6\%$, $p < 0.006$) [6]. Furthermore, in the CGM group, HbA1c remained unchanged, in contrast to SMBG group, in which HbA1c levels increased over the course of pregnancy. Despite the above-mentioned results in five other studies, no significant differences in HbA1c concentration between CGM and SMBG groups were observed [9,11,17,19,20].

3.4. Gestational Weight Gain

Gestational weight gain was analysed in three publications [14,18,20]. Two of them revealed a significantly lower increase in weight gain in the CGM group [14,20]. In addition, there was less incidence of excessive weight gain in the group using continuous glucose monitoring [14,20]. Nevertheless, the third publication, by Kestila et al., did not confirm the impact of CGM on gestational weight gain [18].

3.5. Neonatal Outcomes

Seven studies compared neonatal outcomes, and the results are not conclusive [6,11–13,17,18,20]. In the study by Paramasivan et al., no significant difference in newborn weight between the CGM and SMBG groups was noted (CGM: 2842.4 g ± 448.6 vs. SMBG: 2976.0 g ± 473.5; $p = 0.311$) [6]. Another two prospective studies confirmed their result [18,20]. In the study by Kestilla et al., the incidence of macrosomia was similar in both groups ($p = 0.33$) [18]. In contrast, Yu F et al. observed significantly lower neonatal weight in the CGM group (an average difference of 207 g; $p < 0.001$) and higher incidence of macrosomia or LGA in the SMBG group ($p < 0.05$) [12]. The authors also analysed other neonatal outcomes, but the results were inconclusive. There was a significantly lower incidence of neonatal hypoglycaemia and hyperbilirubinemia in the CGM group; however, NICU admission rates did not differ between the groups [12]. In four other studies, the authors showed no differences in any analysed neonatal outcomes [11,17,18,20].

4. Discussion

In this systematic review, we aimed to assess the efficacy of CGM on glycaemic control in GDM. Overall, the results of our review provide clear evidence for the superiority of CGM over SMBG in dysglycaemia assessment. In the majority of studies, it was shown that, in the CGM group, there was a better detection of dysglycaemia than in the SMBG group [6,7,9,12,15]. However, few studies did not confirm the statistical difference between those two methods [11,13,17]. The difference in outcomes might be the consequence of different methodologies used in the studies, including the number of patients recruited or study duration (for example, too short a period of time to reveal a statistical difference between the groups).

An interesting outcome analysed in the review was the role of CGM in detecting nocturnal hypoglycaemia. In four studies, CGM performed better in the assessment of hypoglycaemic events [6,7,9,16]. Yu et al. revealed that CGM shortens the time spent in hypoglycaemia as compared to SMBG [12]. Moreover, the authors observed that CGM had an impact on diet control, weight monitoring and appropriate exercise. Thus, shorter time spent in hypoglycaemia was correlated with better health behaviour patterns and patient compliance. Overall, it is believed that improved nocturnal hypoglycaemia detection by CGM might have implications for better modification of GDM treatment, not only better qualification for insulin therapy, but also diet modifications [6,12]. It might play a particular role for patients requiring pharmacological treatment.

HbA1c levels, widely used as an assessment tool for patients with diabetes compliance, did not differ between the groups in almost all analysed articles [11,19,20]. Only one study noted the role of CGM in improving HbA1c levels throughout pregnancy [6]. Consequently, these outcomes might confirm that HbA1c is not the most reliable parameter used for gestational diabetes management.

Regarding insulin therapy, almost all studies demonstrated CGM's superiority over SMBG in predicting adequate antihyperglycaemic treatment [8,18–20]. Continuous glucose monitoring not only enabled better qualifications of patients for insulin therapy, but also had an impact on dose modification. CGM improved adjustments in the insulin dosage that, in consequence, could minimalize complications associated with improper treatment [20].

Regarding neonatal outcomes, in most of the included studies, there was no statistical difference between the CGM and SMBG groups [6,18,20]. Only one study, including over 300 patients, revealed a significantly lower incidence of LGA and lower birth weight in the CGM than in the SMBG group [12]. As a result, further studies need to be conducted to elucidate whether lack of differences in neonatal outcomes may be a consequence of methodological shortcomings. It seems likely that if continuous glucose monitoring better detects dysglycaemia and improves pharmacological treatment, it should have an impact on neonatal outcomes.

A few studies revealed the role of CGM in improving health behaviour patterns [14,20]. Zhang et al. noted its role, especially with regard to lower gestational weight gain compared to the SMBG group [14]. However, there is limited data available in other analysed studies about this maternal outcome. The possible cause of this ambiguous result might be a short period of CGM usage in the majority of the included articles (less than 7 days of measurements per patient).

Several methodological flaws limit the internal validity of this systematic review. First, the main limitation of the analysed studies is that they included small study groups (there was only one study including >150 patients). For example, Paramasivan et al. studied the impact of CGM on maternal and neonatal outcomes with a relatively small group of patients ($n = 25$ in CGM and $n = 25$ in SMBG group) [6]. Hence, some of their results do not merge together—the study revealed the impact of continuous glucose monitoring on improving glycaemia control, but it revealed no significant differences in neonatal outcomes. Secondly, not all of the studies were randomized, controlled trials; therefore, some of the results might have been prone to recall bias. Thirdly, the periods planned for conducting the study were relatively short (median: 5 days), which may not allow the demonstration of significant differences in certain perinatal outcomes. Furthermore, there were not many studies that analysed additional maternal outcomes.

The strengths of this systematic review include study selection from five major databases and their further analysis based on clearly defined inclusion and exclusion criteria.

5. Conclusions

This systematic review supports the thesis that CGM is superior to SMBG in the management of dysglycaemia in GDM. Our findings suggest that CGM better detects hyper- and hypolgycaemic events and is a more appropriate predictor of qualification for insulin therapy. Therefore, these results provide justification for the idea that CGM plays an important role in glycaemia management in GDM. CGM improves the detection of fasting and postprandial hyperglycaemia. Additionally, it better assesses nocturnal hypoglycemia episodes. Improved identification of dysglycaemia allows for better patient compliance as well as decreases the rate of unnecessary interventions, including qualification for insulin therapy and further improper dose adjustment.

On the other hand, the results for neonatal outcomes, including LGA incidence in both methods of measurement, were inconclusive. There is limited evidence that CGM improves any of the analysed neonatal outcomes. Furthermore, it will be essential to elucidate the role of CGM in changing patient health behaviour patterns.

To conclude, more prospective studies focusing on maternal and neonatal outcomes in GDM-complicated pregnancies monitored by CGM need to be conducted to support the existing evidence and to solve the inconclusive findings.

Author Contributions: A.M. and P.J.S. drafted the manuscript. P.J.S., M.W., and D.B.-O. participated in the revision of the manuscript. All authors have read and agreed to the published version of the manuscript.

Funding: This research received no external funding.

Institutional Review Board Statement: Not applicable.

Informed Consent Statement: Not applicable.

Data Availability Statement: The data that support the findings of this study are available from the corresponding author on reasonable request. The data are not publicly available due to privacy or ethical restrictions.

Conflicts of Interest: The authors declare no conflict of interest.

References

1. Ogurtsova, K.; da Rocha Fernandes, J.D.; Huang, Y.; Linnenkamp, U.; Guariguata, L.; Cho, N.H.; Cavan, D.; Shaw, J.E.; Makaroff, L.E. IDF Diabetes Atlas: Global estimates for the prevalence of diabetes for 2015 and 2040. *Diabetes Res. Clin. Pract.* **2017**, *128*, 40–50. [CrossRef] [PubMed]
2. International Association of Diabetes; Pregnancy Study Groups Consensus Panel. International association of diabetes and pregnancy study groups recommendations on the diagnosis and classification of hyperglycemia in pregnancy. *Diabetes Care* **2010**, *33*, 676–682. [CrossRef] [PubMed]
3. American Diabetes Association. Diagnosis and classification of diabetes mellitus. *Diabetes Care* **2009**, *32* (Suppl. 1), S62–S67. [CrossRef]
4. American Diabetes Association. 2. Classification and Diagnosis of Diabetes: Standards of Medical Care in Diabetes—2021. *Diabetes Care* **2021**, *44* (Suppl. 1), S15–S33. [CrossRef] [PubMed]
5. Deputy, N.P.; Kim, S.Y.; Conrey, E.J.; Bullard, K.M. Prevalence and Changes in Preexisting Diabetes and Gestational Diabetes Among Women Who Had a Live Birth—United States, 2012–2016. *MMWR Morb. Mortal. Wkly. Rep.* **2018**, *67*, 1201–1207. [CrossRef] [PubMed]
6. Paramasivam, S.S.; Chinna, K.; Singh, A.K.K.; Ratnasingam, J.; Ibrahim, L.; Lim, L.L.; Tan, A.T.B.; Chan, S.P.; Tan, P.C.; Omar, S.Z.; et al. Continuous glucose monitoring results in lower HbA1c in Malaysian women with insulin-treated gestational diabetes: A randomized controlled trial. *Diabet. Med.* **2018**, *35*, 1118–1129. [CrossRef] [PubMed]
7. Afandi, B.; Hassanein, M.; Roubi, S.; Nagelkerke, N. The value of Continuous Glucose Monitoring and Self-Monitoring of Blood Glucose in patients with Gestational Diabetes Mellitus during Ramadan fasting. *Diabetes Res. Clin. Pract.* **2019**, *151*, 260–264. [CrossRef] [PubMed]

8. Marquez-Pardo, R.; Torres-Barea, I.; Cordoba-Dona, J.A.; Cruzado-Begines, C.; Garcia-Garcia-Doncel, L.; Aguilar-Diosdado, M.; Baena-Nieto, M.G. Continuous Glucose Monitoring and Glycemic Patterns in Pregnant Women with Gestational Diabetes Mellitus. *Diabetes Technol. Ther.* **2020**, *22*, 271–277. [CrossRef] [PubMed]
9. Chen, R.; Yogev, Y.; Ben-Haroush, A.; Jovanovic, L.; Hod, M.; Phillip, M. Continuous glucose monitoring for the evaluation and improved control of gestational diabetes mellitus. *J. Matern. Fetal Neonatal. Med.* **2003**, *14*, 256–260. [CrossRef] [PubMed]
10. Murphy, H.R.; Rayman, G.; Lewis, K.; Kelly, S.; Johal, B.; Duffield, K.; Fowler, D.; Campbell, P.J.; Temple, R.C. Effectiveness of continuous glucose monitoring in pregnant women with diabetes: Randomised clinical trial. *BMJ* **2008**, *337*, a1680. [CrossRef] [PubMed]
11. Lane, A.S.; Mlynarczyk, M.A.; de Veciana, M.; Green, L.M.; Baraki, D.I.; Abuhamad, A.Z. Real-Time Continuous Glucose Monitoring in Gestational Diabetes: A Randomized Controlled Trial. *Am. J. Perinatol.* **2019**, *36*, 891–897. [CrossRef] [PubMed]
12. Yu, F.; Lv, L.; Liang, Z.; Wang, Y.; Wen, J.; Lin, X.; Zhou, Y.; Mai, C.; Niu, J. Continuous glucose monitoring effects on maternal glycemic control and pregnancy outcomes in patients with gestational diabetes mellitus: A prospective cohort study. *J. Clin. Endocrinol. Metab.* **2014**, *99*, 4674–4682. [CrossRef] [PubMed]
13. Cypryk, K.; Pertynska-Marczewska, M.; Szymczak, W.; Wilcynski, J.; Lewinski, A. Evaluation of metabolic control in women with gestational diabetes mellitus by the continuous glucose monitoring system: A pilot study. *Endocr. Pract.* **2006**, *12*, 245–250. [CrossRef] [PubMed]
14. Zhang, X.; Jiang, D.; Wang, X. The effects of the instantaneous scanning glucose monitoring system on hypoglycemia, weight gain, and health behaviors in patients with gestational diabetes: A randomised trial. *Ann. Palliat. Med.* **2021**, *10*, 5714–5720. [CrossRef] [PubMed]
15. Buhling, K.J.; Kurzidim, B.; Wolf, C.; Wohlfarth, K.; Mahmoudi, M.; Wascher, C.; Siebert, G.; Dudenhausen, J.W. Introductory experience with the continuous glucose monitoring system (CGMS; Medtronic Minimed) in detecting hyperglycemia by comparing the self-monitoring of blood glucose (SMBG) in non-pregnant women and in pregnant women with impaired glucose tolerance and gestational diabetes. *Exp. Clin. Endocrinol. Diabetes* **2004**, *112*, 556–560. [PubMed]
16. Zaharieva, D.P.; Teng, J.H.; Ong, M.L.; Lee, M.H.; Paldus, B.; Jackson, L.; Houlihan, C.; Shub, A.; Tipnis, S.; Cohen, O.; et al. Continuous Glucose Monitoring Versus Self-Monitoring of Blood Glucose to Assess Glycemia in Gestational Diabetes. *Diabetes Technol. Ther.* **2020**, *22*, 822–827. [CrossRef] [PubMed]
17. Alfadhli, E.; Osman, E.; Basri, T. Use of a real time continuous glucose monitoring system as an educational tool for patients with gestational diabetes. *Diabetol. Metab. Syndr.* **2016**, *8*, 48. [CrossRef] [PubMed]
18. Kestila, K.K.; Ekblad, U.U.; Ronnemaa, T. Continuous glucose monitoring versus self-monitoring of blood glucose in the treatment of gestational diabetes mellitus. *Diabetes Res. Clin. Pract.* **2007**, *77*, 174–179. [CrossRef] [PubMed]
19. Yogev, Y.; Ben-Haroush, A.; Chen, R.; Kaplan, B.; Phillip, M.; Hod, M. Continuous glucose monitoring for treatment adjustment in diabetic pregnancies—A pilot study. *Diabet. Med.* **2003**, *20*, 558–562. [CrossRef] [PubMed]
20. Wei, Q.; Sun, Z.; Yang, Y.; Yu, H.; Ding, H.; Wang, S. Effect of a CGMS and SMBG on Maternal and Neonatal Outcomes in Gestational Diabetes Mellitus: A Randomized Controlled Trial. *Sci. Rep.* **2016**, *6*, 19920. [CrossRef] [PubMed]

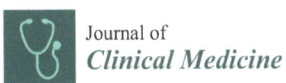

Article

Characterization of the *MG828507* lncRNA Located Upstream of the *FLT1* Gene as an Etiology for Pre-Eclampsia

Hikari Yoshizawa [1,2], Haruki Nishizawa [1,*], Hidehito Inagaki [2], Keisuke Hitachi [3], Akiko Ohwaki [1,2], Yoshiko Sakabe [1,2], Mayuko Ito [1,2], Kunihiro Tsuchida [3], Takao Sekiya [1], Takuma Fujii [1] and Hiroki Kurahashi [2]

[1] Department of Obstetrics and Gynecology, School of Medicine, Fujita Health University, Toyoake 470-1192, Japan
[2] Division of Molecular Genetics, Institute for Comprehensive Medical Science, Fujita Health University, Toyoake 470-1192, Japan
[3] Division for Therapies against Intractable Diseases, Institute for Comprehensive Medical Science, Fujita Health University, Toyoake 470-1192, Japan
* Correspondence: nharuki@fujita-hu.ac.jp

Abstract: Background: *FLT1* is one of the significantly overexpressed genes found in a pre-eclamptic placenta and is involved with the etiology of this disease. Methods: We conducted genome-wide expression profiling by RNA-seq of placentas from women with pre-eclampsia and those with normotensive pregnancy. Results: We identified a lncRNA gene, *MG828507*, located ~80 kb upstream of the *FLT1* gene in a head-to-head orientation, which was overexpressed in the pre-eclamptic placenta. *MG828507* and *FLT1* are located within the same topologically associated domain in the genome. The *MG828507* mRNA level correlated with that of the *FLT1* in placentas from pre-eclamptic women as well as in samples from uncomplicated pregnancies. However, neither the overexpression nor knockdown of *MG828507* affected the expression of *FLT1*. Analysis of pre-eclampsia-linking genetic variants at this locus suggested that the placental genotype of one variant was associated with the expression of *MG828507*. The *MG828507* transcript level was not found to be associated with maternal blood pressure, but showed a relationship with birth and placental weights, suggesting that this lncRNA might be one of the pivotal placental factors in pre-eclampsia. Conclusion: Further characterization of the *MG828507* gene may elucidate the etiological roles of the *MG828507* and *FLT1* genes in pre-eclampsia in a genomic context.

Keywords: lncRNA; FLT1; placenta; pre-eclampsia

1. Introduction

Pre-eclampsia is a syndrome defined by the onset of hypertension with proteinuria and is one of the most common obstetric problems, accounting for almost 15% of pregnancy-associated disorders [1]. It is not a simple complication of pregnancy, however, rather it is a syndrome of multiple organ failures involving the liver, kidneys, and lungs, in addition to coagulation and neural-system difficulties. Since cases of severe pre-eclampsia have a considerably poorer prognosis for both the mother and fetus than an uncomplicated pregnancy, it is potentially one of the most devastating pregnancy-associated disorders faced by gynecologists. There is now an emerging consensus that pre-eclampsia is a multifactorial disease, in which the pathogenetic processes underlying this disorder involve numerous factors such as oxidative stress, endothelial dysfunction, vasoconstriction, metabolic changes, thrombotic disorders, and inflammatory responses, although the precise mechanisms have continued to remain elusive [2,3].

It is generally accepted now that the placenta plays a primary role in the etiology of this disorder. A two-stage disease hypothesis has been proposed, in which an initiating reduction in placental perfusion by abnormal vascular remodeling leads to the maternal symptoms in individuals who have a genetic predisposition to this disease [4]. A considerable body of evidence indicates that placenta-derived anti-angiogenic factors, such as soluble fms-like tyrosine kinase-1 (sFlt-1) and soluble endoglin, are found at high concentrations in the maternal circulation in pre-eclampsia and significantly contribute to disease onset [5–7]. sFlt-1 is a truncated soluble form of this protein lacking the tyrosine kinase domain and acts as an anti-angiogenic factor, by neutralizing proangiogenic factors such as VEGF (vascular endothelial growth factor) or PlGF (placental growth factor), possibly leading to the abnormal placentation in the onset of pre-eclampsia. Assuming that pre-eclampsia is a polygenic disease, several lines of evidence suggest that genetic variants that increase the expression of the *FLT1* gene likely predispose the individual to pre-eclampsia. As the *FLT1* gene is located at chromosome 13q12.3, an elevated sFlt-1 and reduced placental growth factor (PlGF) are associated with trisomy 13 pregnancies, leading to a greater susceptibility to pre-eclampsia [8]. Nucleotide variants that are proximal to the *FLT1* gene in the placenta are also associated with this disease [9–11].

The fine-tuning of gene expression that contributes to the onset of polygenic diseases is often regulated by genetic variants, which act as an expression quantitative trait locus (eQTL). These variants might affect their target gene's expression level via structural changes to a topologically associated domain (TAD) or via expression changes in lncRNAs (>200 nt) or miRNAs (<200 nt), which also regulate the expression of genes associated with disease [12,13]. Nearly 98% of human genome generates many species of non-coding RNAs, and it is now appreciated that many types of DNA regulatory elements, such as enhancers and promoters, produce lncRNAs to regulate the transcription of the relevant gene. Global gene-expression profile analysis is a powerful tool for the elucidation of the mechanistic pathway underlying the disease or identification of its diagnostic or prognostic markers. RNA-seq technology allows us to identify differentially expressed genes, including those genes that have not been well-characterized yet, such as lncRNAs [14–16]. In our current study, we conducted global-expression profiling using RNA-seq in women with uncomplicated pregnancies and in women with severe pre-eclampsia. Our comparative analyses focused on lncRNA species that might potentially regulate the expression of genes associated with pre-eclampsia.

2. Materials and Methods

2.1. Samples

All of the clinical samples analyzed in this study were collected at the Department of Obstetrics and Gynecology, Fujita Health University Hospital, Japan, from 2005 to 2014. Placental biopsy samples were obtained during Caesarean sections from both normotensive patients and women with severe pre-eclampsia (n = 39). Severe pre-eclampsia was defined by a blood pressure of greater than 160/110 mmHg and by proteinuria of more than 2 g over a 24 h collection period, according to the criteria used in Japan at that time, although these criteria have been revised, so the latest version is currently used [17,18]. Normotensive subjects (n = 38) were matched for both maternal and gestational age and for maternal body mass index at pre-pregnancy. Normotensive subjects underwent a Caesarean section due to a breech presentation or a previous Caesarean section. In addition, we collected preterm normotensive control samples from pregnancies with a premature rupture of the membrane that underwent a Caesarean section due to a breech presentation or with a previous Caesarean section without evidence of intrauterine infection. We calculated the birthweight coefficient by dividing the measured birthweight by the expected standard birthweight at the gestational week in the general Japanese population [19]. The clinical details of our study subjects are presented in Table 1.

Table 1. Characteristics of the normotensive and pre-eclamptic study subjects.

	Normotensive Pregnancy	Pre-Eclampsia	p Value
	$n = 38$	$n = 39$	
Maternal age (y)	30 (28–36) [†]	30 (28–32)	n.s
Gestational age (weeks)	37 (31–38)	33 (32–36)	n.s
Systolic BP (mmHg)	114 (107–118)	163 (157–175)	<0.05
Diastolic BP (mmHg)	70 (60–76)	103 (93–110)	<0.05
Proteinuria [‡]	0 (0%)	39 (100%)	<0.05
Body mass index (BMI) [§]	21.2 (19.7–22.8)	21.0 (19.0–23.9)	n.s
Birth weight (g)	2649 (1827–3105)	1494 (1146–1974)	<0.05
Birth weight coefficient	1.000 (0.919–1.112)	0.717 (0.640–0.813)	<0.05
Placental weight (g)	540 (485–630)	300 (240–398)	<0.05

[†] Data are the median (interquartile range). [‡] ≥2 g in a 24-h collection. [§] pre-pregnancy.

To avoid any possible confounding effects of labor on gene expression, only placental samples that were obtained through Caesarean section from women who had not undergone labor were included in the analyses. A central area of chorionic tissue was then dissected, and the maternal deciduae and amnionic membranes were removed. We then dissected 1 cm sections of placental villi from the four different central areas between the basal and chorionic plates [20,21]. After vigorous washing of the maternal blood with saline, the tissues were immediately frozen in liquid nitrogen and stored until use. Informed consent was obtained from each patient, and this study was approved by the Ethical Review Board for Clinical Studies at Fujita Health University.

2.2. RNA-Seq

We performed RNA-seq analyses of placental tissues from severe pre-eclamptic ($n = 6$) and normotensive ($n = 6$) pregnancies. Total RNA was extracted from chorionic villous tissue samples using an RNeasy mini-kit (Qiagen, Valencia, CA, USA), in accordance with the instructions of the manufacturer. Briefly, approximately 1 µg of each total RNA sample was applied for library preparation using the NEBNext Ultra RNA Library Prep Kit for Illumina (#E7530; New England Biolabs, Inc., Ipswich, MA, USA), in accordance with the instructions of the manufacturer, except for the use of AMPure XP beads (A63880; Beckman Coulter, Indianapolis, IN, USA) in the clean-up steps. The NEBNext Poly(A) mRNA Magnetic Isolation Module upstream and the NEBNext Multiplex Oligos for Illumina downstream (#E7500, #E7335; New England Biolabs) were also used for poly(A) RNA purification and multiplex library production steps, respectively. The samples were sequenced using a high-throughput platform (HiSeq2500, Illumina) with a 100 bp single-end strategy.

We obtained about 40 million raw reads for each sample. These sequence data were quality-trimmed using FASTQX-Toolkit v0.0.13 (http://hannonlab.cshl.edu/fastx_toolkit/ accessed on 10 April 2022) with the command "-Q 33 -t 20 -l 30". The reads were aligned to hg38 using Hisat2 ver. 2.0.5 with default parameters. Potential transcripts were assembled and read-counted using StringTie ver. 1.3.3 and TACO ver. 0.7.3 with gencode_v27_annotation.gtf file. The resulting counting data were used for the statistical analyses of differentially expressed genes by DESeq2 ver. 1.14.1 with the Wald test (cut-offs: baseMean > 10, false discovery rate (FDR; adjusted p-value, padj) < 0.05, and log2 fold change of >1 or <−1) [22].

2.3. Quantitative Real-Time RT-PCR

RNA recovered from the placental samples was subjected to quantitative real-time RT-PCR to quantify *MG828507* and *FLT1* gene expression. A Superscript III First-Strand Synthesis SuperMix for RT-PCR (Invitrogen, Grand Island, NY, USA) using random primers was employed to produce single-stranded cDNA from the total RNA. The 18S rRNA housekeeping gene 18S rRNA (Hs99999901_s1) was used to normalize the mRNA concentrations, because other genes commonly used as such a control are often regulated by estrogen [23]. RT-

PCR reactions were performed in triplicate using a THUNDERBIRD Probe qPCR Mix (Toyobo, Osaka, Japan) in a final volume of 20 µL. The cycling conditions for PCR amplification were 1 min at 95 °C, followed by 40 cycles of 15 s at 95 °C, and 1 min at 60 °C. PCR primers and TaqMan probes for the *FLT1* gene were purchased commercially (Hs0105296_m1, Thermo Fisher Scientific, Tokyo, Japan), and those for the *MG828507* gene were custom-designed as follows: forward (5′-AAGTCAGCACACAGCTTGAAAGC-3′), reverse (5′-GTCTTGTGCTGTTTGACAAATGG-3′), and Taqman probe (5′-ACTACAGGCCTTTCTT-3′).

2.4. Overexpression of MG828507 in Cells

Almost the entire cDNA encoding *MG828507* was produced by RT-PCR and cloned into the pEGFP-N1 vector equipped with a CMV promoter. HTR-8/SVneo, a widely-used first trimester human trophoblast cell line, was purchased from Dr. Charles Graham at Queen's University (Kingston, ON, Canada). The HTR-8 cells were seeded at 3.0×10^5 cells per 2 mL in 30 mm dishes. After 24 h, 3.2 µg of the vector was transfected using Lipofectamine 3000 (Thermo Fisher Scientific, Tokyo, Japan). HTR-8 cells that transiently overexpressing the *MG828507* gene were harvested at 48 h after transfection. Expression levels were assayed by qRT-PCR.

2.5. RNAi Knockdown of the MG828507 and FLT1 Genes

HTR-8 cells were seeded at 3.0×10^5 cells per 2 mL in 30 mm dishes. After 24 h, siRNAs were transfected at a 40 nM concentration using Lipofectamine RNAiMax (Invitrogen, Grand Island, NY, USA). The Silencer™ Select siRNAs for the MG828507 gene were designed as follows; sense: 5′-UCUUUUUGUGAUGUAUGUGGC-3′, antisense: 5′-CACAUACAUCACAAAAAGAGG-3′. The siRNAs for the *FLT1* (Silencer™ Select Pre-Designed siRNA 4392420) and scrambled siRNA (Silencer™ Select Negative Control No. 1 siRNA 4390843) were purchased from Thermo Fisher. The HTR-8 cells were harvested at 96 h after transfection. Expression levels for the *MG828507* gene and the *FLT1* were assayed by qRT-PCR.

2.6. Genomic Analysis

Genomic DNA was extracted from the sampled placentas using a commercially available kit in accordance with the protocol of the manufacturer (Qiagen, Frankfurt, Germany). A total of 34 control samples from a normotensive pregnancy and 37 pre-eclampsia samples were used. Two single nucleotide variants (SNVs) (rs4769613, rs12050029) and one short tandem repeat (STR) variant (rs149427560), tag variants of each haplotype block located upstream of the *FLT1* gene, were genotyped. TaqMan primers and probes were purchased to genotype the rs4769613, rs12050029 SNVs, in accordance with the protocol of the manufacturer (C_32231378_10, C_1445411_10, Applied Biosystems, Foster City, CA, USA). For the STR variant, rs149427560, forward primers were labeled with FAM. The PCR products were analyzed by capillary electrophoresis (ABI3730 Genetic Analyzer; Applied Biosystems, Tokyo, Japan). Genotype deviations from a Hardy–Weinberg equilibrium (HWE) were first evaluated using the chi-squared test. Genotype and allele frequency differences between the pre-eclamptic and control groups were then evaluated using chi-squared analysis. All of these calculations were performed using SNPAlyze software (Dynacom, Chiba, Japan). Power calculations were performed using a genetic-power calculator.

To analyze the topologically associated domain (TAD) surrounding the *FLT1* gene and the variants at that site, we used published Hi-C data for the trophoblast cell line (http://promoter.bx.psu.edu/hi-c/view.php accessed on 15 April 2022).

2.7. Statistical Analysis

Intergroup comparisons were made using the Mann–Whitney U test or one way analysis of variance method, and *p* values of less than 0.05 were considered statistically significant. Correlations were evaluated using a Spearman's test. In significant difference tests, *p* values were calculated with the z conversion of Fisher's r. *p* values of less than 0.05 were again considered statistically significant.

3. Results

3.1. Identification of a lncRNA Gene Upregulated in Pre-Eclampsia

To further understand the molecular mechanisms underlying the symptoms of preeclampsia, we performed RNA-seq on pre-eclamptic placentas and normal uncomplicated pregnancies to compare their expression profiles. In comparisons of the data from six pre-eclamptic and six normotensive samples, we extracted 240 transcripts that were differentially expressed in the pre-eclamptic placenta (log2 fold-change >1 or <−1, FDR < 0.05). Since we focused on lncRNAs, we omitted protein-coding genes using annotation data in ref_gene_type and, thereby, obtained a gene set comprising 41 transcripts enriched for these nucleic acids. We manually characterized each transcript, examining the location and annotation information individually. We noted that one of the lncRNA genes in our panel, *MG828507*, was previously identified as being expressed in the placenta [24]. qRT-PCR confirmed that MG828507 was more abundant in the six pre-eclamptic placentas used for RNA-seq than in the controls.

MG828507 contains two exons and encodes a 6489 bp lncRNA. It is located ~80 kb upstream of the *FLT1* gene in a head-to-head orientation (Figure 1). The 5′ upstream region and 3′ end of the first exon is conserved among mammals, but all other regions are conserved only among primates. *MG828507* is known to be abundant in the placenta, and RNA-seq data of various organs in the public database reveals that the expression is scarcely found in other tissues than placenta [24]. Since the *MG828507* and *FLT1* genes are located within the same TAD, we hypothesized that *MG828507* may affect the expression of *FLT1* and, thereby, have an impact on susceptibility to pre-eclampsia.

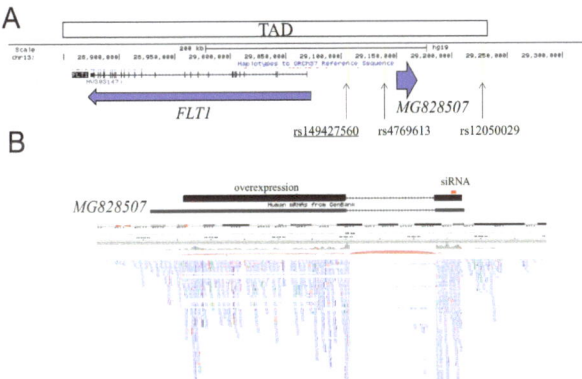

Figure 1. Genomic structure of the *FLT1* upstream region. (**A**) Location of the *MG828507* and *FLT1* genes. The horizontal arrows indicate their transcription direction. The extent of the TAD that incorporates these genes is indicated by the large box. The vertical arrows indicate the location of the three variants tested in this study. The STR, s149427560, is underlined. (**B**) RNA-seq of *MG828507*. The horizontal bar indicates the *MG828507* gene registered in the public database with its exon-intron structure. The upper panel indicates the position of the cDNA for overexpression experiments as well as the position targeted by the siRNA oligonucleotide used in this study.

3.2. Comparison of MG828507 and FLT1 Expression in Pre-Eclamptic and Normotensive Placentas

To validate the differential expression observed in our RNA-seq data, we increased the sample numbers and performed qRT-PCR (Figure 2A). We confirmed the overexpression of *MG828507* in our pre-eclamptic placental samples (*n* = 39), compared to those from the uncomplicated normotensive control pregnancies (*n* = 38), and found that this difference was statistically significant ($p < 0.01$). We also examined the expression level of the *FLT1* gene and found it to be significantly high in our pre-eclamptic samples, as reported previously [5]. Notably, the expression of *MG828507* appeared to be linearly correlated with that of *FLT1* (Figure 2B).

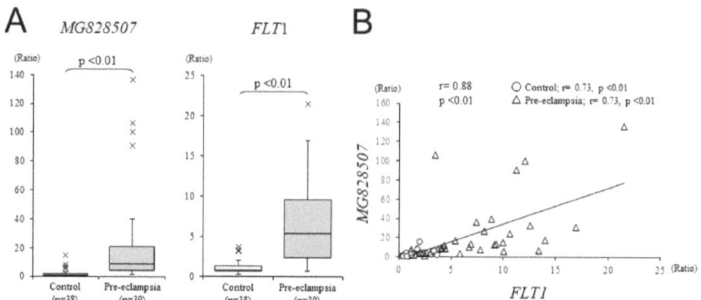

Figure 2. *MG828507* and *FLT1* expression in pre-eclamptic and normotensive placentas. (**A**) Differential expression of *MG828507* and *FLT1* in uncomplicated pregnancies (left) and in the pre-eclampsia samples (right). The boxes indicate the 25th and 75th percentiles, whilst the bands near the middle indicate the median values. The bars indicate the 1.5 interquartile ranges, with the outliers specifically marked. (**B**) Analysis of *MG828507* and *FLT1* correlations. Open circles indicate the uncomplicated pregnancy controls, and open triangles indicate pre-eclampsia. Regression lines are shown with correlation coefficients and *p* values.

3.3. Analysis of MG828507 and FLT1 Expression in the HTR-8 Trophoblast Cell Line

To test the possibility that the *MG828507* lncRNA may regulate the *FLT1* gene, we exogenously overexpressed it in the HTR-8 trophoblast cell line using a transfected vector but observed no impact on the *FLT1* expression level (Figure 3A). We then knocked down the *MG828507* gene in these same cells via siRNA transfection but again saw no changes in *FLT1* expression (Figure 3B).

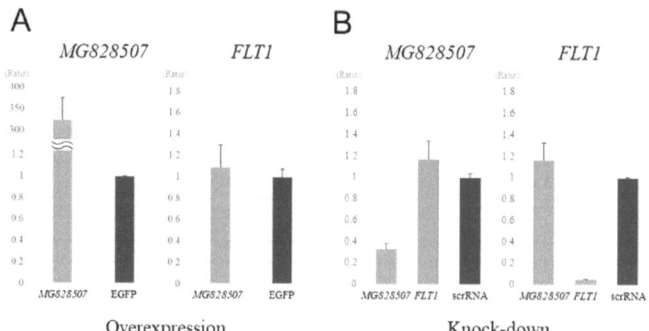

Figure 3. Analysis of the overexpression and knockdown of *MG828507*. (**A**) Expression of *MG828507* and *FLT1* after the exogenous overexpression of *MG828507*. HTR-8 trophoblast cells were transfected with an *MG828507* expression vector. The *MG828507* and *FLT1* transcript levels were analyzed by qRT-PCR. The vertical axis indicates the ratio relative to the data of cells transfected with control vector. (**B**) Expression of *MG828507* and *FLT1* after the knockdown of *MG828507*. HTR-8 trophoblast cells were transfected with an siRNA targeting *MG828507*. The *MG828507* and *FLT1* transcript levels were again analyzed by qRT-PCR. The siRNA for *FLT1* as well as a scrambled siRNA control were also used independently as control transfection experiments. The vertical axis indicates the ratio relative to the data of cells transfected with control oligonucleotides.

3.4. Analysis of MG828507 Expression in the Genetic Variants

Next, we genotyped our placental samples for two SNPs (rs4769613 and rs12050029) and one STR (rs149427560) that are located around the *MG828507* gene and examined whether there was any association between the expression of this lncRNA and these variants. The genotype frequencies in our samples were comparable to those reported in East Asian populations, and the distribution satisfied the HWE. When we analyzed the association between *MG828507* gene expression and rs4769613 and rs12050029, via allele wise and genotype wise analysis, no association was observed (Figure 4). We then examined the STR repeat numbers. Among the four size variants (472, 474, 476, and 478) identified in our samples, the 474 and 476 alleles were observed more frequently than the others. In the genotype-wise analysis, the pre-eclamptic samples of the 476/476 homozygotes showed significantly higher *MG828507* expression ($p < 0.05$). The 476 allele was significantly more frequent than the 474 allele in the allele-wise analysis (Figure 4).

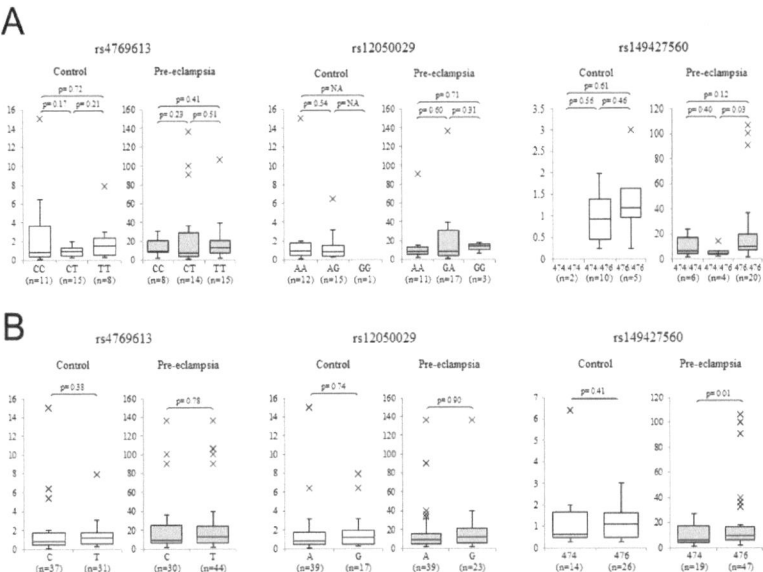

Figure 4. Correlations between *MG828507* expression and the indicated genetic variants. (**A**) Comparison of the placental mRNA levels by variant genotype. Data for rs4769613 (left), rs12050029 (center), and rs149427560 (right) are shown. In each panel, data for the normotensive placental controls are shown on the left, and those from pre-eclamptic cases are shown on the right. (**B**) Comparison of the placental mRNA levels by variant allele type. The boxes indicate the 25th and 75th percentiles. The bands near the middle indicate the median values. The bars indicate the 1.5 interquartile ranges, with the outliers specifically marked. Sample numbers and *p* values are shown in each panel.

3.5. Correlations between MG828507 Expression and Clinical Parameters

We finally assessed whether there were any correlations between *MG828507* expression and various clinical parameters that might reflect the severity of pre-eclampsia. With regard to disease onset, no significant difference in this expression was observed between the severe early onset group (earlier than 34 weeks of gestation, $n = 22$) and late onset group (34 weeks of gestation or later, $n = 17$) (Supplementary Figure S1). The *MG828507* levels appeared to correlate, however, with both the systolic and diastolic blood pressure (Figure 5A,B). However, when these analyses were performed separately for each group, no correlation was observed within either the pre-eclamptic or normotensive groups. These findings suggest that the correlation between *MG828507* level and blood pressure simply reflects an association between this lncRNA and the presence or absence of pre-eclampsia.

On the other hand, a negative correlation was observed between the *MG828507* level and the normalized birth or placental weights (Figure 5C,D). Even after stratification by group, this negative correlation was still evident. In addition, we analyzed the correlation between the *MG828507* level and other clinical parameters that indicate disease severity, including platelet count, serum transaminases, and creatinine levels. However, they did not correlate with the *MG828507* level (Supplementary Figure S2).

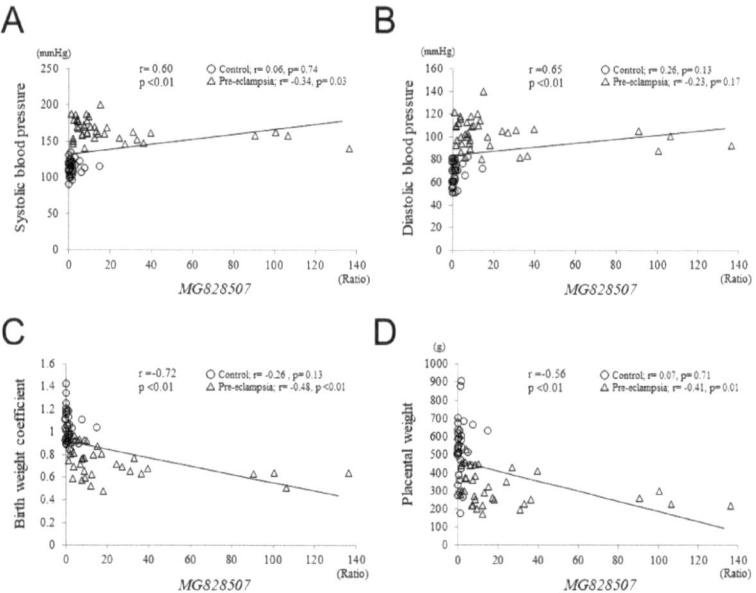

Figure 5. Correlations between *MG828507* expression and systolic blood pressure (**A**), diastolic blood pressure (**B**), normalized birth weight (**C**), or placental weight (**D**). Open circles indicate control uncomplicated pregnancies, and open triangles indicate pre-eclampsia. Regression lines are shown with correlation coefficients and *p* values.

4. Discussion

There is growing evidence that the unbalanced expression of specific lncRNA is involved in the pathogenesis of pre-eclampsia, and several important lncRNA genes have been identified via RNA-seq strategy [15,25,26]. We have reported here that *MG828507* lncRNA is expressed in the placenta, in tandem with the *FLT1* gene, and is highly expressed in a pre-eclamptic placenta compared to that of an uncomplicated normotensive pregnancy. It has been amply documented that lncRNAs play diverse regulatory roles in gene expression [27]. A growing body of evidence now indicates that the lncRNAs act as regulators of placental development and differentiation [28]. Since the expression of *MG828507* lncRNA was found in our current analyses to be linearly associated with that of the *FLT1* gene, we postulated that *MG828507* lncRNA may have a regulatory role in the expression of *FLT1*.

The *MG828507* and *FLT1* genes are located within the same TAD. The TADs are megabase-scale genomic domains, in which certain DNA regions show a significantly higher interaction frequency with other DNA regions within the domain, compared with those outside of the domain [29,30]. TADs are generally separated by an insulating protein complex, including CTCF, and build a common framework for contact between regulatory elements and genes within the domain [31]. One possibility in relation to our current investigation is that *MG828507* is an enhancer of regulatory RNA for the *FLT1* gene. Hence, the promoter of the *FLT1* gene and *MG828507* may interact within the TAD, forming a transcriptional complex via a loop conformation. Although Genhancer analysis did not indicate any interaction between *MG828507* and *FLT1*, the public databases indicate a positive acetylation of H3K27 at the 5′ end of *MG828507* exon, suggesting a possible enhancer function of *MG828507* (data not shown).

As regulatory lncRNAs or enhancer RNAs generally regulate their downstream target genes in either a cis or trans manner, we conducted an overexpression experiment with *MG828507* as a gain-of-function analysis and also, in parallel, a knockdown using siRNA as a loss-of-function experiment [32]. The expression of the *FLT1* gene was unaffected in both instances, however, which did not support our hypothesis. One notable limitation of these experiments was the possibility that HTR-8 cells have already lost the fine regulation of *FLT1* expression that is predicted in normal trophoblasts, since the *FLT1* mRNA level is low and the *MG828507* level is quite high in these cells relative to a normal placenta (data not shown). Alternatively, synergistic action of other genetic modifiers might be required to observe the effects of *MG828507* on *FLT1*.

We analyzed three *FLT1* upstream genomic variants that were previously reported to be associated with pre-eclampsia [9]. In our previous study, two of the SNPs we again tested here did not show such an association, but the rs149427560 STR showed a weak association with pre-eclampsia [11]. Although it was not unreasonable to speculate that the association was possibly based on an eQTL effect by the STR upon *FLT1* expression, we did not observe any association between this genotype and the *FLT1* expression level in our previous investigation [11]. Notably, however, this STR was found in our current analyses to be associated with *MG828507* expression in the pre-eclamptic placentas. The 476/476 genotype, showing a higher *MG828507* level, was frequent in pre-eclampsia, while the 474/476 genotype, showing a lower *MG828507* expression in our present analysis, was found in our prior study to be less frequent in the pre-eclamptic population [11]. This suggests that this STR may serve as an eQTL for *MG828507* and, thereby, lead to a higher susceptibility to pre-eclampsia via the modification of *FLT1* expression. Further validation with an increased sample number will be necessary.

When we analyzed the correlation here between *MG828507* expression and the clinical parameters of our study subjects, no association was found with the maternal blood pressure, but a correlation was observed with both the birth and placental weights. Based on our observation that the expression of *MG828507* correlates that of *FLT1* anti-angiogenic factor, an augmented *MG828507* expression may induce sFlt-1 and, thus, suppress angiogenic factors such as VEGF or PlGF and cause abnormal placentation. It is generally accepted that the initial event in pre-eclampsia is a reduction in placental perfusion via abnormal vascular remodeling, which later leads to symptoms in the women who have a genetic predisposition to the disease [4]. It is not unreasonable, therefore, to speculate that an increase in *MG828507* or *FLT1* expression may be a fundamental placental event that leads to both fetal and placental symptoms, which might not correlate with maternal symptom severity. This would suggest that *MG828507* lncRNA may be a pivotal placental factor in the pathophysiology of pre-eclampsia.

There are some limitations in this study. First, the sample size is small in the association study between *MG828507* expression and the genetic variants. To demonstrate that these genetic variants act as an eQTL, further studies involving a large sample size are required. Second, in the functional experimental study, although overexpression of exogenous *MG828507* did not affect the *FLT1* expression level, it is still possible that induction of endogenous *MG828507* expression might increase the *FLT1* expression. Altogether, it is still noteworthy that the strong correlation of expression levels of *MG828507* and *FLT1* genes might implicate a presence of a common, underlying regulatory mechanism between the *MG828507* and *FLT1* genes.

In summary, genomic variants located between the *MG828507* and *FLT1* genes may affect their expression and, thus, exert influence on the severity of the fetal and placental symptoms in pre-eclampsia. Further characterization of this lncRNA gene is likely to elucidate the etiological role of the *FLT1* gene in pre-eclampsia within a genomic context.

Supplementary Materials: The following supporting information can be downloaded at: https://www.mdpi.com/article/10.3390/jcm11154603/s1, Figure S1: Correlations between *MG828507* expression and disease onset; Figure S2: Correlations between *MG828507* expression and clinical parameters.

Author Contributions: Conceptualization, H.N. and H.K.; investigation, H.Y., H.I., K.H., A.O., Y.S., M.I. and Y.S.; methodology and formal analysis, H.I. and K.H.; drafting of the first version of the manuscript, H.N. and H.K.; critical revision and approval of the final version of the manuscript, K.T., T.S. and T.F. All authors have read and agreed to the published version of the manuscript.

Funding: This work was supported by the Ogyaa Donation Foundation of the Japan Association of Obstetricians and Gynecologists and by grants-in-aid for scientific research from the Ministry of Education, Culture, Sports, Science, and Technology, Japan (16K11117, 15H04710), and the Ministry of Health, Labour and Welfare, Japan (H27-nanchitou (nan)-ippan-024).

Institutional Review Board Statement: The study was conducted in accordance with the Declaration of Helsinki and was approved by the Ethical Review Board for Clinical Studies at Fujita Health University (HG19-003 and 22 April 2019).

Informed Consent Statement: Informed consent was obtained from all the subjects involved in the study.

Data Availability Statement: The data presented in this study are available on request from the corresponding author.

Conflicts of Interest: The authors declare no conflict of interest.

References

1. Lenfant, C. Working group report on high blood pressure in pregnancy. *J. Clin. Hypertens.* **2001**, *3*, 75–88.
2. Laresgoiti-Servitje, E. A leading role for the immune system in the pathophysiology of preeclampsia. *J. Leukoc. Biol.* **2013**, *94*, 247–257. [CrossRef] [PubMed]
3. Goulopoulou, S.; Davidge, S.T. Molecular mechanisms of maternal vascular dysfunction in preeclampsia. *Trends Mol. Med.* **2015**, *21*, 88–97. [CrossRef] [PubMed]
4. Roberts, J.M.; Gammill, H.S. Preeclampsia: Recent insights. *Hypertension* **2005**, *46*, 1243–1249. [CrossRef]
5. Maynard, S.E.; Min, J.Y.; Merchan, J.; Lim, K.H.; Li, J.; Mondal, S.; Libermann, T.A.; Morgan, J.P.; Sellke, F.W.; Stillman, I.E.; et al. Excess placental soluble fms-like tyrosine kinase 1 (sFlt1) may contribute to endothelial dysfunction, hypertension, and proteinuria in preeclampsia. *J. Clin. Investig.* **2003**, *111*, 649–658. [CrossRef]
6. Levine, R.J.; Maynard, S.E.; Qian, C.; Lim, K.H.; England, L.J.; Yu, K.F.; Schisterman, E.F.; Thadhani, R.; Sachs, B.P.; Epstein, F.H.; et al. Circulating angiogenic factors and the risk of preeclampsia. *N. Engl. J. Med.* **2004**, *350*, 672–683. [CrossRef]
7. Venkatesha, S.; Toporsian, M.; Lam, C.; Hanai, J.I.; Mammoto, T.; Kim, Y.M.; Bdolah, Y.; Lim, K.H.; Yuan, H.T.; Libermann, T.A.; et al. Soluble endoglin contributes to the pathogenesis of preeclampsia. *Nat. Med.* **2006**, *12*, 642–649. [CrossRef]
8. Dotters-Katz, S.K.; Humphrey, W.M.; Senz, K.L.; Lee, V.R.; Shaffer, B.L.; Kuller, J.A.; Caughey, A.B. Trisomy 13 and the risk of gestational hypertensive disorders: A population-based study. *J. Matern. Fetal Neonatal. Med.* **2018**, *31*, 1951–1955. [CrossRef]
9. McGinnis, R.; Steinthorsdottir, V.; Williams, N.O.; Thorleifsson, G.; Shooter, S.; Hjartardottir, S.; Bumpstead, S.; Stefansdottir, L.; Hildyard, L.; Sigurdsson, J.K.; et al. Variants in the fetal genome near FLT1 are associated with risk of preeclampsia. *Nat. Genet.* **2017**, *49*, 1255–1260. [CrossRef]
10. Gray, K.J.; Saxena, R.; Karumanchi, S.A. Genetic predisposition to preeclampsia is conferred by fetal DNA variants near FLT1, a gene involved in the regulation of angiogenesis. *Am. J. Obstet. Gynecol.* **2018**, *218*, 211–218. [CrossRef]
11. Ohwaki, A.; Nishizawa, H.; Kato, A.; Kato, T.; Miyazaki, J.; Yoshizawa, H.; Noda, Y.; Sakabe, Y.; Ichikawa, R.; Sekiya, T.; et al. Placental Genetic Variants in the Upstream Region of the FLT1 Gene in Pre-eclampsia. *J. Reprod. Infertil.* **2020**, *21*, 240–246. [CrossRef] [PubMed]
12. Jung, I.; Schmitt, A.; Diao, Y.; Lee, A.J.; Liu, T.; Yang, D.; Tan, C.; Eom, J.; Chan, M.; Chee, S.; et al. A compendium of promoter-centered long-range chromatin interactions in the human genome. *Nat. Genet.* **2019**, *51*, 1442–1449. [CrossRef]
13. De Goede, O.M.; Nachun, D.C.; Ferraro, N.M.; Gloudemans, M.J.; Rao, A.S.; Smail, C.; Eulalio, T.Y.; Aguet, F.; Ng, B.; Xu, J.; et al. Population-scale tissue transcriptomics maps long non-coding RNAs to complex disease. *Cell* **2021**, *184*, 2633–2648.e19. [CrossRef]
14. Gong, S.; Gaccioli, F.; Dopierala, J.; Sovio, U.; Cook, E.; Volders, P.J.; Martens, L.; Kirk, P.D.W.; Richardson, S.; Smith, G.C.S.; et al. The RNA landscape of the human placenta in health and disease. *Nat. Commun.* **2021**, *12*, 2639. [CrossRef] [PubMed]
15. He, J.; Liu, K.; Hou, X.; Lu, J. Identification and validation of key non-coding RNAs and mRNAs using co-expression network analysis in pre-eclampsia. *Medicine* **2021**, *100*, e25294. [CrossRef] [PubMed]

16. Rasmussen, M.; Reddy, M.; Nolan, R.; Camunas-Soler, J.; Khodursky, A.; Scheller, N.M.; Cantonwine, D.E.; Engelbrechtsen, L.; Mi, J.D.; Dutta, A.; et al. RNA profiles reveal signatures of future health and disease in pregnancy. *Nature* **2022**, *601*, 422–427. [CrossRef] [PubMed]
17. Takagi, K.; Yamasaki, M.; Nakamoto, O.; Saito, S.; Suzuki, H.; Seki, H.; Takeda, S.; Ohno, Y.; Sugimura, M.; Suzuki, Y.; et al. A review of best practice guide 2015 for care and treatment of hypertension in pregnancy. *Hypertens. Res. Pregnancy* **2015**, *3*, 65–103.
18. Watanabe, K.; Matsubara, K.; Nakamoto, O.; Ushijima, J.; Ohkuchi, A.; Koide, K.; Makino, S.; Mimura, K.; Morikawa, M.; Naruse, K.; et al. Outline of the new definition and classification of "Hypertensive Disorders of Pregnancy (HDP)"; a revised JSSHP statement of 2005. *Hypertens. Res. Pregnancy* **2018**, *6*, 33–37. [CrossRef]
19. Ogawa, Y.; Iwamura, T.; Kuriya, N.; Nishida, H.; Takeuchi, H.; Takada, M.; Itabashi, K.; Imura, S.; Isobe, K. Birth size standards by gestational age for Japanese neonates. *Acta Neonat. Jap.* **1998**, *34*, 624–632.
20. Nishizawa, H.; Pryor-Koishi, K.; Kato, T.; Kowa, H.; Kurahashi, H.; Udagawa, Y. Microarray analysis of differentially expressed fetal genes in placental tissue derived from early and late onset severe pre-eclampsia. *Placenta* **2007**, *28*, 487–497. [CrossRef]
21. Nishizawa, H.; Ota, S.; Suzuki, M.; Kato, T.; Sekiya, T.; Kurahashi, H.; Udagawa, Y. Comparative gene expression profiling of placentas from patients with severe pre-eclampsia and unexplained fetal growth restriction. *Reprod. Biol. Endocrinol.* **2011**, *9*, 107. [CrossRef] [PubMed]
22. Hitachi, K.; Nakatani, M.; Kiyofuji, Y.; Inagaki, H.; Kurahashi, H.; Tsuchida, K. An Analysis of Differentially Expressed Coding and Long Non-Coding RNAs in Multiple Models of Skeletal Muscle Atrophy. *Int. J. Mol. Sci.* **2021**, *22*, 2558. [CrossRef] [PubMed]
23. Patel, P.; Boyd, C.A.; Johnston, D.G.; Williamson, C. Analysis of GAPDH as a standard for gene expression quantification in human placenta. *Placenta* **2002**, *23*, 697–698. [CrossRef] [PubMed]
24. Majewska, M.; Lipka, A.; Paukszto, L.; Jastrzebski, J.P.; Gowkielewicz, M.; Jozwik, M.; Majewski, M.K. Preliminary RNA-Seq Analysis of Long Non-Coding RNAs Expressed in Human Term Placenta. *Int. J. Mol. Sci.* **2018**, *19*, 1894. [CrossRef] [PubMed]
25. Sun, N.; Qin, S.; Zhang, L.; Liu, S. Roles of noncoding RNAs in preeclampsia. *Reprod. Biol. Endocrinol.* **2021**, *19*, 100. [CrossRef]
26. Gong, R.Q.; Nuh, A.M.; Cao, H.S.; Ma, M. Roles of exosomes-derived lncRNAs in preeclampsia. *Eur. J. Obstet. Gynecol. Reprod. Biol.* **2021**, *263*, 132–138. [CrossRef]
27. Kopp, F.; Mendell, J.T. Functional Classification and Experimental Dissection of Long Noncoding RNAs. *Cell* **2018**, *172*, 393–407. [CrossRef]
28. Basak, T.; Ain, R. Long non-coding RNAs in placental development and disease. *Non Coding RNA Investig.* **2019**, *3*, 14. [CrossRef]
29. Dixon, J.R.; Selvaraj, S.; Yue, F.; Kim, A.; Li, Y.; Shen, Y.; Hu, M.; Liu, J.S.; Ren, B. Topological domains in mammalian genomes identified by analysis of chromatin interactions. *Nature* **2012**, *485*, 376–380. [CrossRef]
30. Nora, E.P.; Lajoie, B.R.; Schulz, E.G.; Giorgetti, L.; Okamoto, I.; Servant, N.; Piolot, T.; van Berkum, N.L.; Meisig, J.; Sedat, J.; et al. Spatial partitioning of the regulatory landscape of the X-inactivation centre. *Nature* **2012**, *485*, 381–385. [CrossRef]
31. Huang, H.; Zhu, Q.; Jussila, A.; Han, Y.; Bintu, B.; Kern, C.; Conte, M.; Zhang, Y.; Bianco, S.; Chiariello, A.M.; et al. CTCF mediates dosage- and sequence-context-dependent transcriptional insulation by forming local chromatin domains. *Nat. Genet.* **2021**, *53*, 1064–1074. [CrossRef] [PubMed]
32. Sartorelli, V.; Lauberth, S.M. Enhancer RNAs are an important regulatory layer of the epigenome. *Nat. Struct. Mol. Biol.* **2020**, *27*, 521–528. [CrossRef] [PubMed]

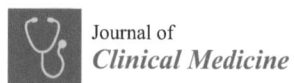

Article

Screening of Gestational Diabetes and Its Risk Factors: Pregnancy Outcome of Women with Gestational Diabetes Risk Factors According to Glycose Tolerance Test Results

Ele Hanson [1,2,*], Inge Ringmets [3], Anne Kirss [1,2], Maris Laan [4] and Kristiina Rull [1,2,4]

1. Department of Obstetrics and Gynaecology, Institute of Clinical Medicine, University of Tartu, Puusepa St. 8, 50406 Tartu, Estonia
2. Women's Clinic, Tartu University Hospital, Puusepa St. 8, 50406 Tartu, Estonia
3. Institute of Family Medicine and Public Health, University of Tartu, Ravila St. 19, 50411 Tartu, Estonia
4. Institute of Biomedicine and Translational Medicine, University of Tartu, Ravila St. 19, 50411 Tartu, Estonia
* Correspondence: ele.hanson@kliinikum.ee; Tel.: +372-555-48033

Abstract: *Background*: Gestational diabetes mellitus (GDM) can cause maternal and neonatal health problems, and its prevalence is increasing worldwide. We assessed the screening of GDM during a 7-year period and compared the outcome of pregnancies at high risk for GDM. *Methods*: We analyzed non-selected pregnant women (n = 5021) receiving antenatal care in Tartu University Hospital, Estonia in 2012–2018. Pregnant women were classified based on the absence or presence of GDM risk factors as low risk (n = 2302) or high risk for GDM (n = 2719), respectively. The latter were divided into subgroups after the oral glycose tolerance test (OGTT): GDM (n = 423), normal result (n = 1357) and not tested (n = 939). *Results*: The proportion of women with GDM risk factors increased from 43.5% in 2012 to 57.8% in 2018, and the diagnosis of GDM more than doubled (5.2% vs. 13.7%). Pregnancies predisposed to GDM but with normal OGTT results were accompanied by an excessive gestational weight gain and increased odds to deliver a LGA baby (AOR 2.3 (CI 1.8–3.0)). *Conclusions*: An increasing number of pregnancies presenting GDM risk factors are diagnosed with GDM. Pregnant women with GDM risk factors are, despite normal OGTT, at risk of increased weight gain and LGA newborns.

Keywords: gestational diabetes; screening test; hyperglycemia; macrosomia; oral glycose tolerance test

1. Introduction

Gestational diabetes mellitus (GDM), glycose tolerance disorder with onset or first recognition during pregnancy, is the most frequent complication of gestation. According to a report from the International Diabetes Federation, every 6th birth was complicated by GDM in 2019 [1].

GDM increases the risk of delivering a large for gestational age newborn (LGA) and related complications such as operative delivery, lacerations in the birth canal, birth trauma and the poor adaptation of the newborn [2]. Additionally, impaired glucose metabolism during the pregnancy is associated with preeclampsia and premature delivery [3,4]. In the long term, approximately half of women with GDM will develop type 2 diabetes later in life [5]. Therefore, screening, early initiation of counselling and treatment remains crucial [6].

Currently there is no generally accepted screening group or "gold standard" test to define the disease status. In most centers, the oral glucose tolerance test (OGTT) is applied but the testing strategy and diagnostic criteria vary [7,8]. In 2010, the International Association of Diabetes and Pregnancy Study Groups (IADPSG) recommended the use of 75 g OGTT at 24–28 gestational weeks with a cut-off point of fasting venous plasma glucose ≥5.1 mmol/L and/or after 1 h and 2 h level of ≥10.0 mmol/L and ≥8.5 mmol/L, respectively [9]. The recommendations are based on the results of the Hyperglycemia and Adverse Pregnancy Outcome (HAPO) study, which demonstrated a continuous relationship between maternal hyperglycemia and adverse perinatal outcome [3].

As in many countries, in Estonia, the decision of OGTT referral is based on the presence of GDM risk factors [10]. The most commonly recognized risk factors for GDM are obesity (BMI >30 kg/m^2), GDM and/or of birth baby >4500 g during any of the previous pregnancies, diabetes mellitus (DM) among first-degree relatives, ethnicity with a high prevalence of diabetes and previous polycystic ovary syndrome (PCOS) [10,11].

After the diagnosis of hyperglycemia, a pregnant woman is referred to diet counselling and if the blood glucose level exceeds the target, metformin and/or insulin, are administered. Treatment of GDM, lifestyle changes and timing of delivery have shown to reduce serious perinatal complications such as the rate of macrosomia and the long-term consequences of GDM [12,13].

The pregnancy outcome of women presenting GDM risk factors who skip the OGTT or whose glycose levels remain below the GDM diagnostic cutoff and therefore continue usual follow-up without additional dietary restrictions is addressed less. High risk untested pregnant women include those with possible undiagnosed GDM and prone to poor gestational outcome [14].

The aim of this study is to assess the prevalence of GDM and its risk factors in 2012–2018 in Estonia and to compare the outcome of pregnancies predisposed to GDM in cases with and without subsequent GDM diagnosis.

2. Materials and Methods

2.1. Study Population

We performed a retrospective observational study including 5735 pregnant women receiving antenatal care in Women's Clinic Tartu University Hospital (TUH), Estonia in 2012–2018.

The study participants were recruited during three time periods. The first study cohort was compiled to assess the compliance to the GDM screening algorithm, and it incorporated data of all women starting antenatal follow-up visits between January and December 2012 ($n = 1373$) [15]. The second set of women ($n = 2334$) originated from a monocentric prospective "Happy Pregnancy" (HP) study (full name "Development of novel non-invasive biomarkers for fertility and healthy pregnancy": principal investigator Prof. Maris Laan). The recruited women included approximately two thirds of unselected pregnant women receiving antenatal care in TUH between March 2013 and August 2015 [16–18]. The third dataset comprised all women whose antenatal follow-up in TUH started between January and December 2018 ($n = 2028$).

The considered GDM risk factors included pre-pregnancy overweight/obesity (BMI 25–29.9/>30 kg/m^2), GDM and/or of birth newborn >4500 g during any of the previous pregnancies, DM among first-degree relatives, PCOS, fasting glucose >5.1 mmol/L, glycosuria, excessive weight gain, suspicion of a LGA fetus or polyhydramnion during the index pregnancy. The information about the GDM risk factors, course and outcome of the pregnancy was collected by midwives and/or extracted from electronic hospital medical records (Supplementary Table S1).

The women with pregestational DM including type 2 DM diagnosed at the 1st trimester (fasting plasma glycose $\geq$7.0 mmol/l or any plasma glycose above 11.1 mmol/L) [19], multiple pregnancy or termination of pregnancy before 22 gestational weeks (g.w.), and those who had missing delivery data were excluded from the analysis.

The final dataset included a total of 5021 pregnancies: 1073 women represented the first (2012), 2176 women the second (2013–2015) and 1772 women the third (2018) recruitment cohort. All participants were of white European ancestry and Estonian residents.

2.2. Patient Grouping and Diagnostic Criteria

The GDM screening algorithm applied in Estonia since 2011 is shown in Figure 1 [19]. According to the current algorithm and clinical guidelines, OGTT is not mandatory to all pregnant women. Only women presenting any GDM risk factor are referred to OGTT.

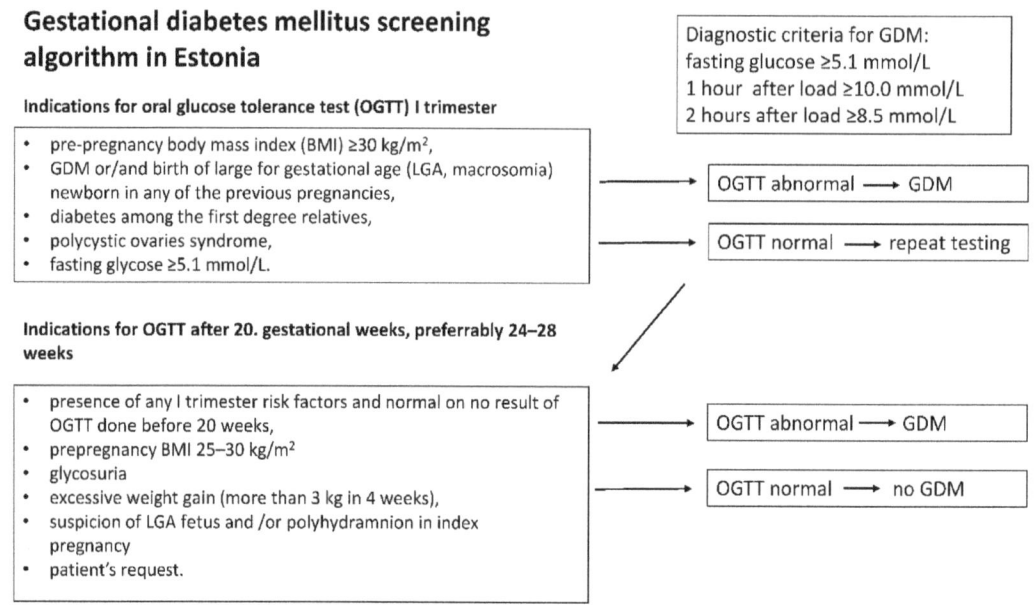

Figure 1. Gestational diabetes mellitus screening algorithm in Estonia.

GDM was diagnosed when any of the three consecutive measurements of oral glucose tolerance test (OGTT) were abnormal. Values were considered abnormal if the fasting venous plasma glucose level was ≥ 5.1 mmol/L and/or 1 h or 2 h after administration of 75 g oral glucose orally resulted in plasma glucose levels of ≥ 10.0 mmol/l and/or ≥ 8.5 mmol/L glucose, respectively [19].

Women were further categorized into four subgroups according to the presence of GDM risk factors and OGTT results: (1) low risk (group 1): women without risk factors and no indication to OGTT (n = 2302, 46%); (2) no OGTT (group 2): women with risk factors but no OGTT or only one normal test result before 20 weeks (n = 939, 19%); (3) normal OGTT (group 3): women with risk factors and a normal OGTT result obtained after 20 g.w. (n = 1357, 27%); (4) GDM (group 4): women with an abnormal OGTT result at any time during the gestation (n = 423, 8%).

For the assessment of a newborn's weight, a growth calculator based on INTERGROWTH-21st Project [20] data was applied to convert the newborn birthweight into gestational age and sex-adjusted centiles. Large-for-gestational-age (LGA) newborns were diagnosed as birthweight $\geq$95th centile and small-for-gestational-age (SGA) newborns as birthweight $\leq$10th centile.

Birth <37th g.w. was defined as preterm birth (PTB). Gestational hypertension (GH) was diagnosed if a patient exhibited after 20 g.w. new-onset isolated hypertension ($\geq$140 mmHg and/or $\geq$90 mmHg). Preeclampsia (PE) was diagnosed if a patient exhibited hypertension after 20 g.w. accompanied by any of the following new-onset conditions: proteinuria, renal insufficiency, impaired liver function; hematological or neurological complications and eclampsia [21]. Only perineal ruptures after vaginal delivery involving anal sphincter (3rd grade) and/or anal epithelium (4th grade) were analyzed.

Total weight gain during the pregnancy was considered excessive when it exceeded the widely accepted recommendations: >9.0 kg for obese (pre-pregnancy BMI 30.0 kg/m^2 or higher); >11.5 kg for overweight (25.0–29.9 kg/m^2), >16.0 kg for normal weight (18.5–24.9 kg/m^2) and >18.0 kg for underweight women (less than 18.5 kg/m^2) [22].

2.3. Statistical Analysis

Summary estimates of the data (median, 5th–95th centile) were calculated and all statistical tests were implemented using the STATA software ver. 13.1 (StataCorp, College Station, TX, USA). To compare groups, the Wilcoxon rank-sum test was used for continuous variables and Chi^2 test for categorical variables. A significance level of 0.05 was used. Bonferroni correction for multiple testing was applied according to the number of tests performed. One-way ANOVA was used for continuous variables to detect the differences in multiple group comparisons. In case of significant difference for post hoc pairwise comparisons, the Wilcoxon rank-sum test was applied. Binary logistic regression analysis was used to examine the association between pregnancy outcome and allocated GDM risk group. The adjusted odds ratios with 95% confidence intervals were calculated. The odds ratios (OR) were adjusted for previous births, LGA baby, pre-pregnancy BMI, age, cohort, or gestational age at delivery depending on pregnancy outcome variable.

2.4. Ethical Approval

The data collection and analysis was approved by the Research Ethics Committee of the University of Tartu, Estonia (permissions no. 225/T-6, 06.05.2013; 221/T-6, 17.12.2012, 286/M-18, 15.10.2018; 291/T-3, 18.03.2019 and 322/M-17, 17.08.2020) and the study was carried out in compliance with the guidelines of the Declaration of Helsinki.

3. Results

3.1. The Prevalence of Gestational Diabetes and Its Risk Factors Has Increased during Seven Years

The study population comprised 5021 unselected pregnant women from three recruitment periods across seven years (Table 1).

Table 1. Maternal characteristics of three datasets [1].

Parameter [2]	I (n = 1073)	II (n = 2176)	III (n = 1772)	p Value [6]		
				I vs. II	I vs. III	II vs. III
Basic characteristics						
Maternal age (years)	28 (20–38)	28 (20–38)	29 (21–38)	n.s	1.9×10^{-7}	1.2×10^{-6}
Pre-pregnancy BMI (kg/m^2)	22.5 (18.0–32.8)	22.3 (18.1–31.5)	22.7 (18.5–33.6)	n.s	n.s	1.9×10^{-5}
Multiparous [3]	NA	1190 (54.7%)	1114 (62.9%)	NA	NA	2.2×10^{-7}
GDM risk factors						
Risk factor carriers	467 (43.5%)	1227 (56.4%)	1025 (57.8%)	5.1×10^{-12}	1.2×10^{-13}	n.s
Correctly tested among risk factor carriers	291 (62.3%)	702 (57.2%)	787 (76.8%)	n.s	1.5×10^{-4}	3.5×10^{-9}
BMI 25–30 kg/m^2 n (% of carriers)	198 (42.4%)	394 (32.1%)	320 (31.2%)	n.s	n.s	n.s
BMI >30 kg/m^2	92 (19.7%)	185 (15.1%)	210 (20.5%)	n.s	n.s	2.0×10^{-4}
GDM previously [3]	13 (2.8%)	26 (2.1%)	28 (2.7%)	n.s	n.s	n.s
Previous baby 4500 g	30 (6.4%)	36 (2.9%)	39 (3.8%)	n.s	n.s	n.s
DM among first degree relatives	78 (16.7%)	224 (18.3%)	161 (15.7%)	n.s	n.s	n.s
PCOS	24 (5.1%)	24 (2.0%)	9 (0.9%)	n.s	3.0×10^{-5}	n.s
Fasting glycose >5.1 mmol/L	48 (10.3%)	471 (38.4%)	235 (22.9%)	3.3×10^{-36}	1.6×10^{-14}	6.0×10^{-10}

Table 1. Cont.

Parameter [2]	I (n = 1073)	II (n = 2176)	III (n = 1772)	p Value [6]		
				I vs. II	I vs. III	II vs. III
Basic characteristics						
Polyhydramnion	19 (4.1%)	42 (3.4%)	40 (3.9%)	n.s	n.s	n.s
Other [4]	68 (14.6%)	116 (9.5%)	245 (23.9%)	n.s	6.1×10^{-10}	3.2×10^{-20}
Pregnancy outcome						
Gestational diabetes	56 (5.2%)	124 (5.7%)	243 (13.7%)	n.s	8.05×10^{-13}	6.4×10^{-18}
Preterm birth	50 (4.7%)	110 (5.1%)	87 (4.9%)	n.s	n.s	n.s
Gestational age at delivery (days)	280 (259–287)	281 (258–293)	279 (259–291)	1.38×10^{-17}	3.69×10^{-10}	n.s
Birthweight (grams)	3596 (2680–4360)	3569 (2680–4366)	3590 (2660–4302)	n.s	n.s	n.s
Cesarean section	181 (16.9%)	363 (16.7%)	342 (19.3%)	n.s	n.s	n.s
LGA [5]	202 (18.8%)	341 (15.7%)	286 (16.1%)	n.s	n.s	n.s
LGA + GDM	23 (11.4%)	30 (8.8%)	57 (9.4%)			
SGA [5]	17 (1.6%)	52 (2.4%)	43 (2.4%)	n.s	n.s	n.s

[1] I dataset represented women recruited for antenatal care in 2012; II dataset in 2013–2015 and III dataset in 2018. [2] Data are given as median (5th–95th percentiles) or number (percentage) when appropriate. Groups were compared using chi-squared test for categorical and Wilcoxon rank-sum test for continuous variables. [3] Missing detailed data for number of previous pregnancies in 2012 cohort. [4] Risk factors: glycosuria, excessive weight gain (more than 3 kg in 4 weeks) suspicion of LGA fetus in index pregnancy were classified as "other" risk factors. [5] For the assignment of a large or small-for-gestational-age (LGA or SGA, respectively) diagnosis, the fetal growth calculator based on INTERGROWTH-21st Project was applied to convert the newborn birthweight into gestational age and sex-adjusted centiles [20]. Newborns were categorized as LGA in cases where the sex-and gestational age adjusted birth centile was more than 95 and SGA in cases where the sex-and gestational age adjusted birth centile was less than 10. centiles [6] p value was adjusted according to Bonferroni correction for 22 tests and 3 subgroups $0.05/3 \times 22 < 7.6 \times 10^{-4}$. DM, diabetes mellitus; GDM, gestational diabetes mellitus; LGA, large for gestational age; NA, not available; n.s, non-significant; PCOS, polycystic ovary syndrome; SGA, small for gestational age.

Between 2012 and 2018, the proportion of pregnant women presenting any of the GDM risk factors increased from 43.5% to 57.8%. The most prevalent GDM risk factor was overweight (BMI 25–29.9 kg/m^2; >30% of high-risk women), followed by women with a high fasting glycose level (10.3–38.3% of pregnancies) and "other" risk factors (9.5–23.9%): glycosuria, excessive weight gain and suspicion of LGA fetus. In 2018, more high-risk women were subjected to the GDM screening algorithm compared to 2012 and 2013–2015 cohorts (Table 1). In addition, compared to the first two cohorts, the women in 2018 were older: 29 (5–95th percentile 21–38) years versus 28 (20–38) years in both 2012 and 2013–2015 cohort, and had a higher BMI compared to the 2013–2015 cohort (22.7 vs. 22.3) (Table 1).

Women with obesity and/or GDM in a previous pregnancy were more frequently subjected to the correct GDM screening algorithm (75.1–88.1% of risk factor carriers) (Table 2) and were more likely to receive a GDM diagnosis: obesity (OR 6.3 (5.0–8.9)), previous GDM (OR 12.5 (95% CI 7.5–20.6)). Although women with "other" risk factors were most often tested, only 14.7% received a GDM diagnosis (Table 2).

While the proportion of LGA babies has slightly decreased since 2012 from 18.8% to 16.1% in 2018 ($p = 3.4 \times 10^{-2}$), it remains not statistically significant after Bonferroni correction ($p < 7.6 \times 10^{-4}$). Additionally, the occurrence of pregnancy complications (preterm delivery and birth of SGA babies) and C-section rate has not changed notably during the examined period (Table 1).

Table 2. Adherence to GDM screening algorithm [1] among high-risk women and odds to receive GDM diagnosis.

Risk Factor	Carrier (n)	Tested Correctly (n/% of Carriers)	GDM (n/% of Correctly Tested)	OR (95% CI)	p-Value [3]
BMI 25.0–29.9 kg/m^2	1385	857 (61.9%)	252 (29.4%)	1.7 (1.4–2.2)	3.2×10^{-6}
BMI ≥ 30.0 kg/m^2	482	362 (75.1%)	139 (62.3%)	6.3 (5.0–8.9)	2.9×10^{-47}
GDM in previous pregnancy	67	59 (88.1%)	36 (62.7%)	12.5 (7.5–20.6)	6.0×10^{-21}
LGA [2] in previous pregnancy	105	88 (83.8%)	32 (38.2%)	4.7 (3.1–7.2)	3.0×10^{-10}
PCOS	57	41 (71.9%)	14 (53.3%)	3.6 (2.0–6.9)	2.4×10^{-4}
DM in relatives	463	305 (65.9%)	78 (25.6%)	2.5 (1.9–3.2)	6.1×10^{-10}
Fasting glycose >5.1 mmol/L	755	436 (57.7%)	175 (40.1%)	5.0 (4.0–6.1)	2.0×10^{-44}
Polyhydramnion	97	63 (64.9%)	16 (26.2%)	2.1 (1.2–3.6)	1.4×10^{-2}
Other	431	402 (93.3%)	59 (14.7%)	1.8 (1.3–2.4)	2.1×10^{-4}

[1] Schematic representation of GDM screening algorithm is presented in Figure 1. [2] For the assignment of large-for-gestational-age (LGA) diagnosis, the fetal growth calculator based on INTERGROWTH-21st Project was applied to convert the newborn birthweight into gestational age and sex-adjusted centiles [20]. Newborn was categorized as LGA in case the sex-and gestational age adjusted birth centile was more than 95. [3] p value was adjusted according to Bonferroni correction for 9 tests and 2 groups 0.05/18 is 2.7×10^{-3}. BMI, body mass index; DM, diabetes mellitus; GA, gestational age; GDM, gestational diabetes mellitus; LGA, large for gestational age; OR, odds ratio; PCOS, polycystic ovary syndrome.

3.2. The Largest Babies Are Born to Mothers Who Undergo Correct GDM Screening Algorithm

The pregnancy outcome was assessed comparatively in the four subgroups formed based on the presence of GDM risk factors and outcome of the OGTT test.

Compared to other subgroups, mothers with GDM (group 4) had the lowest gestational age at delivery, were more likely to deliver a LGA baby and more often via C-section (Tables 3 and 4). Gestational hypertension has also been more frequently reported among the GDM cases (Table 3).

Table 3. Pregnancy outcome in women allocated into four subgroups according to GDM risk factors and OGTT result.

Outcome [1]	Low Risk Pregnancies [5]	High Risk Pregnancies			Pairwise Comparisons
	(Group 1)	No OGTT (Group 2)	OGTT Normal (Group 3)	GDM (Group 4)	Between Groups [6] $p < 7.6 \times 10^{-4}$
Number of women	2302	939	1357	423	1 vs. 4, 2 vs. 4, 3 vs. 4
GA at delivery (days)	280 (259–292)	280 (255–292)	280 (260–293)	276 (252–289)	
Birthweight (grams)	3502 (2644–4233)	3576 (2642–4320)	3705 (2808–4468)	3635 (2695–4430)	1 vs. 2, 1 vs. 3, 1 vs. 4, 2 vs. 3
Birth centile	70.7 (13.7–97.3)	75.7 (18.4–98.2)	82.2 (25.0–99.3)	82.6 (26.5–99.3)	1 vs. 2, 1 vs. 3, 1 vs. 4, 2 vs. 3, 2 vs. 4
LGA [2]	243 (10.5%)	160 (17.1%)	315 (23.2%)	110 (26.0%)	1 vs. 2, 1 vs. 3, 1 vs. 4, 2 vs. 3, 2 vs. 4
SGA [2]	70 (3.0%)	15 (1.6%)	23 (1.7%)	4 (0.95%)	n.s
Cesarean section	322 (14.0%)	175 (18.7%)	274 (20.2%)	114 (27.0%)	1 vs. 3, 1 vs. 4; 2 vs. 4
Preterm delivery	104 (4.5%)	55 (5.9%)	58 (4.3%)	27 (6.4%)	n.s

Table 3. Cont.

Outcome [1]	Low Risk Pregnancies [5]	High Risk Pregnancies			Pairwise Comparisons
	(Group 1)	No OGTT (Group 2)	OGTT Normal (Group 3)	GDM (Group 4)	Between Groups [6] $p < 7.6 \times 10^{-4}$
Shoulder dystocia [3,4]	6/1468 (0.4%)	3/627 (0.5%)	6/883 (0.7%)	1/266 (0.4%)	n.s
Perineal rupture ≥3 grade [3,4]	14/1468 (1.0%)	3/627 (0.5%)	9/883 (1.0%)	2/266 (0.8%)	n.s
Preeclampsia	23 (1.04%)	23 (2.5%)	25 (1.8%)	11 (2.6%)	1 vs. 2, 1 vs. 3, 1 vs. 4
Gestational hypertension [4]	20/1699 (1.2%)	26 (3.4%)	50 (4.5%)	25 (6.8%)	1 vs. 4

[1] Data are given as median (5th–95th percentiles) or number (percentage) when appropriate. [2] For the assignment of large or small-for-gestational-age (LGA or SGA, respectively) diagnosis, the fetal growth calculator based on INTERGROWTH-21st Project was applied to convert the newborn birthweight into gestational age and sex-adjusted centiles [20]. Newborn was categorized as LGA in cases where the sex and gestational age adjusted birth centile was more than 95 and SGA in cases where the sex-and gestational age adjusted birth centile was less than 10 centiles. [3] Percentage is calculated from vaginal deliveries only. [4] Data available for 2013–2015 and 2018 cohorts. [5] Low risk pregnancies for GDM were defined as absence of GDM risk factors, for those individuals OGTT is not indicated. High-risk pregnancies for GDM were defined as the presence of any of the following risk factors: BMI > 25 kg/m^2, GDM or LGA in previous pregnancy, fasting glycose >5.1 mmol/L, PCOS, polyhydramnion, DM in family history, "other" risk factors (glycosuria, excessive weight gain (more than 3 kg in 4 weeks) suspicion of LGA fetus in index pregnancy). Presence of any risk factor is indication for OGTT. [6] Wilcoxon rank-sum test was used for continuous variables and Chi2 test for categorical variables, statistical significance level adjusted according to Bonferron correction for 11 parameters and 4 groups $0.05/66 < 7.6 \times 10^{-4}$. DM, diabetes mellitus; GA, gestational age; GDM, gestational diabetes mellitus; LGA, large for gestational age; OGTT, oral glucose tolerance test; PCOS, polycystic ovary syndrome, SGA, small for gestational age.

Table 4. Crude and adjusted odds ratios for selected pregnancy outcomes between groups devided according to GDM risk factors and OGTT result.

Outcome	Group	Number of Women	OR (95% CI)	AOR (95% CI)
LGA newborn [1,2]				
	Low risk	243	1	1
	No OGTT	160	1.8 (1.4–2.2) ***	1.6 (1.2–2.2) ***
	Normal OGTT	315	2.6 (2.1–3.1) ***	2.3 (1.8–3.0) ***
	GDM	110	3.0 (2.3–3.9) ***	2.4 (1.7–3.4) ***
SGA [2,3]				
	Low risk	70	1	1
	No OGTT	15	0.5 (0.3–0.9) *	0.6 (0.3–1.1)
	Normal OGTT	23	0.5 (0.3–0.9) *	0.6 (0.4–1.0) *
	GDM	4	0.3 (0.1–0.8) *	0.3 (0.1–0.9) *
Preeclampsia [4]				
	Low risk	23	1	1
	No OGTT	23	2.5 (1.4–4.5) **	1.4 (0.7–2.7)
	Normal OGTT	25	1.9 (1.2–3.3) *	1.1 (0.6–2.1)
	GDM	11	2.6 (1.3–5.5) *	1.3 (0.5–3.1)
Cesarean Section [5]				
	Low risk	322	1	1
	No OGTT	175	1.4 (1.2–1.7) **	1.2 (0.9–1.5)
	Normal OGTT	274	1.6 (1.3–1.9) ***	1.3 (1.1–1.7) *
	GDM	114	2.3 (1.8–2.9) ***	1.5 (1.1–2.1) *

[1] Adjusted to previous births, previous LGA baby, BMI, age, cohort and gestational age at delivery. [2] For the assignment of large or small-for-gestational-age (LGA or SGA, respectively) diagnosis, the fetal growth calculator based on INTERGROWTH-21st Project was applied to convert the newborn birthweight into gestational age and sex-adjusted centiles [20]. Newborn was categorized as LGA in case the sex-and gestational age adjusted birth centile was more than 95 and SGA in case the sex-and gestational age adjusted birth centile was less than 10 centile. [3] Adjusted to cohort, previous births and gestational age at delivery. [4] Adjusted to previous births, BMI, and cohort, [5] Adjusted to previous births, previous LGA baby, BMI, age, cohort and gestational age at delivery. * $p < 0.05$, ** $p < 0.005$; *** $p < 0.001$. GDM, gestational diabetes mellitus; GH, gestational diabetes; OGTT, oral glycose tolerance test; OR, odds ratio; AOR, adjusted odds ratio.

The median birthweight of newborns was highest among women with risk factors to GDM, but a normal OGTT result (group 3) compared to other non GDM groups. Birthweight centiles were similar in women presenting risk factors to GDM and receiving OGTT irrespective of the OGTT result (~82 percentile), but significantly higher compared to those with risk factors but no OGTT (group 2) (Table 3).

Additionally, the C-section rate of low-risk women (group 1) was lower compared to women with normal OGTT (group 3) and GDM (group 4) (Table 3).

Birthweight and the proportion of LGA babies was the lowest among low-risk women (group 1) compared to all high-risk women (groups 2, 3 and 4) (Table 3). An inverse trend, however, not significant, was noted in the prevalence of SGA newborns (3% vs. ≤1.7%).

3.3. Comparison of Maternal Characteristics and Pregnancy Course among High-Risk Pregnant Women with Normal or No OGTT Result

Women presenting GDM risk factors but a normal OGTT result had significantly more LGA babies compared to those with no OGTT result and, therefore, their GDM status was unknown (Tables 3 and 5). Among women presenting risk factors to GDM, the odds to deliver a LGA baby after a normal OGTT result was nearly as high as in the GDM diagnosis group (Table 4).

Table 5. Maternal characteristics and pregnancy course among high-risk pregnant women without GDM diagnosis.

	OGTT Normal N = 1357	No OGTT N = 939	p-Value [5]
Basic characteristics [1]			
Age (years)	28 (20–38)	29 (21–39)	n.s
BMI (kg/m^2)	24.4 (18.7–34.6)	25.3 (18.6–32.9)	n.s
Multiparous [2]	48.5%	49.3%	n.s
Risk factors n (% of carriers)			
Previous baby 4500 g	60 (4.4%)	13 (1.4%)	1.2×10^{-4}
GDM previously	25 (1.8%)	4 (0.4%)	n.s
DM among first degree relatives	243 (17.9%)	142 (15.1%)	n.s
PCOS	30 (2.2%)	13 (1.4%)	n.s
Fasting glycose >5.1 mmol/L	267 (19.7%)	311 (33.1%)	7.0×10^{-14}
Polyhydramnion	47 (3.5%)	38 (4.0%)	n.s
Other	358 (26.4%)	35 (3.7%)	1.3×10^{-57}
Pregnancy course and outcome			
Weight gain (0–23 g.w) (kg)	7 (0–16)	6 (−1–14)	2.2×10^{-6}
Weight gain (24–42 g.w) (kg)	11 (3.6–22)	10 (2.9–17)	2.0×10^{-5}
Total weight gain (kg)	17.7 (4–36.5)	15.8 (3–29.6)	3.6×10^{-5}
Excessive weight gain [3]	62.4%	53.9%	2.9×10^{-4}
GA at delivery (days)	280 (260–293)	280 (255–292)	n.s
Male newborn	52.5%	50.0%	n.s
Birthweight (grams)	3705 (2808–4468)	3578 (2642–4320)	5.8×10^{-9}
LGA [4]	315 (23.2%)	161 (17.1%)	4.2×10^{-4}
Birthweight centile	82.2 (25–99.1)	75.7 (18.4–98.2)	5.2×10^{-9}
Cesarean section	274 (20.2%)	175 (18.6%)	n.s
If LGA (% of Cesarean sections)	87 (31%)	32 (18%)	2.0×10^{-3}

[1] Data are given as median (5th–95th percentiles) or number (percentage) when appropriate. Groups were compared using chi-squared test for categorical and Wilcoxon rank-sum test for continuous variables. [2] Data not available for 2012 cohort. [3] Total weight gain during the pregnancy was considered excessive when it exceeded recommendations by Rasmussen [22]. [4] For the assignment of large or small-for-gestational-age (LGA or SGA, respectively) diagnosis, the fetal growth calculator based on INTERGROWTH-21st Project was applied to convert the newborn birthweight into gestational age and sex-adjusted centiles [20]. Newborn was categorized as LGA in cases where the sex-and gestational age adjusted birth centile was more than 95 and SGA in cases where the sex-and gestational age adjusted birth centile was less than 10 centiles. [5] p value was adjusted for multiple testing according to Bonferroni correction for 2 groups $0.05/21 < 2.4 \times 10^{-3}$. DM, diabetes mellitus; GA, gestational age; g.w, gestational weeks; GDM, gestational diabetes mellitus; LGA, large for gestational age; n.s, non-significant; OGTT, oral glucose tolerance test; PCOS, polycystic ovary syndrome; SGA, small for gestational age.

Both birthweight and centile of newborns were significantly lower in high-risk non-OGTT women (group 2) in contrast to the high-risk but normal OGTT group (group 3) (Tables 3 and 5). However, in both groups approximately every fifth woman delivered by C-section; 31% of operative deliveries among women with normal OGTT (group 3) resulted in the birth of a LGA baby compared to 18% in the no OGTT subgroup (group 2).

There was no difference in maternal age and pre-pregnancy BMI between these two groups.

Although the birth of a LGA baby in any of the previous pregnancies accounted for a small number of women as a risk factor, more of them had normal OGTT (group 3). The percentage of women with "other" risk factors was considerably higher in the normal OGTT group (26.4% vs. 3.6%). However, women with increased fasting glycose level detected in the first trimester were in the no OGTT group (group 2).

There was higher total weight gain among women with a normal OGTT (group 3) result compared to non-OGTT women (group 2). Weight gain difference was observed especially after 24 g.w. when OGTT is usually scheduled. Women with normal OGTT (group 3) gained, on average, 11.6 ± 5.7 kg, median 11 kg, compared to 10.2 ± 4.6 kg, median 10 kg in the no OGTT group (group 2) (Table 5). In comparison, the total weight gain in women with GDM 12.7 ± 8.7 kg, median 11.7 kg, and after 24 gestational week 8.3 ± 5.1 kg, median 8 kg.

3.4. Pregnancy Course and Outcome of Women with GDM According to Treatment

In our study, out of 423 women with a GDM diagnosis, 82 (19.4%) needed medical treatment (metformin and/or insulin) in addition to dietary measures. The women receiving medication delivered earlier compared to women whose GDM was controlled with diet (274.5 vs. 277 g.d, $p = 1.3 \times 10^{-3}$). Apart from gestational age at delivery, we did not detect any differences in pregnancy course and outcome between different treatment modalities (Supplementary Table S2).

4. Discussion

We evaluated the pregnancy course and outcome of low and high-risk women with and without GDM diagnosis after the OGTT test at Women's Clinic of Tartu University Hospital, Estonia in 2012–2018. Our study shows sharp increase in GDM risk factor carriers, almost doubling the women diagnosed with GDM over the seven-year period. Additionally, we observed a high fraction of LGA newborns among women carrying GDM risk factors but defined as unaffected based on the current GDM screening algorithm. These women also underwent excessive weight gain during the second half of pregnancy.

In Estonia, the risk factor-based testing of GDM is applied and the reported prevalence of the disease is influenced by the testing activity. Referral to OGTT is dependent on the subjective assessment of risk factors by midwives or obstetricians, as well as the patient's consent and understanding of the necessity of the test. By 2018, more than half of pregnant women had at least one risk factor but only three of four (76.8%) received the OGTT test, as suggested by the guidelines in [19]. Those who remain untested may have undiagnosed GDM and are therefore prone to GDM-related complications, including stillbirth [23]. A study in Finland found that even mild untreated hyperglycemia resulted in an increased Cesarean section rate and larger birth weight [24].

Benhalima et al. studied selective screening for GDM in European countries and found that by using the risk factor-based screening algorithm, more than a third of GDM cases would be missed [10]. They also suggested that to improve testing, the selection of risk factors should be simplified: by screening all women at age 30 or more and/or BMI ≥ 25 kg/m^2, 70% of pregnant women would need OGTT with missed GDM cases of 18.6% [10]. Furthermore, OGTT testing is conducted between 20 and 30 g.w., adding additional OGTT after that period could help to determine late onset GDM with increased risk of operative delivery. Sasson et al. found that pathological OGTT at term due to the suspicion of LGA resulted in a higher rate of Cesarean section [25].

Another option to improve GDM diagnostics would be universal screening, ensuring that every woman is at least offered testing. Universal testing would result in the maximum number of GDM cases at the expense of increased healthcare costs and the workload of clinical personnel; however, overall, this tends to be cost-effective [26]. As GDM also bears responsibility for long-term complications, mothers and offspring would benefit from universal screening and lifestyle interventions when considering their health risks in later life. [27–29].

The aim of detecting most GDM cases would be lowering the risk of complications after successful intervention. The most frequent complication of poorly controlled GDM is a birth of a LGA neonate [3]. In addition to the GDM group, we could expect larger newborns in a high-risk group who have skipped OGTT, possibly due to undiagnosed GDM. However, our data showed a comparable number of LGA neonates between the GDM group and women with a normal OGTT result. This could be explained by the fact that GDM is not the only factor resulting in fetal macrosomia; other known risk factors are multiparity, older age, previous LGA and a male newborn. In addition, pregnancy weight gain and pre-pregnancy BMI have been shown in previous studies to be related to GDM but also to isolated LGA newborns [30–32]. In our cohort, the most noticeable difference among high-risk women with no OGTT and a normal OGTT result was extensive weight gain and a more frequent need for operative delivery due to LGA neonate among the normal OGTT group. We may assume that weight gain was the reason for the referral to OGTT. However, we can also speculate that by relating LGA newborns only to GDM, the normal OGTT result could offer false reassurance of a normal pregnancy course and less motivation for weight management after testing.

Women with a GDM diagnosis receive dietary advice or medication (metformin and/or insulin), monitor their blood sugar carefully, and are referred to labor induction more easily. Although, in our study, the number of GDM patients receiving medical treatment was not enough to assess the effect of different treatment modalities on pregnancy outcome, studies have shown the positive effect of GDM treatment on maternal gestational weight gain, perinatal outcome and the possible long term effects on lifestyle changes [33].

However, high-risk women with normal OGTT results should not receive less attention as they are at increased risk of gestational weight gain and a LGA newborn. As a large proportion of these women are overweight, focusing on a healthy diet and exercise have been shown to significantly reduce gestational weight gain [34]. Dodd et al. assessed the addition of metformin to lifestyle interventions; however, they found no complementary benefits from the medication [35]. More targeted prospective studies are needed to determine if quality of diet and additional testing later in pregnancy would add benefits such as timing the delivery and preventing the birth of a LGA among groups of women with GDM risk factors but a normal OGTT result [36–38].

A limitation of our study is the small sample size to assess the prevalence of less frequent pregnancy and delivery complications such as preeclampsia, shoulder dystocia and III and IV grade perineal tear in different groups.

5. Conclusions

As the number of GDM risk factor carriers is increasing, more women are referred to OGTT and will be diagnosed with GDM with respective pregnancy follow-up. However, we would like to highlight our findings that pregnant women with GDM risk factors are, despite normal OGTT, still at risk of increased weight gain and LGA newborns.

Supplementary Materials: The following supporting information can be downloaded at: https://www.mdpi.com/article/10.3390/jcm11174953/s1, Table S1: Data acquisition for the study in three time periods. Table S2: Comparison of pregnancy course and outcome in GDM patients according to treatment modalities.

Author Contributions: E.H., K.R. and A.K. contributed to the recruitment of the women and collection and analysis of medical data. E.H. drafted the first manuscript. E.H. and K.R. wrote the final manuscript. I.R. contributed to the data analysis. M.L. contributed by design of Happy Pregnancy Study and critical revision of the article. All authors have read and agreed to the published version of the manuscript.

Funding: The study was supported by EU through the European Regional Development Fund (project HAPPY PREGNANCY, 3.2.0701.12-0047; for M.L and K.R), Estonian Research Council (grants IUT34-12 and PRG1021 for M.L) and Institute of Clinical Medicine (target funding for K.R).

Institutional Review Board Statement: The data collection and analysis was approved by the Research Ethics Committee of the University of Tartu, Estonia (permissions no. 225/T-6, 6 May 2013; 221/T-6, 17 December 2012, 286/M-18, 15 October 2018; 291/T-3, 18 March 2019 and 322/M-17, 17 August 2020) and study was carried out in compliance with the guidelines of the Declaration of Helsinki.

Informed Consent Statement: In Happy Pregnancy Study, a written consent was obtained from each participant. For 2012 and 2018 cohort data about GDM risk factors was derived from electronic medical health records.

Data Availability Statement: The datasets used and/or analyzed during the current study are available from the corresponding author on reasonable request.

Acknowledgments: The clinical personnel at the Women's Clinic of Tartu University Hospital are acknowledged for the assistance in recruitment of women.

Conflicts of Interest: The authors declare no conflict of interest. The funders had no role in the design of the study; in the collection, analyses, or interpretation of data; in the writing of the manuscript; or in the decision to publish the results.

References

1. Hyperglycemia in pregnancy: International Diabetes Federation. In *IDF Diabetes Atlas*, 9th ed.; International Diabetes Federation: Brussels, Belgium, 2019.
2. He, X.J.; Qin, F.Y.; Hu, C.L.; Zhu, M.; Tian, C.Q.; Li, L. Is gestational diabetes mellitus an independent risk factor for macrosomia: A meta-analysis? *Arch Gynecol. Obstet.* **2015**, *291*, 729–735. [CrossRef]
3. HAPO Study Cooperative Research Group. The Hyperglycemia and Adverse Pregnancy Outcome (HAPO) Study. *Int. J. Gynaecol. Obstet.* **2002**, *78*, 69–77. [CrossRef]
4. HAPO Study Cooperative Research Group; Metzger, B.E.; Lowe, L.P.; Dyer, A.R.; Dyer, A.R.; Trimble, E.R.; Sheridan, B.; Hod, M.; Chen, R.; Yogev, Y.; et al. Hyperglycemia and adverse pregnancy outcomes. *N. Engl. J. Med.* **2008**, *358*, 1991–2002.
5. Auvinen, A.M.; Luiro, K.; Jokelainen, J.; Järvelä, I.; Knip, M.; Auvinen, J.; Tapanainen, J.S. Type 1 and type 2 diabetes after gestational diabetes: A 23-year cohort study. *Diabetologia* **2020**, *63*, 2123–2128. [CrossRef]
6. Tobias, D.K.; Hu, F.B.; Chavarro, J.; Rosner, B.; Mozaffarian, D.; Zhang, C. Healthful dietary patterns and type 2 diabetes mellitus risk among women with a history of gestational diabetes mellitus. *Arch. Intern. Med.* **2012**, *172*, 1566–1572. [CrossRef]
7. Benhalima, K.; Mathieu, C.; Van Assche, A.; Damm, P.; Devlieger, R.; Mahmood, T.; Dunne, F. Survey by the European Board and College of Obstetrics and Gynaecology on screening for gestational diabetes in Europe. *Eur. J. Obstet. Gynecol. Reprod. Biol.* **2016**, *201*, 197–202. [CrossRef]
8. Minschart, C.; Beunen, K.; Benhalima, K. An Update on Screening Strategies for Gestational Diabetes Mellitus: A Narrative Review. *Diabetes Metab. Syndr. Obes.* **2021**, *14*, 3047–3076. [CrossRef]
9. International Association of Diabetes and Pregnancy Study Groups Consensus Panel. International association of diabetes and pregnancy study groups recommendations on the diagnosis and classification of hyperglycemia in pregnancy. *Diabetes Care* **2010**, *33*, 676–682. [CrossRef]
10. Benhalima, K.; Van Crombrugge, P.; Moyson, C.; Verhaeghe, J.; Vandeginste, S.; Verlaenen, H.; Vercammen, C.; Maes, T.; Dufraimont, E.; De Block, C.; et al. Risk factor screening for gestational diabetes mellitus based on the 2013 WHO criteria. *Eur. J. Endocrinol.* **2019**, *180*, 353–363. [CrossRef]
11. Diabetes in Pregnancy: Management from Preconception to the Postnatal Period: NICE Guideline. Updated: 16 December. Available online: https://www.nice.org.uk/guidance/ng3/chapter/Recommendations (accessed on 13 June 2021).
12. Yamamoto, J.M.; Kellett, J.E.; Balsells, M.; García-Patterson, A.; Hadar, E.; Solà, I.; Gich, I.; van der Beek, E.M.; Castañeda-Gutiérrez, E.; Heinonen, S.; et al. Gestational Diabetes Mellitus and Diet: A Systematic Review and Meta-analysis of Randomized Controlled Trials Examining the Impact of Modified Dietary Interventions on Maternal Glucose Control and Neonatal Birth Weight. *Diabetes Care* **2018**, *41*, 1346–1361. [CrossRef]
13. Thayer, S.M.; Lo, J.O.; Caughey, A.B. Gestational Diabetes: Importance of Follow-up Screening for the Benefit of Long-term Health. *Obstet. Gynecol. Clin. N. Am.* **2020**, *47*, 383–396. [CrossRef] [PubMed]

14. Avalos, G.E.; Owens, L.A.; Dunne, F.; ATLANTIC DIP Collaborators. Applying current screening tools for gestational diabetes mellitus to a European population: Is it time for change? *Diabetes Care* **2013**, *36*, 3040–3044. [CrossRef] [PubMed]
15. Kirss, A.; Lauren, L.; Rohejärv, M.; Rull, K. Gestatsioonidiabeet: Riskitegurid, esinemissagedus, perinataalne tulem ja sõeluuringu vastavus juhendile Tartu Ülikooli Kliinikumi naistekliinikus ajavahemikul 01.01.2012–19.06. *Eesti Arst* **2015**, *94*, 75–82. (In Estonian)
16. Ratnik, K.; Rull, K.; Hanson, E.; Kisand, K.; Laan, M. Single-Tube Multimarker Assay for Estimating the Risk to Develop Preeclampsia. *J. Appl. Lab. Med.* **2020**, *5*, 1156–1171. [CrossRef]
17. Kikas, T.; Inno, R.; Ratnik, K.; Rull, K.; Laan, M. C-allele of rs4769613 Near FLT1 Represents a High-Confidence Placental Risk Factor for Preeclampsia. *Hypertension* **2020**, *76*, 884–891. [CrossRef]
18. Hanson, E.; Rull, K.; Ratnik, K.; Vaas, P.; Teesalu, P.; Laan, M. Value of soluble fms-like tyrosine kinase-1/placental growth factor test in third trimester of pregnancy for predicting preeclampsia in asymptomatic women. *J. Perinat. Med.* **2022**. epub ahead of print. [CrossRef]
19. Vaas, P.; Rull, K.; Põllumaa, S.; Kirss, A.; Meigas, D. Guideline for Antenatal Care (Raseduse Jälgimise Juhend). Estonian Gynaecologists Society 2011; vEstonian. Available online: https://www.ens.ee/ravijuhendid (accessed on 23 June 2019).
20. Villar, J.; Papageorghiou, A.T.; Pang, R.; Ohuma, E.O.; Ismail, L.C.; Barros, F. The likeness of fetal growth and new-born size across non-isolated populations in the INTERGROWTH-21st Project: The Fetal Growth Longitudinal Study and Newborn Cross-Sectional Study. *Lancet* **2014**, *2*, 781–792.
21. Brown, M.A.; Magee, L.A.; Kenny, L.C.; Karumanchi, S.A.; McCarthy, F.P.; Saito, S.; Hall, D.R.; Warren, C.E.; Adoyi, G.; Ishaku, S.; et al. Hypertensive Disorders of Pregnancy: ISSHP Classification, Diagnosis, and Management Recommendations for International Practice. *Hypertension* **2018**, *72*, 24–43. [CrossRef]
22. Rasmussen, K.M.; Abrams, B.; Bodnar, L.M.; Butte, N.F.; Catalano, P.M.; Maria Siega-Riz, A. Recommendations for weight gain during pregnancy in the context of the obesity epidemic. *Obstet. Gynecol.* **2010**, *116*, 1191–1195. [CrossRef]
23. Muin, D.A.; Pfeifer, B.; Helmer, H.; Oberaigner, W.; Leitner, H.; Kiss, H.; Neururer, S. Universal gestational diabetes screening and antepartum stillbirth rates in Austria-A population-based study. *Acta Obstet. Gynecol. Scand.* **2022**, *101*, 396–404. [CrossRef]
24. Koivunen, S.; Viljakainen, M.; Männistö, T.; Gissler, M.; Pouta, A.; Kaaja, R.; Eriksson, J.; Laivuori, H.; Kajantie, E.; Vääräsmäki, M. Pregnancy outcomes according to the definition of gestational diabetes. *PLoS ONE* **2020**, *15*, e0229496. [CrossRef] [PubMed]
25. Mohr Sasson, A.; Shats, M.; Goichberg, Z.; Mazaki-Tovi, S.; Morag, I.; Hendler, I. Oral glucose tolerance test for suspected late onset gestational diabetes. *J. Matern. Fetal. Neonatal. Med.* **2021**, *34*, 3928–3932. [CrossRef] [PubMed]
26. Mo, X.; Gai Tobe, R.; Takahashi, Y.; Arata, N.; Liabsuetrakul, T.; Nakayama, T.; Mori, R. Economic Evaluations of Gestational Diabetes Mellitus Screening: A Systematic Review. *J. Epidemiol.* **2021**, *31*, 220–230. [CrossRef] [PubMed]
27. Xiang, A.H.; Kjos, S.L.; Takayanagi, M.; Trigo, E.; Buchanan, T.A. Detailed physiological characterization of the development of type 2 diabetes in Hispanic women with prior gestational diabetes mellitus. *Diabetes* **2010**, *59*, 2625–2630. [CrossRef] [PubMed]
28. Tuomilehto, J.; Lindstrom, J.; Eriksson, J.G.; Valle, T.T.; Hämäläinen, H.; Ilanne-Parikka, P.; Keinänen-Kiukaanniemi, S.; Laakso, M.; Louheranta, A.; Rastas, M.; et al. Prevention of type 2 diabetes mellitus by changes in lifestyle among subjects with impaired glucose tolerance. *N. Engl. J. Med.* **2001**, *344*, 1343–1350. [CrossRef]
29. Ratner, R.E.; Christophi, C.A.; Metzger, B.E.; Dabelea, D.; Bennett, P.H.; Pi-Sunyer, X.; Fowler, S.; Kahn, S.E.; Diabetes Prevention Program Research Group. Prevention of diabetes in women with a history of gestational diabetes: Effects of metformin and lifestyle intervention. *J. Clin. Endocrinol. Metab.* **2008**, *93*, 4774–4779. [CrossRef]
30. Zhao, R.; Xu, L.; Wu, M.L.; Huang, S.H.; Cao, X.J. Maternal pre-pregnancy body mass index, gestational weight gain influence birth weight. *Women Birth* **2018**, *31*, e20–e25. [CrossRef]
31. Usta, A.; Usta, C.S.; Yildiz, A.; Ozcaglayan, R.; Dalkiran, E.S.; Savkli, A.; Taskiran, M. Frequency of fetal macrosomia and the associated risk factors in pregnancies without gestational diabetes mellitus. *Pan Afr. Med. J.* **2017**, *26*, 62. [CrossRef]
32. Lin, L.H.; Lin, J.; Yan, J.Y. Interactive Affection of Pre-Pregnancy Overweight or Obesity, Excessive Gestational Weight Gain and Glucose Tolerance Test Characteristics on Adverse Pregnancy Outcomes Among Women with Gestational Diabetes Mellitus. *Front. Endocrinol.* **2022**, *13*, 942271. [CrossRef]
33. Rasmussen, L.; Poulsen, C.W.; Kampmann, U.; Smedegaard, S.B.; Ovesen, P.G.; Fuglsang, J. Diet and Healthy Lifestyle in the Management of Gestational Diabetes Mellitus. *Nutrients* **2020**, *12*, 3050. [CrossRef]
34. Peaceman, A.M.; Clifton, R.G.; Phelan, S.; Gallagher, D.; Evans, M.; Redman, L.M.; Knowler, W.C.; Joshipura, K.; Haire-Joshu, D.; Yanovski, S.Z.; et al. Lifestyle Interventions Limit Gestational Weight Gain in Women with Overweight or Obesity: LIFE-Moms Prospective Meta-Analysis. *Obesity* **2018**, *26*, 1396–1404. [CrossRef] [PubMed]
35. Dodd, J.M.; Louise, J.; Deussen, A.R.; Grivell, R.M.; Dekker, G.; McPhee, A.J.; Hague, W. Effect of metformin in addition to dietary and lifestyle advice for pregnant women who are overweight or obese: The GRoW randomised, double-blind, placebo-controlled trial. *Lancet Diabetes Endocrinol.* **2019**, *7*, 15–24. [CrossRef]
36. Zhu, Y.; Hedderson, M.M.; Sridhar, S.; Xu, F.; Feng, J.; Ferrara, A. Poor diet quality in pregnancy is associated with increased risk of excess fetal growth: A prospective multi-racial/ethnic cohort study. *Int. J. Epidemiol.* **2019**, *48*, 423–432. [CrossRef]
37. Han, S.; Crowther, C.A.; Middleton, P. Interventions for pregnant women with hyperglycaemia not meeting gestational diabetes and type 2 diabetes diagnostic criteria. *Cochrane Database Syst. Rev.* **2012**, *1*, CD009037. [CrossRef] [PubMed]
38. Munda, A.; Starčič Erjavec, M.; Molan, K.; Ambrožič Avguštin, J.; Žgur-Bertok, D.; Pongrac Barlovič, D. Association between pre-pregnancy body weight and dietary pattern with large-for-gestational-age infants in gestational diabetes. *Diabetol. Metab. Syndr.* **2019**, *11*, 68. [CrossRef] [PubMed]

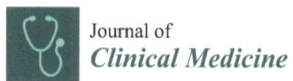

Article

Ultrasonographic Prediction of Placental Invasion in Placenta Previa by Placenta Accreta Index

Keita Hasegawa [1], Satoru Ikenoue [1,*], Yuya Tanaka [1], Maki Oishi [1], Toyohide Endo [1], Yu Sato [1], Ryota Ishii [2], Yoshifumi Kasuga [1], Daigo Ochiai [3] and Mamoru Tanaka [1]

1. Department of Obstetrics and Gynecology, Keio University School of Medicine, 35 Shinanomachi, Sinjuku, Tokyo 1608582, Japan
2. Department of Clinical Trial and Clinical Epidemiology, University of Tsukuba Faculty of Medicine, 1-1-1 Tennodai, Tsukuba 305-8577, Japan
3. Department of Obstetrics and Gynecology, Kitasato University School of Medicine, 1-15-1 Kitazato, Minami, Sagamihara 252-0375, Japan
* Correspondence: sikenoue.a3@keio.jp; Tel.: +81-3-3353-1211; Fax: +81-3-3226-1667

Citation: Hasegawa, K.; Ikenoue, S.; Tanaka, Y.; Oishi, M.; Endo, T.; Sato, Y.; Ishii, R.; Kasuga, Y.; Ochiai, D.; Tanaka, M. Ultrasonographic Prediction of Placental Invasion in Placenta Previa by Placenta Accreta Index. *J. Clin. Med.* **2023**, *12*, 1090. https://doi.org/10.3390/jcm12031090

Academic Editor: Rinat Gabbay-Benziv

Received: 12 December 2022
Revised: 27 January 2023
Accepted: 29 January 2023
Published: 31 January 2023

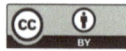

Copyright: © 2023 by the authors. Licensee MDPI, Basel, Switzerland. This article is an open access article distributed under the terms and conditions of the Creative Commons Attribution (CC BY) license (https://creativecommons.org/licenses/by/4.0/).

Abstract: This study aimed to investigate the diagnostic accuracy of the placenta accreta index (PAI) for predicting placenta accreta spectrum (PAS) in women with placenta previa. We analyzed 33 pregnancies with placenta previa at Keio University Hospital. The PAI was assessed in the early third trimester, and PAS was diagnosed histologically or clinically defined as retained placenta after manual removal attempts. The PAI and incidence of PAS were analyzed. Ten women (30%) were diagnosed with PAS and had higher volumes of perioperative bleeding ($p = 0.016$), higher rate of requiring uterine artery embolization ($p = 0.005$), and peripartum hysterectomy ($p = 0.0002$) than women without PAS. A PAI > 2 was the most useful cut-off point for predicting PAS and was more sensitive than prediction values using traditional evaluation (history of cesarean section and placental location). Post-hoc analysis revealed a higher rate of previous history of cesarean delivery (30% vs. 4.4%, $p = 0.038$), severe placental lacunae ($\geq$grade2) (70% vs. 8.7%, $p = 0.0003$), thin myometrial thickness (90% vs. 22%, $p = 0.0003$), anterior placenta (100% vs. 30%, $p = 0.0002$), and presence of bridging vessels (30% vs. 0%, $p = 0.0059$) in PAS women. PAI could help predict the outcomes of women with placenta previa with and without a history of cesarean delivery to reduce PAS-induced perinatal complications.

Keywords: placenta accreta spectrum; placenta previa; ultrasonography; placenta accreta index

1. Introduction

Placenta accreta spectrum (PAS) is first suspected when placenta previa is identified because 9.3% of placenta previa cases are associated with PAS [1]. Although the mortality rate of women with PAS has improved from 6–7% [2] to 0.05% recently [3], PAS is related to an increased risk of perinatal complications and interventions, such as excessive peripartum bleeding requiring blood transfusion, uterine artery embolization, and peripartum hysterectomy. Therefore, predicting PAS in the antepartum period is crucial because it is a means to decrease maternal morbidity/mortality.

Ultrasonography is the mainstay of prenatal diagnosis and monitoring, as well as preoperative prediction of PAS, and has a high accuracy for prenatal diagnosis of invasive placentation in high-risk pregnancies [4]. Rac et al. [5] recently reported using the placenta accreta index (PAI) scored by ultrasonography for predicting PAS; however, validation and replication studies for PAI are limited. Additionally, a previous study on the use of PAI only recruited women with a history of cesarean delivery [5]. It is well known that women without a history of cesarean delivery also have an increased risk of the adherent placenta in case of placenta previa [1].

Therefore, we aimed to investigate and validate the clinical utility of the PAI to predict PAS in women with placenta previa both with and without a history of cesarean delivery.

2. Materials and Methods

This was a single-center retrospective study. The hospital records of 33 consecutive women with singleton pregnancies, diagnosed with placenta previa at Keio University Hospital from June 2017 to January 2021, were analyzed. Placenta previa was diagnosed using transvaginal ultrasonography and defined as the presence of a placenta that completely covered the internal cervical ostium. Excluded were multiple pregnancies and patients who were referred to our hospital after having delivered elsewhere. All the ultrasonography images of patients with placenta previa have been stored. Women for whom ultrasonography images were unavailable or inadequate to evaluate PAI retrospectively were excluded from the analysis.

Abdominal and vaginal ultrasonography were performed by obstetricians trained in ultrasonography in the early third trimester. The ultrasound images were reviewed by a single observer (K.H.), and a PAI score was assigned preoperatively for each woman. Table 1 shows the parameters of the PAI. The PAI is a composite of the following five parameters: previous history of cesarean delivery, placental lacunae, smallest myometrial thickness, placental location, and bridging vessels [5].

Table 1. Clinical values of obstetric parameters for evaluating the placenta accreta index.

Obstetric Parameter	Value
≥ 2 cesarean delivery	3.0
Lacunae	
Grade 3	3.5
Grade 2	1.0
Sagittal smallest myometrial thickness	
≤ 1 mm	1.0
<1 but ≥ 3 mm	0.5
>3 but ≤ 5 mm	0.25
Anterior placenta previa	1.0
Bridging vessels to the bladder	0.5

PAS was diagnosed histologically after hysterectomy or clinically defined as placenta retained after previous attempts of manual removal according to the FIGO classification [6]. Depends on the predicted severity of the PAS, and for improving the perinatal outcomes, we decided the delivery timing of women with placenta previa between 34 and 37 weeks of gestation [7]. However, when the patient entered labor or had massive vaginal bleeding, emergency cesarean delivery was performed even before 34 weeks of gestation. Blood loss was counted as intraoperative bleeding.

The student's t-test or chi-square test was used to test differences between the groups. The estimates and Clopper–Pearson confidence intervals for sensitivity, specificity, positive predictive value, and negative predictive value for the prediction of PAS were calculated for each cut-off point of the PAI. Receiver operating characteristic curve (ROC) analysis was performed for PAS prediction using the PAI; the area under the curve (AUC) was calculated, and the cut-off value of the PAI was calculated by using the Youden index. All statistical analyses were performed using SAS, version 9.4 (SAS Institute, Cary, NC, USA). Two-sided p-values < 0.05 were considered to indicate statistical significance.

The study was approved by the Ethics Committee of Keio University School of Medicine (No. 20030107). As all information was anonymous in the institutional database, informed consent from each patient was not needed.

3. Results

Maternal characteristics and perinatal outcomes are summarized in Table 2. Of the 33 women with placenta previa, 10 (30%) were diagnosed with PAS, and 23 did not have PAS. The PAS group showed a significantly larger volume of perioperative bleeding and higher rates of uterine artery embolization and peripartum hysterectomy than the non-PAS group.

Table 2. Maternal characteristics and perinatal outcomes.

	PAS $n = 10$	Non-PAS $n = 23$	p-Value
Maternal age, years	39 ± 3.3	38 ± 5.2	0.59
BMI, kg/m^2	20 ± 3.0	22 ± 3.6	0.12
Nulliparas	4 (40%)	15 (65%)	0.17
Gestational age at delivery, weeks	35.2 ± 1.5	35.5 ± 2.4	0.51
Perioperative blood loss, g	2913 ± 1314	1650 ± 841	**0.01**
Uterine artery embolization	6 (60%)	3 (13%)	**<0.01**
Blood transfusion	9 (90%)	14 (61%)	0.09
Peripartum hysterectomy	5 (50%)	0 (0%)	**<0.01**
Birth weight, g	2372 ± 427	2333 ± 505	0.83
Apgar score at 1 min < 7	2 (20%)	7 (30%)	0.54
Apgar score at 5 min < 7	0 (0%)	3 (13%)	0.23

Continuous variables are presented as means ± standard deviations. Categorical variables are presented as n (%). Statistically significant p-values are shown in **bold** text. Abbreviations: BMI, body mass index, PAS, placental accreta spectrum.

The ROC curve predicting PAS using the PAI showed an AUC of 0.974 (95% confidence interval [CI], 0.925–1.00). A PAI > 2 was indicated as the most useful cut-off point for PAS prediction, with a sensitivity of 0.900 (95% CI, 0.555–0.997); specificity, 0.957 (95% CI, 0.781–0.999); positive predictive value, 0.900 (95% CI, 0.555–0.997); negative predictive value, 0.957 (95% CI, 0.781–0.999) (Table 3). These values were higher than the prediction rate of PAS based on the traditionally evaluated information (history of cesarean delivery and anterior placental location: sensitivity, 0.300; specificity, 0.957; positive predictive value, 0.750; negative predictive value; 0.759). Seven (70%) out of 10 women with PAS had no previous cesarean delivery, all of whom had a PAI > 2. Of the seven women with PAS without a history of cesarean delivery, five (71%) were aged above 35, three (43%) received infertility treatments, and only one (14%) had a history of uterine artery embolization.

Table 3. Sensitivity, specificity, and positive and negative predictive values corresponding to each PAI score.

PAI	Non-PAS	PAS	Sensitivity (95% CI)	Specificity (95% CI)	PPV (95% CI)	NPV (95% CI)
>0	9	10	100.0 [69.2–100.0]	60.9 [38.5–80.3]	52.6 [28.9–75.6]	100.0 [76.8–100.0]
≤0	14	0				
>1	5	10	100.0 [69.2–100.0]	78.3 [56.3–92.5]	66.7 [38.4–88.2]	100.0 [81.5–100.0]
≤1	18	0				
>2	1	9	90.0 [55.5–99.7]	95.7 [78.1–99.9]	90.0 [55.5–99.7]	95.7 [78.1–99.9]
≤2	22	1				
>3	1	5	50.0 [18.7–81.3]	95.7 [78.1–99.9]	83.3 [35.9–99.6]	81.5 [61.9–93.7]
≤3	22	5				
>4	1	5	50.0 [18.7–81.3]	95.7 [78.1–99.9]	83.3 [35.9–99.6]	81.5 [61.9–93.7]
≤4	22	5				
>5	0	2	20.0 [2.5–55.6]	100.0 [85.2–100.0]	100.0 [15.8–100.0]	74.2 [55.4–88.1]
≤5	23	8				

Values are presented as median (Interquartile range). Abbreviations: PAI, placenta accreta index, PAS, placental accreta spectrum, PPV, positive predictive value, NPV, negative predictive value, CI, confidence interval.

The post-hoc analysis of the five parameters of the PAI score revealed significantly higher rates of previous cesarean deliveries ≥ 2 (30% vs. 4.4%, $p = 0.038$), placental lacunae $\geq$ Grade 2 (70% vs. 8.7%, $p = 0.0003$), myometrial thickness ≤ 5 mm (90% vs. 22%, $p = 0.0003$), placenta adhering to the anterior wall of the uterus (100% vs. 30%, $p = 0.0002$), and presence of bridging vessels to the bladder (30% vs. 0%, $p = 0.0059$) in the PAS group than in the non-PAS group.

4. Discussion

As previously reported, our study replicated the finding that PAS is associated with an increased risk of perinatal complications and requiring uterine artery embolization. Moreover, the present study indicated the clinical utility and significance of the PAI to predict PAS preoperatively in women with placenta previa both with and without a previous history of cesarean delivery, whereas previous study applied PAI only for women with a history of cesarean delivery [5]. In particular, a PAI > 2 indicated a practical cut-off point to predict PAS in women with placenta previa.

As expected, in the present study, the PAS group showed a significantly increased number of perioperative complications, including a larger amount of perioperative bleeding, a higher rate of uterine artery embolization, and peripartum hysterectomy than the non-PAS group. Per previous reports, PAS is associated with a significantly higher risk of blood transfusion (46.9%) and peripartum hysterectomy (52.2%) [3,8,9] which is consistent with this study's findings. The PAI assessment may be clinically important for women with suspected placental invasion to reduce perinatal complications and maternal mortality associated with PAS.

The present study revealed that the PAI has high diagnostic accuracy for PAS. In particular, a PAI > 2 could be a useful cut-off point to predict PAS. Rac et al. [5] did not present a cut-off point for the PAI, but used it to help with risk stratification and counseling. Meanwhile, the present study suggests that PAI > 2 is useful for predicting PAS in women with and without a previous history of cesarean delivery. Of the five parameters comprising the PAI evaluated in this study (history of cesarean delivery, presence of placental lacunae, smallest myometrial thickness, placental location, and presence of bridging vessels to the bladder), significant differences were identified in all parameters between the PAS and non-PAS groups. We also reported on several ultrasonographic parameters that are associated with PAS. The sensitivity of placental lacunae for identifying placenta accreta was reported as 75% [10]. The sensitivity and specificity of the loss of the clear zone for identifying placenta accreta were reported as 74.9% and 76.9%, respectively [10]. Another study showed that the sensitivity, specificity, and positive and negative predictive values of placenta accreta using ultrasound findings were 53.3%, 88.1%, 82.1%, and 64.8%, respectively [11]. The prediction parameters calculated in the present study using the PAI were greater than those calculated in previous reports. On this basis, the diagnostic accuracy of PAI for PAS could be superior to the single ultrasonographic parameter-based method.

Happe et al. validated the predictability of the PAI for PAS by using 79 PAS cases, but only for women who had a history of previous cesarean delivery [12]. In fact, prior cesarean delivery has a large influence on PAI scoring [5], and the higher prevalence of cesarean deliveries has led to an increased incidence of PAS [13]. However, it is well known that women diagnosed with placenta previa even without previous cesarean delivery have an increased risk of PAS [1]. Indeed, the present study included seven (70%) women with PAS without a history of cesarean delivery, all of whom presented with PAI >2 and increased risk of PAS. The present findings potentially expand the utility of PAI for PAS prediction in patients even without a previous history of cesarean delivery.

Magnetic resonance imaging (MRI) is another modality used to predict PAS and MRI findings have been reported to be useful to define the topography and area of placental invasion [14,15]. Berkley et al. [16] reported that the sensitivity of MRI is 80–85% and the specificity is 65–100%. Fiocchi et al. [17] reported that MRI has 100% sensitivity and 92.3%

specificity for the prediction of PAS. However, MRI may also mislead the diagnosis of PAS using ultrasonography [18], and it is not cost-effective as a screening tool for PAS. In this study, we revealed similar sensitivity and specificity of the PAI as for MRI for predicting PAS, indicating that the PAI has a high rate of diagnostic accuracy and exclusive diagnosis. Given these results, predicting PAS using ultrasonography may be preferable to using MRI.

Our study and a previous study have demonstrated the diagnostic accuracy of PAS using the PAI. However, Rac et al. [12] reported that the PAI could not help predict the depth of placental invasion. Recently, machine learning models have been used to predict the clinical outcomes in women with placenta accreta spectrum [19]. Because the severity of PAS (e.g., depth of placental invasion) is associated with increased maternal morbidity [20], further investigations including machine learning method and serum biomarkers are warranted to predict the severity of perioperative complications (blood loss, uterine artery embolization, and hysterectomy).

In our study, there were several strengths and limitations. The first strength was that the PAI was scored preoperatively and reviewed by a single observer, which could avoid observation bias and interobserver differences. The second strength was that the effectiveness of other prediction methods had not been demonstrated. Maternal serum alpha-fetoprotein, free beta-human chorionic gonadotropin [21,22], antithrombin III, PAI-1, soluble Tie2, and soluble vascular endothelial growth factor receptor 2 have been shown as biomarkers to predict PAS [23]. In addition, the maternal serum VEGF and Serum Cripto-1 levels have been reported as novel biomarkers to predict abnormally invasive placenta [24,25]. These biomarkers might aid clinicians additionally to ultrasonography in detecting PAS cases in the early weeks of gestation. Meanwhile, the first limitation was a small sample size, which might affect the statistical power of the present results. In addition, women with PAS in the present study had risk factors besides a history of cesarean delivery. The second limitation of our study was that patients with PAS accounted for approximately 30% of all the placenta previa cases, which is higher than the general frequency [1]. This may be related to the fact that our institution is a tertiary center and that many of our patients are elderly or post-IVF pregnant women. The fact that our institution is a tertiary center also resulted in high rates of blood loss, blood transfusion and embolization in the non-PAS group despite 65% being nulliparas without PAS. The third limitation was that systematic bias may have occurred because the observer could not be blinded to the patients' risk factors completely. The last limitation was that we performed uterine artery embolization to preserve the uterus on maternal request for PAS cases where the placenta was found to be invading the uterine wall at cesarean delivery, where the placenta was retained after attempts at manual removal. Hence, these PAS cases were diagnosed clinically, and there was a lack of pathological evaluation.

In conclusion, the present study confirmed the clinical significance of the PAI in predicting PAS preoperatively in women with placenta previa, regardless of prior history of cesarean delivery. In particular, a PAI >2 was found to be a valid cut-off point to predict PAS in women who had placenta previa with and without a previous history of cesarean delivery. Assigning a PAI score could be clinically important to avoid perinatal complications and reduce maternal mortality associated with PAS.

Author Contributions: All authors accept responsibility for the paper as published. K.H. and S.I. researched data, wrote the manuscript, contributed to discussion, and reviewed/edited the manuscript. Y.T., M.O., T.E., Y.S., Y.K., D.O. and M.T. contributed to the discussion and reviewed the manuscript. R.I. contributed to data analyses and reviewed the manuscript. All authors have read and agreed to the published version of the manuscript.

Funding: This work was supported in the writing of the report by the Japan Society for the Promotion of Science (JSPS) KAKENHI, Grant Number 22K16864.

Institutional Review Board Statement: The study was conducted according to the guidelines of the Declaration of Helsinki, and approved by the Ethics Committee of Keio University School of Medicine (No. 20030107).

Informed Consent Statement: As all information was anonymous in the institutional database, informed consent from each included woman patient was not needed.

Data Availability Statement: The data presented in this study are available on reasonable request from the corresponding author.

Acknowledgments: The authors thank all the medical staff at the Keio University Hospital who contributed to the excellent patient care for patients included in this study.

Conflicts of Interest: The authors declare no conflict of interest.

References

1. Comstock, C.H. Antenatal diagnosis of placenta accreta: A review. *Ultrasound Obstet. Gynecol.* **2005**, *26*, 89–96. [CrossRef] [PubMed]
2. Committee, Publications. Society for Maternal-Fetal Medicine, Belfort M.A. Placenta accreta. *Am. J. Obstet. Gynecol.* **2010**, *203*, 430–439.
3. Jauniaux, E.; Bunce, C.; Grønbeck, L.; Langhoff-Roos, J. Prevalence and main outcomes of placenta accreta spectrum: A systematic review and meta-analysis. *Am. J. Obstet. Gynecol.* **2019**, *221*, 208–218. [CrossRef]
4. D'Antonio, F.; Iacovella, C.; Bhide, A. Prenatal identification of invasive placentation using ultrasound: Systematic review and meta-analysis. *Ultrasound Obstet. Gynecol.* **2013**, *42*, 509–517. [PubMed]
5. Rac, M.W.; Dashe, J.S.; Wells, C.E.; Moschos, E.; McIntire, D.D.; Twickler, D.M. Ultrasound predictors of placental invasion: The placenta accreta Index. *Am. J. Obstet. Gynecol.* **2015**, *212*, 343.e1–343.e7. [CrossRef] [PubMed]
6. Jauniaux, E.; Ayres-de-Campos, D.; Langhoff-Roos, J.; Fox, K.A.; Collins, S.; FIGO Placenta Accreta Diagnosis and Management Expert Consensus Panel. FIGO classification for the clinical diagnosis of placenta accreta spectrum disorders. *Int. J. Gynaecol. Obstet.* **2019**, *146*, 20–24. [CrossRef] [PubMed]
7. Oğlak, S.C.; Ölmez, F.; Tunç, Ş. Evaluation of Antepartum Factors for Predicting the Risk of Emergency Cesarean Delivery in Pregnancies Complicated with Placenta Previa. *Ochsner. J.* **2022**, *22*, 146–153. [CrossRef]
8. Bartels, H.C.; Rogers, A.C.; O'Brien, D.; McVey, R.; Walsh, J.; Brennan, D.J. Association of implementing a multidisciplinary team approach in the management of morbidly adherent placenta with maternal morbidity and mortality. *Obstet. Gynecol.* **2018**, *132*, 1167–1176. [CrossRef] [PubMed]
9. WOMAN Trial Collaborators. Effect of early tranexamic acid administration on mortality, hysterectomy, and other morbidities in women with post-partum haemorrhage (WOMAN): An international, randomised, double-blind, placebo-controlled trial. *Lancet* **2017**, *389*, 2105–2116.
10. Pagani, G.; Cali, G.; Acharya, G.; Trisch, I.T.; Palacios-Jaraquemada, J.; Familiari, A.; Buca, D.; Manzoli, L.; Flacco, M.E.; Fanfani, F.; et al. Diagnostic accuracy of ultrasound in detecting the severity of abnormally invasive placentation: A systematic review and meta-analysis. *Acta Obstet. Gynecol. Scand.* **2018**, *97*, 25–37.
11. Bowman, Z.S.; Eller, A.G.; Kennedy, A.M.; Richards, D.S.; Winter, T.C., 3rd; Woodward, P.J.; Silver, R.M. Accuracy of ultrasound for the prediction of placenta accreta. *Am. J. Obstet. Gynecol.* **2014**, *211*, 177.e1–177.e7. [CrossRef] [PubMed]
12. Happe, S.K.; Yule, C.S.; Spong, C.Y.; Wells, C.E.; Dashe, J.S.; Moschos, E.; Rac, M.W.F.; McIntire, D.D.; Twickler, D.M. Predicting placenta accreta spectrum: Validation of the placenta accreta index. *J. Ultrasound Med.* **2021**, *40*, 1523–1532. [CrossRef] [PubMed]
13. Silver, R.M.; Landon, M.B.; Rouse, D.J.; Leveno, K.J.; Spong, C.Y.; Thom, E.A.; Moawad, A.H.; Caritis, S.N.; Harper, M.; Wapner, R.J.; et al. Maternal morbidity associated with multiple repeat cesarean deliveries. *Obstet. Gynecol.* **2006**, *107*, 1226–1232. [CrossRef] [PubMed]
14. Palacios Jaraquemada, J.M.; Bruno, C.H. Magnetic resonance imaging in 300 cases of placenta accreta: Surgical correlation of new findings. *Acta Obstet. Gynecol. Scand.* **2005**, *84*, 716–724. [PubMed]
15. Familiari, A.; Liberati, M.; Lim, P.; Pagani, G.; Cali, G.; Buca, D.; Manzoli, L.; Flacco, M.E.; Scambia, G.; D'antonio, F. Diagnostic accuracy of magnetic resonance imaging in detecting the severity of abnormal invasive placenta: A systematic review and meta-analysis. *Acta Obstet. Gynecol. Scand.* **2018**, *97*, 507–520. [CrossRef]
16. Berkley, E.M.; Abuhamad, A. Imaging of placenta accreta spectrum. *Clin. Obstet. Gynecol.* **2018**, *61*, 755–765. [CrossRef] [PubMed]
17. Fiocchi, F.; Monelli, F.; Besutti, G.; Casari, F.; Petrella, E.; Pecchi, A.; Caporali, C.; Bertucci, E.; Busani, S.; Botticelli, L.; et al. MRI of placenta accreta: Diagnostic accuracy and impact of interventional radiology on foetal-maternal delivery outcomes in high-risk women. *Br. J. Radiol.* **2020**, *93*, 20200267. [CrossRef]
18. Einerson, B.D.; Rodriguez, C.E.; Kennedy, A.M.; Woodward, P.J.; Donnelly, M.A.; Silver, R.M. Magnetic resonance imaging is often misleading when used as an adjunct to ultrasound in the management of placenta accreta spectrum disorders. *Am. J. Obstet. Gynecol.* **2018**, *218*, 618.e1–618.e7. [CrossRef]
19. Shazly, S.A.; Hortu, I.; Shih, J.C.; Melekoglu, R.; Fan, S.; Ahmed, F.U.A.; Karaman, E.; Fatkullin, I.; Pinto, P.V.; Irianti, S.; et al. Prediction of clinical outcomes in women with placenta accreta spectrum using machine learning models: An international multicenter study. *J. Matern. Fetal. Neonatal. Med.* **2022**, *35*, 6644–6653. [CrossRef]
20. Marcellin, L.; Delorme, P.; Bonnet, M.P.; Grange, G.; Kayem, G.; Tsatsaris, V.; Goffinet, F. Placenta percreta is associated with more frequent severe maternal morbidity than placenta accreta. *Am. J. Obstet. Gynecol.* **2018**, *219*, 193.e1–193.e9. [CrossRef]

21. Hung, T.H.; Shau, W.Y.; Hsieh, C.C.; Chiu, T.H.; Hsu, J.J.; Hsieh, T.T. Risk factors for placenta accreta. *Obstet. Gynecol.* **1999**, *93*, 545–550. [PubMed]
22. Kupferminc, M.J.; Tamura, R.K.; Wigton, T.R.; Glassenberg, R.; Socol, M.L. Placenta accreta is associated with elevated maternal serum alpha-fetoprotein. *Obstet. Gynecol.* **1993**, *82*, 266–269. [PubMed]
23. Shainker, S.A.; Silver, R.M.; Modest, A.M.; Hacker, M.R.; Hecht, J.L.; Salahuddin, S.; Dillon, S.T.; Ciampa, E.J.; D'Alton, M.E.; Out, H.H.; et al. Placenta accreta spectrum: Biomarker discovery using plasma proteomics. *Am. J. Obstet. Gynecol.* **2020**, *223*, 433.e1–433.e14. [CrossRef] [PubMed]
24. Schwickert, A.; Chantraine, F.; Ehrlich, L.; Henrich, W.; Muallem, M.Z.; Nonnenmacher, A.; Petit, P.; Weizsäcker, K.; Braun, T. Maternal Serum VEGF Predicts Abnormally Invasive Placenta Better Than NT-proBNP: A Multicenter Case-Control Study. *Reprod. Sci.* **2021**, *28*, 361–370. [CrossRef] [PubMed]
25. Ozkose, Z.G.; Oglak, S.C.; Behram, M.; Ozdemir, O.; Acar, Z.; Ozdemir, I. Maternal Serum Cripto-1 Levels in Pregnancies Complicated with Placenta Previa and Placenta Accreta Spectrum (Pas). *J. Coll. Physicians Surg. Pak.* **2022**, *32*, 1570–1575.

Disclaimer/Publisher's Note: The statements, opinions and data contained in all publications are solely those of the individual author(s) and contributor(s) and not of MDPI and/or the editor(s). MDPI and/or the editor(s) disclaim responsibility for any injury to people or property resulting from any ideas, methods, instructions or products referred to in the content.

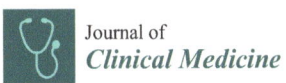

Article

Is There a Correlation between Apelin and Insulin Concentrations in Early Second Trimester Amniotic Fluid with Fetal Growth Disorders?

Dionysios Vrachnis [1,*], Nikolaos Antonakopoulos [2], Alexandros Fotiou [2], Vasilios Pergialiotis [3], Nikolaos Loukas [4], Georgios Valsamakis [5], Christos Iavazzo [6], Sofoklis Stavros [2], Georgios Maroudias [4], Periklis Panagopoulos [2], Nikolaos Vlahos [7], Melpomeni Peppa [8], Theodoros Stefos [9] and George Mastorakos [5]

1. Department of Clinical Therapeutics, Alexandra Hospital, Medical School, National and Kapodistrian University of Athens, 115 28 Athens, Greece
2. Third Department of Obstetrics and Gynecology, General University Hospital "Attikon", Medical School, National and Kapodistrian University of Athens, 124 62 Athens, Greece
3. First Department of Obstetrics and Gynecology, Alexandra Hospital, Medical School, National and Kapodistrian University of Athens, 115 28 Athens, Greece
4. Department of Obstetrics and Gynecology, Tzaneio Hospital, 185 36 Piraeus, Greece
5. Unit of Endocrinology, Diabetes Mellitus and Metabolism, Aretaieio Hospital, Medical School, National and Kapodistrian University of Athens, 115 28 Athens, Greece
6. Department of Gynecologic Oncology, Metaxa Memorial Cancer Hospital, 185 37 Piraeus, Greece
7. Second Department of Obstetrics and Gynecology, Aretaieio Hospital, Medical School, National and Kapodistrian University of Athens, 115 28 Athens, Greece
8. Endocrine Unit, 2nd Propaedeutic Department of Internal Medicine, Research Institute & Diabetes Center, General University Hospital "Attikon", Medical School, National and Kapodistrian University of Athens, 124 62 Athens, Greece
9. Department of Obstetrics and Gynecology, University of Ioannina, 45500 Ioannina, Greece
* Correspondence: dionisisvrachnis@gmail.com

Abstract: Introduction: Fetal growth disturbances place fetuses at increased risk for perinatal morbidity and mortality. As yet, little is known about the basic pathogenetic mechanisms underlying deranged fetal growth. Apelin is an adipokine with several biological activities. Over the past decade, it has been investigated for its possible role in fetal growth restriction. Most studies have examined apelin concentrations in maternal serum and amniotic fluid in the third trimester or during neonatal life. In this study, apelin concentrations were examined for the first time in early second-trimester fetuses. Another major regulator of tissue growth and metabolism is insulin. Materials and Methods: This was a prospective observational cohort study. We measured apelin and insulin concentrations in the amniotic fluid of 80 pregnant women who underwent amniocentesis in the early second trimester. Amniotic fluid samples were stored in appropriate conditions until delivery. The study groups were then defined, i.e., gestations with different fetal growth patterns (SGA, AGA, and LGA). Measurements were made using ELISA kits. Results: Apelin and insulin levels were measured in all 80 samples. The analysis revealed statistically significant differences in apelin concentrations among groups ($p = 0.007$). Apelin concentrations in large for gestational age (LGA) fetuses were significantly lower compared to those in AGA and SGA fetuses. Insulin concentrations did not differ significantly among groups. Conclusions: A clear trend towards decreasing apelin concentrations as birthweight progressively increased was identified. Amniotic fluid apelin concentrations in the early second trimester may be useful as a predictive factor for determining the risk of a fetus being born LGA. Future studies are expected/needed to corroborate the present findings and should ideally focus on the potential interplay of apelin with other known intrauterine metabolic factors.

Keywords: apelin; insulin; amniotic fluid; second trimester; SGA; LGA; fetal growth; fetal macrosomia; FGR; fetal metabolism

1. Introduction

Despite considerable scientific progress having been achieved in the field of fetal monitoring, fetal growth evaluation and surveillance are still challenging. Meanwhile, the underlying regulatory mechanisms continue to be under investigation given that it has long been known that fetal growth disturbances have a major impact on both short-term and long-term pregnancy outcomes. Perinatal morbidity and mortality are increased in small for gestational age (SGA) and large for gestational age (LGA) fetuses [1,2]. Growth-restricted fetuses (fetal growth restriction—FGR) that fail to reach their growth potential and the majority of severe cases of SGA fetuses (those below the 3rd centile) are most affected and at greater risk for adverse perinatal outcomes [3,4]. The same applies to fetuses with weight over the 90th centile partly due to labor complications [2,5,6]. Although the pathogenic mechanisms involved in both impaired and excessive fetal growth are still to be fully clarified, the majority of the existing literature on the topic implicates impaired uterine artery remodeling during early placental invasion and/or preterm placental insufficiency at a later gestational age [7,8].

In the current literature, several biomarkers have been investigated as possible markers of fetal growth aberrations, including apelin and insulin [9–17]. Apelin is an adipokine mainly produced in white adipose tissue and lung tissue, but also in the placenta. Apelin is encoded by the APLN gene located on the long arm of the X chromosome at position Xq25-26. Expression of the APLN gene produces pre-proapelin, which, after translational modification, is transformed into several apelin isoforms with different biological activities. A large number of published studies have highlighted the role of apelin in the cardiovascular as well as female reproductive systems. Interestingly, recent studies have investigated the expression of the apelinergic system in the placenta and its possible effects on specific pregnancy pathologies, such as preeclampsia, fetal growth restriction, and gestational diabetes mellitus [18–25].

Insulin is an essential hormone produced by the pancreas that contributes to the regulation of blood glucose levels. During pregnancy, maternal insulin production rises and exogenous administration may be needed to maintain normal maternal serum concentrations and prevent the consequences of gestational diabetes. Insulin is transferred to the amniotic fluid via fetal urine and its concentrations increase as pregnancy progresses. At present, there is some evidence demonstrating decreased amniotic fluid insulin concentrations in pregnancies complicated by placental insufficiency, fetal growth restriction, fetal malformations, or intrauterine fetal death [17]. Importantly, data exist showing that maternal glucose intolerance can impact the production of fetal insulin prior to 20 weeks gestation. Moreover, evidence published in the literature has pointed to an association between elevated amniotic fluid insulin concentration at 14–20 weeks gestation and both maternal glucose intolerance and fetal macrosomia, which were determined postnatally [26] Other studies have failed to reveal a correlation between amniotic fluid insulin concentrations and fetal growth [27].

This prospective observational study investigates the possible associations between apelin and insulin concentrations in the amniotic fluid of early second-trimester gestations with fetal growth abnormalities in the third trimester with regard to birthweight.

2. Subjects and Methods

2.1. Subjects

This is a prospective observational cohort study of 80 pregnant women consecutively recruited according to the inclusion criteria. The inclusion criteria were as follows: singleton pregnancies; pregnancies with indication for amniocentesis in the second trimester of pregnancy; advanced maternal age; increased nuchal translucency; and previous history of birth defects. The exclusion criteria were the following: pregnancies with major congenital abnormalities or chromosomal abnormalities as diagnosed by amniocentesis; multiple pregnancies; pregnancies occurring by in vitro fertilization; and pregnancies complicated by pregestational diabetes. All cases underwent amniocentesis after informed consent in the second trimester of pregnancy (15th to 22nd gestational week). Gestational age was estimated based on the date of the last period and was verified by a crown-rump length measurement taken from weeks 12 through 14. The maternal characteristics are shown in Table 1. Follow-up was carried out for all pregnancies until delivery. None of the participants classified within the AGA or the LGA groups were diagnosed with gestational diabetes during the current pregnancy, while only two cases belonging to the SGA group developed gestational diabetes out of the 80 women who were included in this study.

Table 1. Maternal characteristics and neonatal birthweight among the study groups. Maternal age, maternal weight, maternal height, maternal parity, fetal sex, gestational age in weeks, and birthweight are expressed using the median (25th quartile–75th quartile); statistical significance was set at $p < 0.05$ (bold values). Discrete variables were analyzed with the chi-square test using Fisher's exact test; continuous variables were analyzed with the Mann–Whitney non-parametric test, as described in Section 2.

	AGA (n = 31)	LGA (n = 18)	SGA (n = 31)	p-Value
Maternal age (years)	35 (32–37)	35 (32–37)	37 (36–38)	**0.01**
Maternal weight (kg)	61.5 (56.25–72)	60.5 (55–64.75)	66 (59–78.5)	0.15
Maternal BMI	22.5 (18.4–34.1)	22.0 (18.5–29.6)	23.9 (17.9–40.3)	0.82
Maternal height (cm)	167 (165–171.5)	166 (158–170)	168 (163–170)	0.60
Maternal parity	1 (0–1.5)	1 (0–1)	0 (0–1)	0.24
Fetal sex (female)	11 (36.7%)	4 (23.5%)	19 (63.3%)	**0.02**
Gestational age (week)	38 (37–39)	38 (37–39)	38 (38–39)	0.11
Birthweight (gr)	3300 (3200–3510)	3870 (3667–4185)	2580 (2420–2775)	**0.01**

AGA: appropriate weight for gestational age, LGA: large weight for gestational age, SGA: small weight for gestational age, BMI: body-mass index.

2.2. Protocol

At the first medical visit, the past medical histories of the pregnant women were taken. Following amniocentesis, amniotic fluid samples were collected. The latter were centrifuged immediately after amniocentesis and the supernatant was stored in polypropylene tubes at −80 °C. At delivery, neonatal birthweight was recorded, and gestational age-related fetal weight software allocated the exact weight centile of each fetus. Based on this calculation, the neonates were divided into three groups, as follows: fetuses with birthweight below the 10th centile (n = 31) were defined as small for gestational age (SGA); fetuses with birthweight between the 10th and 90th centile (n = 31) were defined as appropriate for gestational age (AGA); and fetuses with birthweight above the 90th centile (n = 18) were defined as large for gestational age (LGA). The group of AGA fetuses represents the control group. The study was approved by the Ethical Committee of Aretaieion University Hospital, Athens, Greece (143/291119), and was conducted in compliance with the Declaration of Helsinki guidelines.

2.3. Hormone Measurements

Amniotic fluid apelin concentrations were measured using the Apelin-12 (Human, Rat, Mouse, Bovine) extraction-free ELISA (enzyme immunoassay) kit (Phoenix Pharmaceuticals, Inc., Burlingame, CA, USA) according to the manufacturer's instructions. Apelin is synthesized as the single peptide, preproapelin, which consists of 77 amino acids; these are converted into active fragments, including apelin-12, apelin-13, and apelin-36, which contain a range of amino acids formed by cleavage at specific sites. Most are bioactive. Standard immunoassays quantify apelin bioactivity as a whole and cannot specifically quantify each apelin peptide. The cross-reactivity of the kit for human peptides Apelin-12, Apelin-13, and Apelin-36 is 100%. The sensitivity concentration of the kit is 0.07 ng/mL, with a linear range 0.07–0.79 ng/mL, while the intra- and interassay variation is less than 10% and 15%, respectively. This ELISA kit has been used for human serum/plasma/cerebrospinal fluid or tissue extraction. Given the resemblance of early second-trimester composition to that of serum, it was appropriate for use in amniotic fluid. Amniotic fluid insulin concentrations were measured using the Quantikine®™ human insulin enzyme immunoassay (ELISA) kit (R&D Systems Inc., Minneapolis, MN, USA), according to the manufacturer's instructions. The sensitivity concentration of the kit is 2.15 pmol/L, with a linear range 15.6–500 pmol/L, while the intra- and interassay variation is less than 4% and 8%, respectively.

2.4. Statistics

Data were analyzed using the Statistical Package for Social Sciences (SPSS) version 21 (IBM Corp., Armonk, NY, USA; Released 2012. IBM SPSS Statistics for Windows, Version 21) [18]. Assessment of the normality distributions of the quantitive variables was carried out via graphical methods and Kolmogorov–Smirnoff analysis. The Mann–Whitney non-parametric test was employed for the comparison of continuous variables due to their abnormal distribution. For the categorical variables, the chi-square test was used with Fisher's exact test as fewer than five observations were available. Differences were considered statistically significant if the null hypothesis could be rejected with >95% confidence ($p < 0.05$). Multiple regression analysis was used to define the independent effect of maternal age, weight, height, parity, gestational age at delivery, fetal sex, and amniotic fluid apelin and insulin concentrations on the possibility of a SGA/AGA or LGA/AGA birth. The Enter method was used for the analysis.

3. Results

3.1. Anthropometrics

No statistically significant difference was detected between the three studied groups (SGA, LGA, and AGA) with regard to maternal weight, height, BMI, or gestational age at birth. Maternal age, fetal sex, and fetal birthweight were significantly different among these groups ($p < 0.05$) (Table 1).

3.2. Apelin and Insulin Concentrations in Amniotic Fluid Samples in Relation to Fetal Growth

Apelin and insulin concentrations in amniotic fluid were examined for potential differences among the three studied groups. The apelin concentrations for each of the three groups are presented in Table 2. Significantly lower concentrations of apelin were observed in LGA fetuses > 95th percentile compared to AGA fetuses. Differences among LGA fetuses > 97th percentile and AGA fetuses were not significant. This finding might be influenced by the small sample size of this group. No differences in apelin concentrations were observed between the SGA and AGA fetuses. Statistically significant differences were found among all the studied groups regarding apelin concentrations ($p = 0.007$). More specifically, apelin concentrations were significantly different between the AGA and LGA groups ($p = 0.002$), while there was no difference in apelin concentrations between the AGA and SGA groups ($p = 0.668$) (Figure 1). Insulin concentrations did not differ significantly among the three groups.

The possible associations between apelin concentrations in amniotic fluid and the severity of fetal growth disturbances were investigated. Table 2 presents the apelin concentrations in the amniotic fluid of pregnancies divided into subgroups according to SGA centile (3rd, 5th), AGA, and LGA centile (95th, 97th). Amniotic fluid apelin concentrations in the SGA fetuses were found to be greater than those in the AGA and LGA fetuses. Apelin concentrations progressively increased as the SGA centiles dropped. The apelin concentrations in the LGA fetuses were significantly lower compared to those in both the SGA and AGA fetuses ($p = 0.015$). By contrast, SGA fetuses below either the 3rd or the 5th percentiles exhibited greater apelin concentrations when compared with those in the AGA group (44.3, 41.5 and 40.2 ng/mL, respectively); however, the differences were not statistically significant.

Table 2. Comparisons of apelin concentrations (median, 25th quartile–75th quartile) of the study subgroups with apelin concentrations of AGA. The asterisk indicates a statistically significant difference from the AGA group (the asterisk indicates the statistical significance). Statistical significance was set at $p < 0.05$.

	No. of Cases	Apelin (ng/mL)
SGA < 10th centile	31	35.80 (15.60, 63.40)
SGA < 3rd centile	16	44.30 (11.28, 70.08)
SGA < 5th centile	22	41.50 (8.82, 62.88)
AGA	31	40.20 (18.90, 63.40)
LGA > 90th centile	18	14.35 * (2.59, 26.075)
LGA > 95th centile	11	17.90 * (2.71, 25.80)
LGA > 97th centile	4	21.15 (5.48, 33.30)

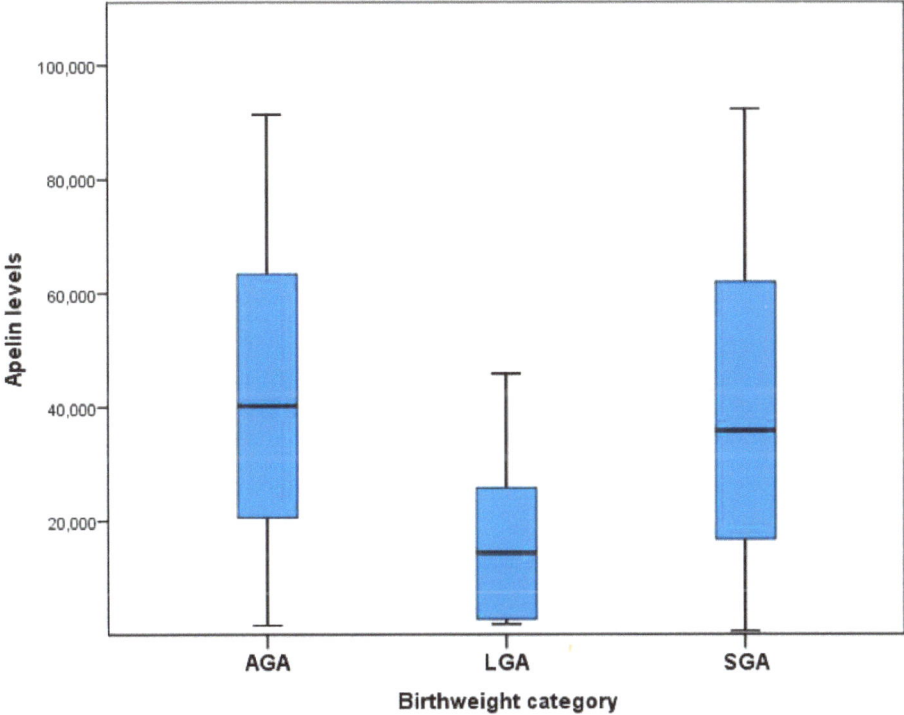

Figure 1. Apelin concentrations in the amniotic fluid of the AGA, SGA, and LGA groups. Box and whisker plot indicates box limits: Q1 and Q3.

In addition, the possible influence of fetal birthweight on the concentration of insulin in amniotic fluid was investigated. Table 3 illustrates insulin concentrations in amniotic fluid at the extremes of fetal birthweight. No statistically significant differences were detected between insulin concentrations in the amniotic fluid of the different fetal growth subgroups.

Table 3. Insulin concentrations (median, 25th quartile–75th quartile) did not differ among the study subgroups.

	No. of Cases	Median (Q1–Q3) (pmol/L)
SGA < 10th centile	24	2.265 (2.00, 3.59)
SGA < 3rd centile	12	2.34 (2.01, 4.45)
SGA < 5th centile	16	2.34 (2.00, 3,75)
AGA	27	2.40 (2.00, 2.88)
LGA > 90th centile	15	2.24 (2.00, 3.74)
LGA > 95th centile	9	2.68 (2.16, 3.78)
LGA > 97th centile	3	2.68 (2.13, 3.75)

3.3. Predictors of SGA, AGA, and LGA Status among Maternal Anthropometrics, Fetal Sex, Gestational Age, and Amniotic Apelin and Insulin Concentrations

Multiple logistic regression of independent parameters such as maternal age, maternal weight, maternal height, fetal sex, and gestational age, which could influence the development of SGA, AGA, or LGA (dependent parameters), revealed that fetal female sex and amniotic insulin concentrations were significantly predictive of LGA fetuses ($p = 0.047$ and 0.042, respectively). The pseudo-$R^2_{Nagelkerke}$ of the regression analysis was 0.247 for the LGA vs. AGA analysis and 0.195 for the SGA vs. AGA analysis. Table 4 summarizes the results of the multiple regression analysis.

Table 4. Multiple regression analysis of parameters with potential influence on fetal growth in SGA and AGA taken together, and LGA and AGA taken together. Statistical significance was set at $p < 0.05$ (bold value). AGA was used as the reference variable and the OR presented relates to the possibility of SGA or LGA for each examined variable.

	SGA and AGA		LGA and AGA	
Maternal age	1.17 (0.88, 1.56)	$p = 0.276$	0.81 (0.63, 1.05)	$p = 0.109$
Maternal weight	1.03 (0.94, 1.13)	$p = 0.504$	0.95 (0.89, 1.01)	$p = 0.075$
Maternal height	1.18 (0.97, 1.14)	$p = 0.105$	1.00 (0.86, 1.15)	$p = 0.957$
Maternal parity	0.83 (0.29, 2.40)	$p = 0.725$	0.93 (0.44, 1.96)	$p = 0.853$
Fetal female sex	8.37 (0.47, 150.27)	$p = 0.149$	0.21 (0.04, 0.98)	$p = 0.047$
Gestational age	1.87 (0.87, 4.05)	$p = 0.110$	1.26 (0.70, 2.26)	$p = 0.449$
Amniotic apelin	1.03 (0.98, 1.08)	$p = 0.236$	1.00 (0.97, 1.03)	$p = 0.848$
Amniotic insulin	1.38 (0.41, 4.57)	$p = 0.601$	0.61 (0.33, 0.94)	**$p = 0.042$**

AGA: appropriate weight for gestational age, LGA: large weight for gestational age, SGA: small weight for gestational age.

4. Discussion

Despite the considerable advances achieved in prenatal medicine, fetal growth abnormalities remain one of the most common causes of maternal and fetal mortality and morbidity; the underlying pathogenesis remains unclear and further investigation is certainly required. The present prospective observational cohort study was conducted in order to determine whether there is any correlation connecting the amniotic fluid apelin and insulin concentrations with fetal growth and birthweight abnormalities. This is, to the best of our knowledge, the first study to scrutinize apelin concentrations in the amniotic fluid of fetuses in the second trimester of pregnancy. The published data concerning apelin in pregnancy include studies in which the bioactive peptide was collected from either maternal blood or placental tissue [16,19–25,28]. Amniotic fluid in the early second trimester of pregnancy reflects fetal serum; therefore, amniotic fluid apelin concentrations correspond to fetal serum apelin concentrations [29,30].

In this study, we found that apelin concentrations were significantly lower in LGA fetuses compared to those in AGA and SGA fetuses, respectively. More specifically, the median apelin concentration in LGA fetuses was found to be 14.35 ng/mL, while in AGA it was 40.2 ng/mL, and in SGA it was 35.8 ng/mL. A progressive increase in apelin concentrations was observed with a reduction in birthweight, even though statistical analysis failed to show any significant difference. On the other hand, a significant effect was observed with increasing birthweight, which implies that the impact of apelin might not be evident until a critical fetal body mass has been attained. When regression analysis was conducted to account for confounding factors, the effect of apelin levels on fetal growth failed to remain significant. It is common that weak correlations, although biologically relevant, may be masked in regression analysis when several factors are included, especially in the case of small study samples. We believe that our study sample is responsible for this result. Moreover, none of the participants in the AGA or the LGA group were, later in pregnancy, diagnosed with gestational diabetes, a variable that can potentially affect fetal growth. Since a statistically significant association was identified between these two groups, gestational diabetes could not have been a factor influencing the results.

Several studies have indicated the positive effect of the apelinergic system on the proliferation of placental cells and trophoblast survival. These processes are essential during the second trimester when fetal growth is determined mainly by cell proliferation [4]. In their study, Van Mieghem et al. investigated apelin concentrations in maternal blood at several gestational ages: their findings revealed a 30% decrease in apelin concentrations in pregnancies with fetal growth restriction compared to normal pregnancies. Moreover, they highlighted that these serum results were also reflected in decreased placental apelin expression and staining. However, since their study included only four IUGR pregnancies their outcomes should be interpreted with caution [11]. In the present study, no such differences were revealed between AGA and SGA amniotic fluid apelin concentrations.

Apelin, which is an adipokine secreted by adipose and other tissues, shows elevated expression in obesity; it plays a central key role in lipid and glucose metabolism and is also implicated in atherosclerosis and oxidative stress. It is of note that pregnancy itself is characterized by hyperlipidemia, oxidative stress, and reduced insulin sensitivity [31,32]. Fetal macrosomia is considered to be the manifestation of an impaired maternal metabolism. Interestingly, cord blood apelin-36 levels are found to be similar in diabetic pregnancies compared to controls [33]. Apelin may be a mediator of fetal growth, but may also serve in protective feedback mechanisms; our finding of reduced apelin concentrations in LGA fetuses compared to AGA and SGA fetuses supports this hypothesis.

Regarding insulin concentrations, no statistically significant differences between the AGA, SGA, and LGA groups were found in the present study. However, paired multivariate regression analysis carried out for the AGA and LGA fetuses revealed that amniotic fluid insulin concentrations comprise an independent factor that affects fetal birthweight. In the past, we have shown that the low demand for nutrient uptake in the second trimester as well as the immaturity of the fetal pancreas could account for the lack of pronounced differences in insulin concentrations [11].

Reviewing the existing literature concerning insulin, the data are controversial. There is evidence that, prior to 20 weeks gestation, fetal insulin production may be impaired by maternal glucose intolerance. Interestingly, an association has been shown between increased amniotic fluid insulin concentration occurring at 14–20 weeks gestation and maternal glucose intolerance and fetal macrosomia observed postnatally [26]. On the other hand, other studies have failed to reveal a correlation between amniotic fluid insulin concentrations and fetal growth [27]. Other data show that prior to routine screening for gestational diabetes mellitus (GDM), exposure of the fetus to altered amniotic fluid glucose, insulin, and insulin-like growth factor-binding protein 1 has occurred [34]. Although a statistically significant difference was expected at least among severe LGA fetuses, subgroup analysis also failed to reach statistical significance, while a trend for higher values was observed. The small size of the specific subgroups may be responsible for this non-statistical significance.

Amniotic fluid insulin is known to be elevated in mothers with GDM versus those without [35–37]. It has also been hypothesized that insulin levels may be more closely associated with glucose intolerance rather than with growth disturbances, and glucose intolerance may be present without overt macrosomia; likewise, mild macrosomia may be present without significant insulin resistance. Hence, previous studies have already reported the considerable importance of amniotic fluid insulin levels as a predictor of fetal macrosomia in mothers suffering from gestational diabetes, as well as the fact that higher concentrations of amniotic fluid insulin levels are a marker of fetal hyperinsulinemia [38]. It is clear that identifying a hyperinsulinemic fetus before birth could lead to intensified maternal insulin therapy, thus reducing both the incidence and severity of diabetic fetopathy (a hormonal and metabolic dysfunction and its morphological sequelae) for the fetus of the diabetic mother.

A limitation of the present study is the small number of cases included, resulting in the small number of cases in the study subgroups. Of note, amniotic fluid is a biological material that is hard to collect, and thus, gathering sufficient cases prospectively is extremely difficult. For the same reason, we did not divide our cases further into subgroups according to the time of the amniocentesis. The exact gestational week of amniocentesis was defined by the indication. Moreover, our purpose was to correlate fetal development at term with apelin and insulin amniotic fluid levels in the early second trimester as a period of pregnancy and not by pregnancy week-by-week. This also allowed for the expansion of the implementation of our findings into clinical practice where the timing of invasive testing is mainly determined by the gestational stage at which the indication is set; this is in most cases after 16 weeks of gestation and usually up until 22–23 weeks, as per our study. Furthermore, we do not expect the levels of the studied substances to differ significantly by week during this time period, as this period of fetal life is characterized by a very shallow fetal growth curve. To the best of our knowledge, this is the first time that amniotic fluid apelin concentrations have been examined in the second trimester; this underlines the need for larger multicenter prospective studies to elucidate the possible associations between fetal growth abnormalities and amniotic fluid mediators, such as apelin and insulin, as well as their predictive value.

On the other hand, a strength of the study is the prospective design employed, which significantly limited the possibility of selection bias, consequently rendering our findings accurate and fully interpretable while being directly relevant to our population.

5. Conclusions

Amniotic fluid apelin concentrations in the early second trimester are likely to be useful as a predictive marker for the determination of the risk of a fetus being born LGA for gestational age. Whereas our study did not detect a statistically significant effect, a clear trend was identified toward decreasing values of apelin as birthweight progressively increased. It remains unknown whether other confounders may affect this association, including fetal gender, maternal age, and maternal weight, as the multiple regression analysis revealed that the coefficient of apelin for the detection of SGA and LGA compared to AGA was rendered non-significant. Larger studies are necessary to corroborate our findings and further expand on variables that could determine the variation of apelin levels; the studies should ideally focus on the potential interplay of apelin with known factors that appear to be predictive of LGA fetuses, including fasting maternal blood glucose concentrations, fasting insulin concentrations, and glucose concentrations in the oral glucose tolerance test. Such an approach could reveal the mechanisms that determine fetal growth and help us to better understand the pathophysiological pathways that place fetuses at risk of being born SGA or LGA.

Author Contributions: Conceptualization, G.M. (George Mastorakos); Methodology, D.V., N.A., G.V., N.V., T.S. and G.M. (George Mastorakos); Validation, D.V.; Formal analysis, D.V. and V.P.; Investigation, N.L., C.I., S.S. and G.M. (Georgios Maroudias); Resources, A.F. and G.M. (Georgios Maroudias); Data curation, T.S.; writing—original draft, D.V., N.A., A.F., N.L., G.V., C.I., S.S., P.P. and M.P.; writing—review & editing, D.V., V.P., N.V. and G.M. (George Mastorakos). All authors have read and agreed to the published version of the manuscript.

Funding: The research received no external funding.

Institutional Review Board Statement: The study was conducted in accordance with the Declaration of Helsinki and approved by the Ethical Committee of Aretaieion University Hospital, Athens, Greece (143/29.11.19).

Informed Consent Statement: Informed consent was obtained from all women involved in the study.

Data Availability Statement: The data presented in this study are available on request from the corresponding author.

Conflicts of Interest: The authors declare no conflict of interest.

References

1. Salomon, L.J.; Alfirevic, Z.; Da Silva Costa, F.; Deter, R.; Figueras, F.; Ghi, T.; Glanc, P.; Khalil, A.; Lee, W.; Napolitano, R.; et al. ISUOG Practice Guidelines: Ultrasound assessment of fetal biometry and growth. *Ultrasound Obs. Gynecol* **2019**, *53*, 715–721. [CrossRef] [PubMed]
2. Vasak, B.; Koenen, S.V.; Koster, M.P.H.; Hukkelhoven, C.W.P.M.; Franx, A.; Hanson, M.A.; Visser, G.H.A. Human fetal growth is constrained below optimal for perinatal survival. *Ultrasound Obstet. Gynecol.* **2015**, *45*, 162–167. [CrossRef] [PubMed]
3. Unterscheider, J.; Daly, S.; Geary, M.P.; Kennelly, M.M.; McAuliffe, F.M.; O'donoghue, K.; Hunter, A.; Morrison, J.J.; Burke, G.; Dicker, P.; et al. Definition and management of fetal growth restriction: A survey of contemporary attitudes. *Eur. J. Obstet. Gynecol. Reprod. Biol.* **2014**, *174*, 41–45. [CrossRef] [PubMed]
4. Savchev, S.; Figueras, F.; Cruz-Martinez, R.; Illa, M.; Botet, F.; Gratacos, E. Estimated weight centile as a predictor of perinatal outcome in small-for-gestational-age pregnancies with normal fetal and maternal Doppler indices. *Ultrasound Obstet. Gynecol.* **2012**, *39*, 299–303. [CrossRef] [PubMed]
5. Vrachnis, N.; Botsis, D.; Iliodromiti, Z. The fetus that is small for gestational age. *Ann. N. Y. Acad. Sci.* **2006**, *1092*, 304–309. [CrossRef] [PubMed]
6. Tsantekidou, I.; Evangelinakis, N.; Bargiota, A.; Vrachnis, N.; Kalantaridou, S.; Valsamakis, G. Macrosomia and fetal growth restriction: Evidence for similar extrauterine metabolic risks but with differences in pathophysiology. *J. Matern. Fetal. Neonatal. Med.* **2021**, *35*, 8450–8455. [CrossRef] [PubMed]
7. Papageorghiou, A.T.; Yu, C.K.; Nicolaides, K.H. The role of uterine artery Doppler in predicting adverse pregnancy outcome. *Best Pract. Res. Clin. Obs. Gynaecol.* **2004**, *18*, 383–396. [CrossRef]
8. Botsis, D.; Vrachnis, N.; Christodoulakos, G. Doppler assessment of the intrauterine growth-restricted fetus. *Ann. N. Y. Acad. Sci.* **2006**, *1092*, 297–303. [CrossRef]
9. Gourvas, V.; Dalpa, E.; Konstantinidou, A.; Vrachnis, N.; Spandidos, D.A.; Sifakis, S. Angiogenic factors in placentas from pregnancies complicated by fetal growth restriction (review). *Mol. Med. Rep.* **2012**, *6*, 23–27.
10. Vrachnis, N.; Kalampokas, E.; Sifakis, S.; Vitoratos, N.; Kalampokas, T.; Botsis, D.; Iliodromiti, Z. Placental growth factor (PlGF): A key to optimizing fetal growth. *J. Matern. Fetal Neonatal Med.* **2013**, *26*, 995–1002. [CrossRef]
11. Vrachnis, N.; Argyridis, S.; Vrachnis, D.; Antonakopoulos, N.; Valsamakis, G.; Iavazzo, C.; Zygouris, D.; Salakos, N.; Rodolakis, A.; Vlahos, N.; et al. Increased Fibroblast Growth Factor 21 (FGF21) Concentration in Early Second Trimester Amniotic Fluid and Its Association with Fetal Growth. *Metabolites* **2021**, *11*, 581. [CrossRef] [PubMed]
12. Antonakopoulos, N.; Iliodromiti, Z.; Mastorakos, G.; Iavazzo, C.; Valsamakis, G.; Salakos, N.; Papageorghiou, A.; Margeli, A.; Kalantaridou, S.; Creatsas, G.; et al. Association between Brain-Derived Neurotrophic Factor (BDNF) Levels in 2nd Trimester Amniotic Fluid and Fetal Development. *Mediat. Inflamm.* **2018**, *2018*, 8476217. [CrossRef]
13. Vrachnis, N.; Dalainas, I.; Papoutsis, D.; Samoli, E.; Rizos, D.; Iliodromiti, Z.; Siristatidis, C.; Tsikouras, P.; Creatsas, G.; Botsis, D. Soluble Fas and Fas-ligand levels in mid-trimester amniotic fluid and their associations with severe small for gestational age fetuses: A prospective observational study. *J. Reprod Immunol.* **2013**, *98*, 39–44. [CrossRef] [PubMed]
14. Vrachnis, N.; Loukas, N.; Vrachnis, D.; Antonakopoulos, N.; Christodoulaki, C.; Tsonis, O.; George, M.; Iliodromiti, Z. Phthalates and fetal growth velocity: Tracking down the suspected links. *J. Matern. Fetal. Neonatal. Med.* **2021**, *35*, 4985–4993. [CrossRef] [PubMed]
15. Vrachnis, N.; Loukas, N.; Vrachnis, D.; Antonakopoulos, N.; Zygouris, D.; Kolialexi, A.; Pergaliotis, V.; Iavazzo, C.; Mastorakos, G.; Iliodromiti, Z. A Systematic Review of Bisphenol A from Dietary and Non-Dietary Sources during Pregnancy and Its Possible Connection with Fetal Growth Restriction: Investigating Its Potential Effects and the Window of Fetal Vulnerability. *Nutrients* **2021**, *13*, 2426. [CrossRef] [PubMed]

16. Dawid, M.; Młyczyńska, E.; Jurek, M.; Respekta, N.; Pich, K.; Kurowska, P.; Gieras, W.; Milewicz, T.; Kotula-Balak, M.; Rak, A. Apelin, APJ, and ELABELA: Role in Placental Function, Pregnancy, and Foetal Development-An Overview. *Cells* **2021**, *11*, 99. [CrossRef]
17. Weiss, P.A.; Pürstner, P.; Winter, R.; Lichtenegger, W. Insulin levels in amniotic fluid of normal and abnormal pregnancies. *Obs. Gynecol.* **1984**, *63*, 371–375.
18. IBM Corp. *IBM SPSS Statistics for Windows, Version 21.0*; IBM Corp: Armonk, NY, USA, 2012.
19. Eberlé, D.; Marousez, L.; Hanssens, S.; Knauf, C.; Breton, C.; Deruelle, P.; Lesage, J. Elabela and Apelin actions in healthy and pathological pregnancies. *Cytokine Growth Factor Rev.* **2019**, *46*, 45–53. [CrossRef]
20. Hamza, R.Z.; Diab, A.A.A.; Zahra, M.H.; Asalah, A.K.; Moursi, S.M.; Al-Baqami, N.M.; Al-Salmi, F.A.; Attia, M.S. Correlation between Apelin and Some Angiogenic Factors in the Pathogenesis of Preeclampsia: Apelin-13 as Novel Drug for Treating Preeclampsia and Its Physiological Effects on Placenta. *Int. J. Endocrinol.* **2021**, *2021*, 5017362. [CrossRef]
21. Deniz, R.; Baykus, Y.; Ustebay, S.; Ugur, K.; Yavuzkir, Ş.; Aydin, S. Evaluation of elabela, apelin and nitric oxide findings in maternal blood of normal pregnant women, pregnant women with pre-eclampsia, severe pre-eclampsia and umbilical arteries and venules of newborns. *J. Obs. Gynaecol.* **2019**, *39*, 907–912. [CrossRef]
22. Młyczyńska, E.; Myszka, M.; Kurowska, P.; Dawid, M.; Milewicz, T.; Bałajewicz-Nowak, M.; Kowalczyk, P.; Rak, A. Anti-Apoptotic Effect of Apelin in Human Placenta: Studies on BeWo Cells and Villous Explants from Third-Trimester Human Pregnancy. *Int. J. Mol. Sci.* **2021**, *22*, 2760. [CrossRef] [PubMed]
23. Gürlek, B.; Yılmaz, A.; Durakoğlugil, M.E.; Karakaş, S.; Kazaz, I.M.; Önal, Ö.; Şatıroğlu, Ö. Evaluation of serum apelin-13 and apelin-36 concentrations in preeclamptic pregnancies. *J. Obs. Gynaecol. Res.* **2020**, *46*, 58–65. [CrossRef] [PubMed]
24. Guo, Y.Y.; Li, T.; Liu, H.; Tang, L.; Li, Y.-C.; Hu, H.-T.; Su, Y.-F.; Lin, Y.; Wang, Y.-Y.; Li, C.; et al. Circulating levels of Elabela and Apelin in the second and third trimesters of pregnancies with gestational diabetes mellitus. *Gynecol. Endocrinol.* **2020**, *36*, 890–894. [CrossRef]
25. Van Mieghem, T.; Doherty, A.; Baczyk, D.; Drewlo, S.; Baud, D.; Carvalho, J.; Kingdom, J. Apelin in Normal Pregnancy and Pregnancies Complicated by Placental Insufficiency. *Reprod. Sci.* **2016**, *23*, 1037–1043. [CrossRef] [PubMed]
26. De Prins, F.A.; Van Assche, F.A. Insulin levels in amniotic fluid and fetal growth. *Padiatr. Padol.* **1982**, *17*, 223–229.
27. Carpenter, M.W.; Canick, J.A.; Hogan, J.W.; Shellum, C.; Somers, M.; Star, J.A. Amniotic Fluid Insulin at 14–20 Weeks' Gestation: Association with later maternal glucose intolerance and birth macrosomia. *Diabetes Care* **2001**, *24*, 1259–1263. [CrossRef]
28. Wang, C.; Liu, X.; Kong, D.; Qin, X.; Li, Y.; Teng, X.; Huang, X. Apelin as a novel drug for treating preeclampsia. *Exp. Ther. Med.* **2017**, *14*, 5917–5923. [CrossRef]
29. Benzie, R.J.; Doran, T.A.; Harkins, J.L.; Jones Owen, V.M.; Porter, C.J. Composition of the amniotic fluid and maternal serum in pregnancy. *Am. J. Obstet. Gynecol.* **1974**, *119*, 798–810. [CrossRef]
30. Brzezinski, A.; Sadovsky, E.; Shafrir, E. Protein composition of early amniotic fluid and fetal serum with a case of bis-albuminemia. *Am. J. Obs. Gynecol.* **1964**, *89*, 488–494. [CrossRef]
31. Paradisi, G.; Biaggi, A.; Ferrazzani, S.; De Carolis, S.; Caruso, A. Abnormal carbohydrate metabolism during pregnancy: Association with endothelial dysfunction. *Diabetes Care* **2002**, *25*, 560–564. [CrossRef]
32. Sanchez-Vera, I.; Bonet, B.; Viana, M.; Quintanar, A.; Martín, M.D.; Blanco, P.; Donnay, S.; Albi, M. Changes in plasma lipids and increased low-density lipoprotein susceptibility to oxidation in pregnancies complicated by gestational diabetes: Consequences of obesity. *Metab. Clin. Exp.* **2007**, *56*, 1527–1533. [CrossRef] [PubMed]
33. Aslan, M.; Celik, O.; Celik, N.; Turkcuoglu, I.; Yilmaz, E.; Karaer, A.; Simsek, Y.; Celik, E.; Aydin, S. Cord blood nesfatin-1 and apelin-36 levels in gestational diabetes mellitus. *Endocrine* **2012**, *41*, 424. [CrossRef] [PubMed]
34. Tisi, D.K.; Burns, D.H.; Luskey, G.W.; Koski, K.G. Fetal exposure to altered amniotic fluid glucose, insulin, and insulin-like growth factor-binding protein 1 occurs before screening for gestational diabetes mellitus. *Diabetes Care* **2011**, *34*, 139–144. [CrossRef] [PubMed]
35. Star, J.; Canick, J.A.; Palomaki, G.E.; Carpenter, M.W.; Saller, D.N., Jr.; Sung, C.J.; Tumber, M.B.; Coustan, D.R. The relationship between second-trimester amniotic fluid insulin and glucose levels and subsequent gestational diabetes. *Prenat. Diagn.* **1997**, *17*, 149–154. [CrossRef]
36. D'Anna, R.; Baviera, G.; Cannata, M.L.; De Vivo, A.; Di Benedetto, A.; Corrado, F. Midtrimester amniotic fluid leptin and insulin levels and subsequent gestational diabetes. *Gynecol. Obs. Invest.* **2007**, *64*, 65–68. [CrossRef]
37. Carpenter, M.W.; Canick, J.A.; Star, J.; Carr, S.R.; Burke, M.E.; Shahinian, K. Fetal hyperinsulinism at 14–20 weeks and subsequent gestational diabetes. *Obs. Gynecol.* **1996**, *87*, 89–93. [CrossRef]
38. Fraser, R.B.; Bruce, C. Amniotic fluid insulin levels identify the fetus at risk of neonatal hypoglycaemia. *Diabet. Med.* **1999**, *16*, 568–572. [CrossRef]

Disclaimer/Publisher's Note: The statements, opinions and data contained in all publications are solely those of the individual author(s) and contributor(s) and not of MDPI and/or the editor(s). MDPI and/or the editor(s) disclaim responsibility for any injury to people or property resulting from any ideas, methods, instructions or products referred to in the content.

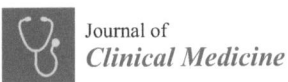

Article

The Accuracy of Sonographically Estimated Fetal Weight and Prediction of Small for Gestational Age in Twin Pregnancy—Comparison of the First and Second Twins

Moran Gawie-Rotman [1,2], Shoval Menashe [2], Noa Haggiag [1,2], Alon Shrim [1,2], Mordechai Hallak [1,2] and Rinat Gabbay-Benziv [1,2,*]

[1] Obstetrics and Gynecology Division, Hillel Yaffe Medical Center, Hadera 3846201, Israel; moran.gawie7@gmail.com (M.G.-R.)
[2] The Ruth and Bruce Rappaport Faculty of Medicine, Technion-Israel Institute of Technology, Haifa 3200003, Israel
[*] Correspondence: gabbayrinat@gmail.com; Tel.: +972-4-7744514

Abstract: Accurate sonographic estimation of fetal weight is essential for every pregnancy, especially in twin gestation. We conducted a retrospective analysis of the sonographically estimated fetal weight (sEFW) of all twin gestations performed within 14 days of delivery in a single center that aimed to evaluate the accuracy of sEFW in predicting neonatal weight and small for gestational age (SGA) by comparing the first fetus to the second. A total of 190 twin gestations were evaluated for the study. There was no statistically significant difference in the sEFW between the first and the second twins, but the second twin had a statistically significant lower birth weight (2434 vs. 2351 g, $p = 0.028$). No difference was found in median absolute systematic error ($p = 0.450$), random error, or sEFW evaluations that were within 10% of the birth weight between the fetuses (65.3% vs. 67.9%, $p = 0.587$). Reliability analysis demonstrated an excellent correlation between the sEFW and the birth weight for both twins; however, the Euclidean distance was slightly higher for the first twin (12.21%). For SGA prediction, overall, there was a low sensitivity and a high specificity for all fetuses, with almost no difference between the first and second twins. We found that sEFW overestimated the birth weight for the second twin, with almost no other difference in accuracy measures or SGA prediction.

Keywords: twin pregnancy; small for gestational age; estimated fetal weight; accuracy of birthweight

1. Introduction

Twin pregnancies are associated with a high incidence of pregnancy complications. One of the most prevalent risks is preterm delivery, which accounts for most of the increased perinatal morbidity and mortality. Additionally, higher rates of fetal growth abnormalities and congenital anomalies contribute to adverse outcomes in twin pregnancies [1].

It has been suggested that neonatal morbidity and mortality tend to be higher for the second-born twin (as compared to the first-born). In a systematic review of observational studies, overall neonatal morbidity, defined as pH < 7.0, Apgar score < 7 at 5 min, or any neonatal birth trauma, was 3.0 and 4.6 percent, respectively (OR 0.53, 95% CI 0.39–0.70), and overall neonatal mortality, defined as death within 28 days, of the first and second twins was 0.3 and 0.6 percent, respectively (OR 0.55, 95% CI 0.38–0.81). The increased risk of adverse neonatal outcomes in the second-born twin was most likely related to a lower birth weight, a higher frequency of malpresentation, cord prolapse, placental abruption, and the need for obstetric maneuvers at delivery [2].

In twin gestation, monitoring the fetus's growth is of utmost importance. According to the International Society of Ultrasound in Obstetrics and Gynecology (ISOUG) guidelines, sonographic evaluation of fetal growth is recommended every four weeks for uncomplicated bichorionic twins and every two weeks for uncomplicated monochorionic twins [3].

Accurate follow-up is imperative for the early detection of peripartum placental insufficiency, ultimately allowing the healthcare provider to prepare for complications that may arise during childbirth. Unfortunately, sonographic estimation of fetal weight (sEFW) has been proven to be less accurate in twins than in singleton pregnancies [4].

For a singleton pregnancy, the mean error between the sEFW and the neonate's birth weight is about 10–20% [5–7]. The degree of accuracy depends on the examiner and on the fetal and maternal parameters, such as fetal presentation, gestational age, amniotic fluid volume, and the level of maternal obesity [8,9]. For twin pregnancies, despite the high incidence of growth abnormalities, only a few studies in the literature have evaluated the accuracy of sEFW. Furthermore, these studies have presented conflicting results [10–13].

This study aims to evaluate the accuracy of ultrasound in the prediction of neonatal birth weight with an emphasis on comparing the first fetus (closer to the cervix) with the second fetus. Moreover, we calculated the accuracy measurements for the determination of small for gestational age (SGA), defined as sEFW under the tenth percentiles for the two fetuses, and compared them.

2. Materials and Methods

2.1. Population

This was a retrospective cohort analysis of women carrying twin gestations who delivered in a single, tertiary, university-affiliated medical center. All twin pregnancies delivered between September 2011 and August 2021, in which sonographic fetal biometry estimation was performed within 14 days before deliveries, were analyzed. The study was approved by the local Institutional Review Board committee (HYMC-0048-22). Due to the retrospective nature of the study, informed consent was waived. Inclusion criteria included all live twin births who had a sonographic evaluation within 14 days before delivery. Cases with any known chromosomal abnormalities or major malformations were excluded. In addition, we excluded women without available full documentation of all biometric measurements (biparietal diameter (BPD), head circumference (HC), abdominal circumference (AC), and femur length (FL)), as well as women who were in active labor or with ruptured membranes at the time of the sonographic assessment. Cases with unclear chorionicity or suspected growth abnormalities were not excluded.

2.2. Data

Data were retrieved from the comprehensive computerized database of sonographic examinations and compared to the perinatal database. Matching was verified by comparing the date of the last menstrual period to avoid mixing data from two different pregnancies of the same woman. The gestational age at the time of the sonographic evaluation was calculated by the last menstrual period or by first-trimester ultrasound if a discrepancy exceeding six days between them was present. Antenatal data, including the gestational age at delivery and the actual birth weights, were obtained from the perinatal database. Small for gestational age was defined as neonates under the 10th percentile using twins, gestational age, and gender-specific customized curves, constructed based on our population [14]. The sonographic sEFW was calculated for every twin using the Hadlock formula: $(EFW(hadlock\_4) = 10^{(1.3596 + 0.0064 \times Q2 + 0.0424 \times R2 + 0.174 \times S2 + 0.00061 \times P2 \times R2 - 0.00386 \times R2 \times S2)})$.

2.3. Measurements

By convention, fetal sonographic evaluations included all standard fetal biometry measurements (AC, FL, BPD, and HC) according to ISUOG guidelines [3], presenting part, placental location, and amniotic fluid estimation for every twin, measured by the largest vertical pocket. All examinations were performed trans-abdominally using a high-quality ultrasound system, GE Voluson E6, Voluson E8, or Voluson E10 (GE Medical Systems, Zipf, Austria), by physicians who are ultrasound specialists or by experienced ultrasound technicians. Twin A (the 1st twin) was defined as the fetus closer to the cervix. The BPD was measured from the proximal echo of the fetal skull to the proximal edge of the deep border (outer–inner) at the level of the cavum septum pellucidum. The HC was measured as an ellipse around the perimeter of the fetal skull at the same level [15]. The AC was measured in the transverse plane of the fetal abdomen at the level of the umbilical vein in the anterior third and the stomach bubble in the same plane; measurements were taken around the perimeter [16]. The FL was measured in a view in which the full femoral diaphysis was seen and was taken from one end of the diaphysis to the other, not including the distal femoral epiphysis [17]. After birth, neonatal birth weight and anthropometric data were immediately documented. Neonate A (1st neonate) was defined as the first twin delivered.

2.4. Accuracy and SGA Evaluation

For every twin fetus, the sEFW was evaluated and compared to the neonatal birth weight. Accuracy was evaluated for every twin and compared between the 1st (closer to the cervix) and 2nd fetus. Measures of accuracy included the systematic error (calculated as the absolute [sEFW − birth weight]/birth weight × 100, reflecting the systematic deviation of the sEFW from the birth weight, expressed as a percentage of the birth weight); the random error (the standard deviation of the systematic error), reflecting the random component of prediction error; and the proportion of estimates within 10% of the birth weight. To further compare the accuracy of EFW between the 1st and 2nd twins, we utilized the Euclidean distance (=square root of [systematic error^2 + random error^2]), representing the geometric average of the systematic and random errors.

Next, to evaluate the sEFW prediction of SGA at birth for every twin, we compared the sEFW and the neonatal birth weight with the 10th percentile for the exact gestational age. Accuracy was then evaluated using the following measures: sensitivity, specificity, positive predictive value (PPV), negative predictive value (NPV), positive likelihood ratio (+LR, defined as sensitivity/(1 − specificity)), and negative likelihood ratio (−LR, defined as (1 − sensitivity)/specificity). Overall accuracy was defined as (true negative + true positive cases)/all cases.

2.5. Statistical Analysis

Statistical analysis was performed using SPSS version 28.0 software (SPSS, Inc., Chicago, IL, USA). $p < 0.05$ was considered significant. Categorical data were analyzed using Fisher's exact test, and continuous variables were compared using the Mann–Whitney–Wilcoxon test as appropriate. Reliability analysis was used to calculate the Cronbach's α value, which measures the power of correlation between sEFW and the neonatal birth weight ($\alpha \geq 0.9$, excellent correlation; $0.7 \leq \alpha < 0.9$, good correlation; $0.6 \leq \alpha < 0.7$, accepted correlation; $0.5 \leq \alpha < 0.6$, poor correlation; and $\alpha < 0.5$, unacceptable correlation).

3. Results

3.1. Demographics

Overall, 28,834 women delivered in our institution during the study period, of which 1064 had twin gestations. After consolidating the database, 190 women with twin gestations had sonographic fetal evaluations performed within 14 days of delivery and were thus eligible for our analysis.

The demographic and obstetrical characteristics of the cohort are shown in Table 1. The median maternal age was 31.34 (26.42–36.2) years. One hundred thirty-six pregnancies were dichorionic-diamniotic (71.57%) twins, 34 (17.8%) were monochorionic-diamniotic twins, and the remaining were monochorionic-monoamniotic (0.52%). Only 38 (20%) pregnancies were complicated by maternal diabetes. For the entire cohort, the median gestational age at ultrasound evaluation was 35.54 (28.29–39.14) weeks, and the median sEFW was 2452 (834–5187) grams. The median gestational age at delivery was 36.37 (29.29–39.14) weeks, with a median birth weight of 2397 (775–3750) g. The median time interval from ultrasound evaluation to delivery was 5 (0–14) days. The majority of women delivered within 7 days of the sonographic evaluation (130/190, 68%), and over a third (82/190, 43.15%) delivered within 3 days of the evaluation.

explained by the high incidence of non-vertex presentation in the second twin group, causing dolichocephaly and smaller-than-anticipated BPD measurements [24,25].

Our results matched previous studies showing a tendency to underestimate the weight of the first twin and overestimate the weight of the second twin [10,22].

For sEFW prediction of SGA, overall we found high accuracy for both twins, as shown in previous studies [10]. We found low sensitivity in the prediction of SGA with high specificity, similar to other studies [10,22,23]. Conflicting results have been shown regarding sensitivity. While Kaouther et al. have shown good sensitivity for SGA prediction, our study, along with others [10,22,23], has found low sensitivity for the prediction of SGA.

Cognitive biases are unconscious mental shortcuts or patterns that can influence how people perceive, interpret, and make decisions about information. Although diagnostic errors arising from cognitive biases are well studied in the radiology field, there remains a lack of research in the obstetric ultrasound field [26]. Our study highlights the importance of acknowledging that cognitive biases exist in the sonographic estimation of fetal weight.

The strength of our study relies on the selection of cases for sonographic evaluation within 14 days of delivery, with the majority performed up to 7 days before delivery. Additionally, sonographic evaluation was undertaken by highly experienced ultrasound technicians or physicians who were ultrasound specialists.

Our study is not free of limitations. First, this study is limited by its retrospective design. For this reason, no data was available regarding patients' body mass index, demographics, or ethnic origin. Additionally, fetal data regarding gender was unavailable, which potentially could have affected the sonographic weight estimation prior to delivery and should have been evaluated as a confounding variable. Secondly, our study included a relatively small sample size of twins at all gestational ages, which could have affected our results. The inclusion of preterm deliveries that are potentially related to placental insufficiency complications during pregnancy may have influenced the proportion of SGA or growth-restricted fetuses. Therefore, future studies are needed to further study and validate our findings. Thirdly, chorionicity was evaluated sonographically without validation using postpartum placental examinations. Lastly, although care was taken to correctly name the first and second twins, we could not retrospectively validate that the presenting twin in ultrasound was always the first delivered, particularly in cases of cesarean section.

5. Conclusions

In conclusion, twin gestations are prone to growth abnormalities, and fetal weights are typically smaller at term than in singleton pregnancies. Our study shows that sEFW has no difference in predicting birth weight for first and second twins, with high accuracy in predicting SGA but low sensitivity.

Author Contributions: R.G.-B.—conception and design, interpretation of data, writing the manuscript; S.M.—analysis and interpretation of data, drafting the article; M.G.-R.—conception and design, writing the manuscript; A.S. and N.H.—data acquisition and drafting the manuscript; M.H.—conception and design, drafting the manuscript. All authors will be accountable for all aspects of the work in ensuring that questions related to the accuracy or integrity of any part of the work are appropriately investigated and resolved. All authors have read and agreed to the published version of the manuscript.

Funding: This research received no external funding.

Institutional Review Board Statement: The study was approved by the local Institutional Review Board committee (HYMC-0048-22).

Informed Consent Statement: Due to the retrospective nature of the study, informed consent was waived.

Data Availability Statement: The data presented in this study are available on request from the corresponding author.

Conflicts of Interest: All authors declare no conflict of interest.

References

1. Santana, D.S.; Silveira, C.; Costa, M.L.; Souza, R.T.; Surita, F.G.; Souza, J.P.; Mazhar, S.B.; Jayaratne, K.; Qureshi, Z.; Sousa, M.H.; et al. Perinatal outcomes in twin pregnancies complicated by maternal morbidity: Evidence from the WHO Multicountry Survey on Maternal and Newborn Health. *BMC Pregnancy Childbirth* **2018**, *18*, 449. [CrossRef] [PubMed]
2. Rossi, A.C.; Mullin, P.M.; Chmait, R.H. Neonatal outcomes of twins according to birth order, presentation and mode of delivery: A systematic review and meta-analysis. *BJOG* **2011**, *118*, 523–532. [CrossRef] [PubMed]
3. Khalil, A.; Rodgers, M.; Baschat, A.; Bhide, A.; Gratacos, E.; Hecher, K.; Kilby, M.D.; Lewi, L.; Nicolaides, K.H.; Oepkes, D.; et al. ISUOG Practice Guidelines: Role of ultrasound in twin pregnancy. *Ultrasound Obstet. Gynecol.* **2016**, *47*, 247–263. [CrossRef] [PubMed]
4. Khalil, A.; D'Antonio, F.; Dias, T.; Cooper, D.; Thilaganathan, B. Ultrasound estimation of birth weight in twin pregnancy: Comparison of biometry algorithms in the STORK multiple pregnancy cohort. *Ultrasound Obstet. Gynecol.* **2014**, *44*, 210–220. [CrossRef]
5. Gabbay-Benziv, R.; Aviram, A.; Bardin, R.; Ashwal, E.; Melamed, N.; Hiersch, L.; Wiznitzer, A.; Yogev, Y.; Hadar, E. Prediction of Small for Gestational Age: Accuracy of Different Sonographic Fetal Weight Estimation Formulas. *Fetal Diagn. Ther.* **2016**, *40*, 205–213. [CrossRef]
6. Shmueli, A.; Aviram, A.; Bardin, R.; Wiznitzer, A.; Chen, R.; Gabbay-Benziv, R. Effect of fetal presentation on sonographic estimation of fetal weight according to different formulas. *Int. J. Gynecol. Obstet.* **2017**, *137*, 234–240. [CrossRef]
7. Aviram, A.; Yogev, Y.; Ashwal, E.; Hiersch, L.; Hadar, E.; Gabbay-Benziv, R. Prediction of large for gestational age by various sonographic fetal weight estimation formulas-which should we use? *J. Perinatol.* **2017**, *37*, 513–517. [CrossRef]
8. Bardin, R.; Gabbay-Benziv, R. Accuracy of Sonographic Estimated Fetal Weight: Is there Still Room for Improvement? *Isr. Med. Assoc. J.* **2019**, *21*, 831–832.
9. Ocer, F.; Aydin, Y.; Atis, A.; Kaleli, S. Factors affecting the accuracy of ultrasonographical fetal weight estimation in twin pregnancies. *J. Matern. Fetal Neonatal Med.* **2011**, *24*, 1168–1172. [CrossRef]
10. Danon, D.; Melamed, N.; Bardin, R.; Meizner, I. Accuracy of ultrasonographic fetal weight estimation in twin pregnancies. *Obstet. Gynecol.* **2008**, *112*, 759–764. [CrossRef]
11. Suzuki, S.; Shimizu, E.; Kinoshita, M.; Araki, S. Accuracy of ultrasonographic fetal weight estimation in Japanese twin pregnancies. *J. Med. Ultrason.* **2009**, *36*, 157–158. [CrossRef] [PubMed]
12. Jensen, O.H.; Jenssen, H. Prediction of fetal weights in twins. *Acta Obstet. Gynecol. Scand.* **1995**, *74*, 177–180. [CrossRef] [PubMed]
13. Lynch, L.; Lapinski, R.; Alvarez, M.; Lockwood, C.J. Accuracy of ultrasound estimation of fetal weight in multiple pregnancies. *Ultrasound Obstet. Gynecol.* **1995**, *6*, 349–352. [CrossRef] [PubMed]
14. Wilkof Segev, R.; Gelman, M.; Maor-Sagie, E.; Shrim, A.; Hallak, M.; Gabbay-Benziv, R. New reference values for biometrical measurements and sonographic estimated fetal weight in twin gestations and comparison to previous normograms. *J. Perinat. Med.* **2019**, *47*, 757–764. [CrossRef]
15. Chitty, L.S.; Altman, D.G.; Henderson, A.; Campbell, S. Charts of fetal size: 2. Head measurements. *Br. J. Obstet. Gynaecol.* **1994**, *101*, 35–43. [CrossRef] [PubMed]
16. Chitty, L.S.; Altman, D.G.; Henderson, A.; Campbell, S. Charts of fetal size: 3. Abdominal measurements. *Br. J. Obstet. Gynaecol.* **1994**, *101*, 125–131. [CrossRef]
17. Chitty, L.S.; Altman, D.G.; Henderson, A.; Campbell, S. Charts of fetal size: 4. Femur length. *Br. J. Obstet. Gynaecol.* **1994**, *101*, 132–135. [CrossRef]
18. Chien, P.F.; Owen, P.; Khan, K.S. Validity of ultrasound estimation of fetal weight. *Obstet. Gynecol.* **2000**, *95*, 856–860. [CrossRef]
19. Benacerraf, B.R.; Gelman, R.; Frigoletto, F.D.J. Sonographically estimated fetal weights: Accuracy and limitation. *Am. J. Obstet. Gynecol.* **1988**, *159*, 1118–1121. [CrossRef]
20. Shamley, K.T.; Landon, M.B. Accuracy and modifying factors for ultrasonographic determination of fetal weight at term. *Obstet. Gynecol.* **1994**, *84*, 926–930.
21. Basha, A.S.; Abu-Khader, I.B.; Qutishat, R.M.; Amarin, Z.O. Accuracy of sonographic fetal weight estimation within 14 days of delivery in a Jordanian population using Hadlock formula 1. *Med. Princ. Pract.* **2012**, *21*, 366–369. [CrossRef] [PubMed]
22. Harper, L.M.; Roehl, K.A.; Tuuli, M.G.; Odibo, A.O.; Cahill, A.G. Sonographic accuracy of estimated fetal weight in twins. *J. Ultrasound Med.* **2013**, *32*, 625–630. [CrossRef] [PubMed]
23. Dimassi, K.; Karoui, A.; Triki, A.; Gara, M.F. Performance de l'estimation échographique du poids fœtal dans les grossesses gémellaires. Performance of ultrasound fetal weight estimation in twins. *La Tunis. Med.* **2016**, *94*, 203–209.
24. Levine, D.; Kilpatrick, S.; Damato, N.; Callen, P.W. Dolichocephaly and oligohydramnios in preterm premature rupture of the membranes. *J. Ultrasound Med.* **1996**, *15*, 375–379. [CrossRef] [PubMed]

25. Kasby, C.B.; Poll, V. The breech head and its ultrasound significance. *Br. J. Obstet. Gynaecol.* **1982**, *89*, 106–110. [CrossRef]
26. Sotiriadis, A.; Odibo, A.O. Systematic error and cognitive bias in obstetric ultrasound. *Ultrasound Obstet. Gynecol.* **2019**, *53*, 431–435. [CrossRef]

Disclaimer/Publisher's Note: The statements, opinions and data contained in all publications are solely those of the individual author(s) and contributor(s) and not of MDPI and/or the editor(s). MDPI and/or the editor(s) disclaim responsibility for any injury to people or property resulting from any ideas, methods, instructions or products referred to in the content.

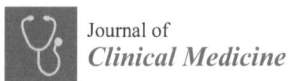

Article

Long-Term Postnatal Follow-Up in Monochorionic TTTS Twin Pregnancies Treated with Fetoscopic Laser Surgery and Complicated by Right Ventricular Outflow Tract Anomalies

Stefano Faiola [1,2,*], Maria Mandalari [2], Chiara Coco [2], Daniela Casati [1,2], Arianna Laoreti [1,2], Savina Mannarino [3], Carla Corti [3], Dario Consonni [4], Irene Cetin [2] and Mariano Lanna [1,2]

[1] Fetal Therapy Unit 'Umberto Nicolini', Buzzi Children's Hospital, 20154 Milan, Italy
[2] Department of Woman, Mother and Neonate, Buzzi Children's Hospital, 20154 Milan, Italy
[3] Pediatric Cardiology Unit, Buzzi Children's Hospital, 20154 Milan, Italy
[4] Epidemiology Unit, Fondazione IRCCS Ca' Granda, Ospedale Maggiore Policlinico, 20122 Milan, Italy
* Correspondence: stefano.faiola@asst-fbf-sacco.it

Abstract: Right ventricular outflow tract anomalies (RVOTAs), such as pulmonary stenosis (PS), pulmonary atresia (PA), and pulmonary insufficiency (PI), are typical cardiac anomalies in monochorionic twins, and they are complicated by twin-to-twin transfusion syndrome (TTTS). The aim of this study was to conduct a long-term postnatal cardiological evaluation of prenatal RVOTAs in monochorionic diamniotic twin pregnancies complicated by TTTS and treated with fetoscopic laser surgery (FLS) and to analyze possible prenatal predictors of congenital heart disease (CHD). Prenatal RVOTAs were retrospectively retrieved from all TTTS cases treated with FLS in our unit between 2009 and 2019. Twenty-eight prenatal cases of RVOTAs (16 PI, 10 PS, 2 PA) were observed out of 335 cases of TTTS. Four cases did not reach the postnatal period. CHD was present in 17 of the remaining 24 cases (70.8%), with 10 being severe (58.8%; 10/17); nine cases of PS required balloon valvuloplasty, and one case required biventricular non-compaction cardiomyopathy. The risk of major CHD increased with prenatal evidence of PS and decreased with the gestational age at the time of TTTS and with the prenatal normalization of blood flow across the pulmonary valve. Despite treatment with FLS, the majority of monochorionic diamniotic twin pregnancies complicated by TTTS with prenatal RVOTAs had CHD at long-term follow-up.

Keywords: monochorionic twin; TTTS; fetoscopic laser surgery; prenatal RVOTA; CHD

1. Introduction

Right ventricular outflow tract anomalies (RVOTAs), such as pulmonary stenosis (PS), pulmonary atresia (PA), and pulmonary insufficiency (PI), have been described as cardiac anomalies that are typical in monochorionic twin (MC) pregnancies complicated by twin-to-twin transfusion syndrome (TTTS), with a prevalence of 7–9% in the recipient twin (RT) in untreated pregnancies [1,2]. RT cardiomyopathy might be the consequence of the passage from donor to recipient of blood volumes and vasoactive peptides of the renin–angiotensin system through placental anastomosis; these increase vascular resistance, leading to higher pre- and afterloads on the left and right sides of RT hearts [3,4]. Fetoscopic laser surgery (FLS) of placental vascular anastomosis has been identified as the best treatment for TTTS [5]. Furthermore, previous studies demonstrated how FLS, which interrupts the passage of blood and vasoactive mediators, leads to an improvement in the right ventricular systolic and diastolic function of the RT [6]. However, in the ex-RT, the persistence or even the appearance of an RVOTA weeks after FLS or transient cardiac involvement in the ex-donor twin (DT) has been reported, despite successful FLS [7]. The primary aim of the present study was to evaluate long-term postnatal cardiological evaluations of cases with a prenatal RVOTA in a group of MC diamniotic (MC/DA) twin pregnancies complicated by TTTS

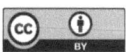

and treated with FLS at a single center. The secondary aim was to analyze possible prenatal predictors of postnatal congenital heart disease (CHD).

2. Materials and Methods

This is a retrospective descriptive analysis of all MC/DA pregnancies complicated by TTTS and treated with FLS at the "Umberto Nicolini" Fetal Therapy Unit of the Vittore Buzzi Children's Hospital in Milan (Italy) between January 2009 and January 2019. TTTS was defined according to the Eurofetus criteria (i.e., polyhydramnios of a ≥ 8 cm maximum vertical pocket in the recipient or ≥ 10 cm from 20 weeks of gestation onwards and oligohydramnios of a ≤ 2 cm maximum vertical pocket in the donor), and the Quintero Staging system was used to classify the severity of TTTS [8].

For each case, a detailed ultrasound anatomical evaluation including echocardiography was carried out for both MC/DA twins by using a GE Voluson 730, Expert, and GE E8, GE Healthcare, Zipf, Austria.

The presence, absence, and types of RVOTAs were noted. Prenatal RVOTAs were classified as pulmonary stenosis (PS) if a forward turbulent flow was detected across the pulmonary valve (PV) with aliasing and a peak systolic velocity (PSV) of >100 cm/sec, as pulmonary insufficiency (PI) if a bidirectional flow was identified across the PV, and as pulmonary atresia (PA) if no flow was detectable across the PV, with exclusive ductal reverse flow in the pulmonary artery [9]. At each ultrasound evaluation, in addition to the blood flow across the PV, the following parameters were recorded to assess the cardiovascular profile: the cardiothoracic circumference ratio (C/T) measured at a cross-sectional section through the fetal chest; tricuspid and mitral regurgitation, which was classified as mild if the jet was protosystolic, moderate if proto-mesosystolic, and moderate if holosystolic [7]; the ductus venosus a-wave flow, which was reported as present, absent, or reversed. The presence or absence of ascites was recorded. Pregnancies were also screened for selective fetal growth restriction (sFGR). sFGR was diagnosed based on an estimated fetal weight (EFW) of less than the 10th percentile in one twin and an intertwin EFW difference of >25%.

FLS was performed by using the selective technique until January 2012 and then with the Solomon technique from that date onwards [10].

Post-FLS fetal assessments were performed 24 and 48 h after the procedure, followed by prenatal echocardiographic assessments, which were performed at our center at 1 week and 1 month after the treatment, and all cardiovascular parameters were recorded. In addition, the patients who were directly followed in our hospital underwent a weekly assessment. All cases of MC/DA twin pregnancies with a prenatal diagnosis of an RVOTA were delivered at our hospital or at tertiary hospitals, allowing the newborns to undergo a formal cardiac assessment within 24 h of delivery. Postnatal examinations of patients delivered in our hospital were carried out by a dedicated pediatric cardiologist. The right outflow tract was evaluated and the transpulmonary mean and maximum gradients were recorded to assess the presence and severity of the abnormality [11]. The postnatal criterion for the presence of PS was an echocardiographic ventricular to pulmonary artery pressure gradient of >20 mmHg. In these patients, a different postnatal cardiological follow-up was scheduled according to the type and severity of the PS; they were monitored particularly closely during the first year of life due to the high risk of progression. After the first year of life, mild cases (peak gradient < 36 mmHg) were evaluated once or twice per year, while moderate cases (peak gradient: 36–64 mmHg; mean gradient: ≤ 50 mmHg) were assessed every 1–3 months. Patients with severe pulmonary stenosis (mean gradient: ≥ 50 mmHg) and pulmonary atresia underwent balloon valvuloplasty (BV) [12]. To ensure optimal follow-ups, in 2022, we contacted the mothers of all of the prenatal RVOTA cases and asked them to send us all pediatric cardiac evaluations, including their last clinical and echocardiographic report. Presence or absence of cardiac involvement and postnatal treatment (BV or medical therapy) was recorded under the supervision of our pediatric cardiologists. The CHD cases were divided into two categories: major if they required surgical or medical treatments or minor if they only required a clinical follow-up.

All women provided written informed consent for further clinical evaluation, and the study was approved by the ethics committee of Milan Area 1.

Survival analyses were performed by calculating the Kaplan–Meier failure functions and performing log-rank tests. Crude Cox models were used to calculate hazard ratios (HRs) and 95% confidence intervals (CIs). Analyses were performed with Stata 17 (StataCorp. 2021).

3. Results

During the study period, 28 prenatal cases of RVOTAs were observed in 335 MC/DA twin pregnancies complicated by TTTS and treated with FLS.

The prenatal data of these fetuses are shown in Table 1. As a type of prenatal RVOTA, PI was present in 16 cases (57.1%, 16/28), PS was present in 10 cases (35.7%, 10/28), and PA was present in 2 cases (7.1%, 2/28). The time at which RVOTAs appeared was related to TTTS and FLS; in three cases (10.7%), RVOTAs developed before TTTS; in 12 cases (42.8%), they developed at the same time as TTTS, and in 13 cases (46.4%), they developed after FLS. RVOTAs involved the RT in 24 cases (85.7%) and the DT in 4 cases (14.2%). All cases in the DTs developed after FLS; among them, there were three PIs and one PA, for an overall RVOTA incidence in DT of 1.5% (4 of the 258 DTs survived from FLS until birth).

Among the RTs, we observed 24 cases of RVOTAs. In three RTs, RVOTAs (two PSs and one PI) were observed before TTTS developed, and in 12 RTs, RVOTAs were observed at the time of the TTTS diagnosis: eight PIs, one PAs, and three PSs. Overall, in 4.5% (15/335) of the RTs, prenatal RVOTAs were present at the time of the TTTS diagnosis.

In nine RTs, RVOTAs were observed only after FLS, with an incidence in this subgroup of 3.5% (9 of the 259 RTs who did not exhibit an RVOTA before FLS and survived until birth). In this subgroup, we recorded four PIs and five PSs and, in four cases (three PIs and one PS), recurrent TTTS was also present.

In our population, the total incidence of prenatal RVOTAs was 8% (4.5% before FLS and 3.5% after FLS).

Out of the 28 prenatal RVOTA cases, we had two cases of fetal death. One death occurred after FLS, and there was one termination of the pregnancy due to the critical condition of both twins (an ex-recipient with hydrops and an ex-donor with sFGR and reversed flow in the umbilical arteries).

We were able to collect the postnatal cardiac long-term follow-up data of all 24 patients who survived the perinatal period, for a median of 9.5 years (range 3–13 years). In 17 patients (70.8%; 17/24), a CHD was present, with a major CHD in 10 cases (58.8%; 10/17); there were nine cases with severe PS requiring BV and one with biventricular non-compaction cardiomyopathy. In the other seven cases (41.1%; 7/17), the long-term FU showed a minor CHD in the form of dysplastic AV valves in five cases, left ventricular hypertrabeculation in one case, and mild pulmonary steno-insufficiency in another case.

The prognostic role of prenatal parameters in major CHDs is shown in Table 2. The risk of a major CHD was almost five times higher in the case of prenatal PS than in the case of PI (HR 4.71, 95° CI: 1.18–18.7). No major CHDs were observed if the DT presented prenatal RVOTAs (P: 0.07). The risk of major CHDs decreased with the gestational age at the time of TTTS (HR 0.69, 95° CI: 0.49–0.96). The prenatal normalization of the blood flow across the pulmonary valve was associated with a strongly reduced risk (HR 0.09, 95° CI: 0.02–0.42). No significant associations were observed between major CHDs at the long-term follow-up and the following prenatal parameters: the onset of an RVOTA (before or at the time of TTTS or after FLS), the TTTS stage, the presence of sFGR, C/T > 0.55, abnormal DV, severe tricuspid valve regurgitation, severe mitral valve regurgitation, gestational age, and weight at delivery.

Table 1. Prenatal outcomes of twins with RVOTAs in MC pregnancies with TTTS.

Case N	RVOTA Type	RVOTA GA (Weeks)	Twin with RVOTA	Onset RVOTA	Severe TV-R	Severe MV-R	DV a-Wave	C/T Ratio ≥ 0.55	TTTS Type	TTTS GA (Weeks)	Additional US Findings Detected during Pregnancy	Last US (Weeks)	Normalization FVW-PV	Pregnancy Outcome
1	PS	15.0	R	Before TTTS	yes	yes	no	yes	3	15.6	IUD D 24 h after FLS. Biventricular hypertrophy	21.6	no	Alive
2	PS	20.3	R	After FLS	yes	no	yes	yes	3	18.2	None	35.2	no	Alive
3	PS	19.6	R	Before TTTS	no	no	yes	no	1	21.4	None	26.0	no	Alive
4	PI	20.6	R	At the time of TTTS	yes	no	no	yes	4	20.6	PA at 23 weeks	24.1	yes	IUD
5	PA	21.0	R	At the time of TTTS	yes	no	no	yes	4	21.0	Dilated cardiomyopathy	NA	yes	Alive
6	PI	21.1	D	After FLS	yes	no	yes	no	2	20.0	Ex-donor tricuspid valve dysplasia 11 weeks after FLS	31.1	no	Alive
7	PS	23.3	R	After FLS	no	no	no	no	2	17.6	PS 5 weeks after FLS	23.3	yes	Alive
8	PI	21.3	R	At the time of TTTS	yes	yes	no	yes	4	21.3	None	27.0	no	Alive
9	PS	17.3	R	At the time of TTTS	yes	yes	no	yes	3	17.3	IUD donor 24 h after FLS.	30.3	yes	Alive
10	PI	23.5	D	After FLS	yes	no	no	yes	2	22.5	Ex-donor hydrops due to heart failure 6 days after FLS	33.1	no	Alive
11	PS	23.0	R	At the time of TTTS	yes	yes	no	yes	4	23.0	Myocardial hypertrophy	35.3	yes	Alive
12	PA	23.6	D	After FLS	no	no	yes	no	2	21.5	Ex-donor: hydrops due to heart failure 13 days after FLS; therapy with Digoxin from 26 weeks. Mirror syndrome	30.0	yes	Alive
13	PS	24.0	R	After FLS	yes	no	yes	yes	1	20.1	TTTS recurrence 3 weeks after FLS; amniodecompression	33.0	yes	Alive
14	PS	18.2	R	After FLS	yes	no	yes	yes	2	16.3	Ex-donor IUD 14 days after FLS	31.0	yes	Alive
15	PI	22.4	D	After FLS	no	no	yes	yes	2	19.6	Hydrops due to heart failure 12 days after FLS, spontaneously resolved	34.4	yes	Alive
16	PS	17.4	R	At the time of TTTS	yes	no	yes	yes	2	17.4	Ex-donor sFGR with AEDF	30.1	no	Alive
17	PS	26.2	R	After FLS	no	yes	yes	yes	3	21.0	IUD ex-donor sFGR with REDF. Myocardial hypertrophy	27.3	yes	Alive
18	PI	26.3	R	Before TTTS	no	no	no	yes	3	26.4	IUD ex-donor 14 days after FLS	34.1	yes	Alive
19	PI	20.0	R	After FLS	yes	yes	no	yes	2	19.0	TTTS persistence after FLS; 2° FLS after 7 days. Heart failure in ex-recipient with hydrops; ex-donor with sFGR	22.1	no	TOP (recurrence of TTTS with hydrops of the recipient and donor severe sFGR with REDF in UA)

Table 1. *Cont.*

Case N	RVOTA Type	RVOTA GA (Weeks)	Twin with RVOTA	Onset RVOTA	Severe TV-R	Severe MV-R	DV a-Wave	C/T Ratio ≥ 0.55	TTTS Type	TTTS GA (Weeks)	Additional US Findings Detected during Pregnancy	Last US (Weeks)	Normalization FVW-PV	Pregnancy Outcome
20	PI	24.4	R	At the time of TTTS	yes	no	no	yes	4	24.4	None	26.0	yes	Alive
21	PI	19.5	R	After FLS	yes	yes	no	yes	1	18.5	Ascites 24 h after FLS	34.5	yes	Alive
22	PI	17.4	R	At the time of TTTS	yes	no	no	yes	4	17.4	Myocardial hypertrophy	31.1	yes	Alive
23	PI	25.1	R	At the time of TTTS	yes	no	no	yes	4	25.1	MRI before FLS: IVH grade 1	30.0	yes	Alive
24	PI	22.2	R	At the time of TTTS	yes	no	no	yes	4	22.2	Myocardial hypertrophy	25.3	yes	Alive
25	PI	22.6	R	After FLS	yes	no	no	yes	2	22.0	Ex-donor with SNC damage. Selective TOP of ex-donor. Amniodecompression 2 days after FLS. Myocardial hypertrophy.	23.2	yes	Alive
26	PI	20.4	R	At the time of TTTS	yes	yes	no	yes	3	20.4	TAPS sequence 48 h after FSL. Myocardial hypertrophy	22.6	yes	Alive
27	PI	26.3	R	After FLS	no	no	no	no	1	20.1	TTTS recurrence 6 weeks after FLS; 3 amniodecompression; heart failure of ex-recipient treated with Digoxin from 26 weeks. Biventricular hypokinesia	28.5	no	Alive
28	PI	23.4	R	At the time of TTTS	yes	yes	no	yes	4	23.4	Ex-recipient heart failure from 26 weeks treated with Digoxin; ex-donor sFGR. Myocardial hypertrophy	33.0	yes	Alive

RVOTA: right ventricle outflow tract abnormality; MC: monochorionic pregnancy; US: ultrasound; GA: gestational age; TV-R: tricuspid valve regurgitation; MV-R: mitral valve regurgitation; C/T: cardiothoracic ratio; sFGR: selective fetal growth restriction; D: donor; R: receiving; pPROM: premature preterm rupture of membranes; IVH: intraventricular hemorrhage; TAPS: twin anemia polycytemia sequence; TTTS: twin–twin transfusion syndrome; PS: pulmonary stenosis; PI: pulmonary insufficiency; PSI: pulmonary steno-insufficiency; PA: pulmonary atresia; FLS: fetoscopic laser surgery; REDF in UA: reverse-end diastolic flow in umbilical artery; TOP: termination of pregnancy; IUD: intrauterine death. The postnatal data of the remaining 26 fetuses are shown in Table 3. In the postnatal population, we recorded two neonatal deaths: one due to prematurity and the other due to heart failure. Overall, among these 28 prenatal RVOTA cases, 24 survived the perinatal period and formed our study population (Figure 1).

Table 2. Prenatal variables in 24 children with RVOTAs.

Variable	N or Median (Range)	Cases with Major CHDs N (%) or Median (Range)	Hazard Ratio (95%CI)
Pulmonary insufficiency	12	3 (25)	1.00 (Reference)
Pulmonary stenosis	10	7 (70)	**4.71 (1.18–18.7)**
Pulmonary atresia	2	0	NC
Recipient twin with an RVOTA	20	10 (50)	1.00 (Reference)
Donor twin with an RVOTA	4	**0**	NC
RVOTA at the time of TTTS	10	5 (50)	1.00 (Reference)
RVOTA before TTTS	3	2 (67)	1.48 (0.28–7.69)
RVOTA developed after FLS	11	3 (27)	0.52 (0.12–2.19)
Gestational age at time of TTTS (weeks)	21.2 (16.4–23.6)	18.1 (15.9–23)	**0.69 (0.50–0.97)**
TTTS Stage 1–2	12	5 (42)	1.00 (Reference)
TTTS Stage 3–4	12	5 (42)	1.28 (0.37–4.43)
No selective fetal growth restriction	12	5 (42)	1.00 (Reference)
Selective fetal growth restriction	12	5 (42)	1.16 (0.33–4.04)
Cardio/thoracic ratio < 0.55	8	3 (37)	1.00 (Reference)
Cardio/thoracic ratio ≥ 0.55	16	7 (43)	1.49 (0.38–5.86)
No reversed a-wave in ductus venosus	8	3 (37)	1.00 (Reference)
Reversed a-wave in ductus venosus	16	7 (43)	1.25 (0.32–4.85)
No severe insufficiency in TV	7	2 (29)	1.00 (Reference)
Severe insufficiency in TV	17	8 (47)	1.62 (0.34–7.79)
No severe insufficiency in MV	13	4 (31)	1.00 (Reference)
Severe insufficiency in MV	11	6 (54)	2.23 (0.63–7.93)
No prenatal normalization of the flow across the pulmonary valve	8	8 (100)	1.00 (Reference)
Prenatal normalization of the flow across the pulmonary valve	16	2 (12)	**0.09 (0.02–0.42)**
Gestational age at delivery (weeks)	33 (24–38)	32 (24–35)	0.89 (0.73–1.08)
Weight at delivery (gr)	1.850 (500–2.960)	1.770 (500–2170)	0.99 (0.99–1.00)

N: numbers; RVOTAs: right ventricular outflow tract anomalies; FLS: fetoscopic laser surgery; TV: tricuspid valve; MV: mitral valve; CI: confidence interval; NC: not calculable.

Table 3. Postnatal outcomes of twins with RVOTAs in MC pregnancies with TTTS.

Case N *	GA at the Delivery	BW (gr)	Neonatal Type of RVOTA	Years of Follow-Up	CHD at Follow-Up
1	32	1850	PS	4	Major CHD: severe PS with BV
2	35	2960	PS	8	Major CHD: severe PS with BV and closure of the ductus arteriosus
3	33	1500	PA	7	Major CHD: PA with intact ventricular septum, BV, iatrogenic hemopericardium during the procedure. Persistence of mild PI; possibility of re-intervention
5	36	1960	0	8	Minor CHD: left ventricular hypertrabeculation
6	34	1490	0	9	Minor CHD: tricuspid dysplasia with mild to moderate TV-R
7	34	2020	PS	5	Major CHD: severe PS with BV. Residual PSI at FU

Table 3. Cont.

Case N *	GA at the Delivery	BW (gr)	Neonatal Type of RVOTA	Years of Follow-Up	CHD at Follow-Up
8	34	1690	0	6	None
9	37	2680	PS	11	Major CHD: severe PS with BV
10	33	1793	0	10	None
11	35	2170	PS	11	Major CHD: severe PS with BV, atrial septal defect closure. Planned replacement of the PV due to the residual severe PI
12	30	1200	0	11	Minor CHD: neonatal correction of patent ductus arteriosus; dysplastic atrioventricular valves; persistence of moderate TV-R and MV-R at the follow-up, without the need for surgical correction
13	33	2150	0	10	Minor CHD: tricuspid dysplasia with moderate TV-R
14	38	2700	PS	10	Minor CHD: mild PSI, gradient 34 mmHg. Stationary follow-up
15	35	2340	0	12	None
16	31	1630	PS	10	Major CHD: severe PS with BV; hypertrophic cardiomyopathy
17	28	1430	NA	11	None
18	35	2285	0	3	None
20	26	1100	NA	NA	NND due to severe prematurity at birth, severe RDS and heart failure with biventricular dilatation and systolic dysfunction
21	34	2660	0	10	None
22	32	1700	PS	5	Major CHD: severe PS with BV
23	33	1800	0	6	None
24	26	1000	PI	4	Minor CHD: mitral dysplasia with MV-R: no intervention
25	24	500	PS	13	Major CHD: severe PS with BV
26	28	690	0	11	Major CHD: cardiomyopathy at 7 years, non-compact myocardium
27	28	990	NA	NA	NND due to heart failure
28	33	1900	0	9	Minor CHD: tricuspid and mitral dysplasia with moderate TV-R and mild MV-R at birth

RVOTA: right ventricle outflow tract abnormality; MC: monochorionic pregnancy; TTTS: twin–twin transfusion syndrome; BW: birth weight; CHD: congenital heart defect; PS: pulmonary stenosis; PI: pulmonary insufficiency; PSI: pulmonary steno-insufficiency; PA: pulmonary atresia; TV-R: tricuspid valve regurgitation; MV-R: mitral valve regurgitation; BV: pulmonary balloon valvuloplasty; ND: neonatal death; * Cases 4 and 19 are not shown as intrauterine deaths.

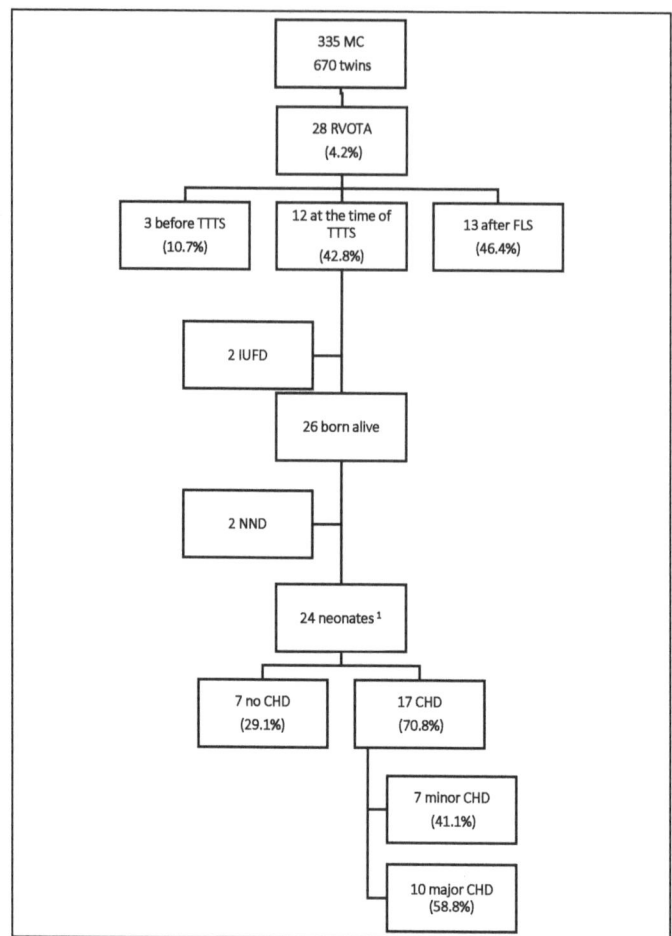

Figure 1. Study population. MC: monochorionic pregnancy; RVOTA: right ventricle outflow tract abnormality; TTTS: twin–twin transfusion syndrome; IUFD: intrauterine fetal demise; NND: neonatal death; CHD: congenital heart defects. [1] Study population.

4. Discussion

To the best of our knowledge, this is the first study to analyze long-term postnatal cardiological evaluations of cases with prenatal RVOTAs in a homogeneous group of MC/DA twin pregnancies complicated by TTTS and treated with FLS. Furthermore, in our series, we checked for RVOTAs in the DT as well, finding an RVOTA incidence in DTs of 1.5%. The RVOTA incidence in DTs has never been investigated before in studies of TTTS. Alterations in the cardiac function of DTs after laser coagulation are common and were previously described by Van Mieghem et al. [13]. They arise due to a relative overload occurring in the DT after FLS in the form of the vasoactive peptides and blood volume previously given to the RT, interrupting the passage through the placental anastomoses, and they must be managed by the DT themselves. However, in four of our DTs, these alterations had a significant impact on cardiac function, causing hydrops in the prenatal period and minor CHDs, such as AV dysplasia, at the long-term follow-up. The incidence of RVOTAs in the RTs in our series (8%) was similar to the value of 7.5% reported by Chang et al. [14], even though PI, as a type of RVOTA, was not considered in that study.

The onset of RVOTAs before TTTS has not previously been described. However, we recently published cases of RVOTAs in MC pregnancies without TTTS, especially in cases of sFGR with amniotic fluid discrepancies [15,16]. A possible pathophysiologic explanation for these findings is that the uneven and mismatched transfer of blood volume and vasoactive peptides is enough to cause cardiac adaptation without TTTS typically being found; this may develop afterwards, as in the three cases described in the present study.

The onset of RVOTAs, especially PS, several weeks after FLS without signs of recurrence was already described in a prospective TTTS series by Eschbach et al., where it was correlated with mild postnatal PS. In our series, in two cases of PS that developed two and five weeks after FLS, severe postnatal PS was observed, requiring BV. Those cases may demonstrate that, even in the second trimester, the processes of valve maturation are still taking place and valvular damage can appear weeks after the adverse event.

Regarding the types of RVOTAs, we found a strong correlation between prenatal PS and the risk of major CHDs, with 70% of prenatal PS cases requiring BV for severe postnatal PS. This finding could be explained by prenatal PS being the expression of an organic valve pathology rather than a functional alteration. Therefore, it is not cured by the improvement of the right ventricular systolic and diastolic function that is visible after the FLS. Furthermore, our finding of a strong risk reduction for major CHDs with the prenatal normalization of blood flow across the pulmonary valve (PV) could be the expression of a prenatal RVOTA as a transient functional abnormality rather than an organic disease. We also found that all patients with a postnatal dysplastic AV valve exhibited a normalization of blood across the PV before birth and never developed PS. We could not find an explanation for this finding. In addition, we found an association between the gestational age at the time of TTTS and a risk of major CHDs, with a risk reduction of 31% for each additional gestational week. This finding is in agreement with those of other studies [14,17] and confirms how alterations in cardiac hemodynamics in the early stages of embryogenesis lead to irreversible organic changes. However, treatment with FLS can ensure the regression of functional RVOTAs before they become organic. This is thoroughly demonstrated by the finding in our recent publication that RVOTA incidence at birth in RTs was halved in the FLS group compared with a TTTS group that was treated before 2004 with amnioreduction (4.5% vs. 9.4%, respectively) [18].

Biventricular non-compaction cardiomyopathy is a rare cardiac abnormality that is characterized by a two-layered myocardium, numerous prominent trabeculations, and deep intertrabecular recesses communicating with the ventricular cavity [19]. To the best of our knowledge, this is the first ventricular non-compaction cardiomyopathy (VNC) to be reported in an MC pregnancy.

VNC is a genetic cardiomyopathy with a multifactorial origin involving mutations of the genes that encode the sarcomeric, cytoskeletal, and nuclear membrane proteins [20]. In our case series, this abnormality was present as a discordant abnormality in an MC recipient twin who exhibited severe biventricular dysfunction as a fetus. This finding points to an underlying epigenetic origin that could act by modifying one of the multiple pathways involved in normal myocardial compaction [21].

Strengths and limitations: This study has many strengths. One major strength is the homogeneity of the population of MC/DA twin pregnancies complicated by TTTS and treated with FLS. Another strength is that all prenatal evaluations were conducted in a third-level center with extensive experience with MC twins. Moreover, a complete postnatal follow-up was conducted in all cases.

The main limitations of this study are its retrospective nature and the lack of centralization or a shared protocol in the postnatal follow-up examinations, as many of these patients were not born in our hospital.

A multicenter prospective study on prenatal RVOTAs in MC/DA twin pregnancies complicated by TTTS and treated with FLS is needed to better understand their incidence, prenatal evolution, and long-term postnatal cardiological outcomes.

5. Conclusions

Our study demonstrates that following fetoscopic laser surgery, the majority of babies born of monochorionic pregnancies complicated by TTTS with a prenatal right ventricular outflow tract anomaly develop a congenital heart disease according to long-term follow-up observations. TTTS cases complicated by right ventricular outflow tract anomalies should be referred to a tertiary care hospital where specialized prenatal and postnatal cardiac evaluations, treatments, and long-term follow-ups are available.

Author Contributions: S.F.: conceptualization and writing—original draft preparation; C.C. (Chiara Coco) and M.M.: data curation; D.C. (Daniela Casati), A.L., C.C. (Carla Corti), S.M. and I.C.: writing—review and editing; D.C. (Dario Consonni): formal analysis; M.L. writing—review and editing and supervision. All authors have read and agreed to the published version of the manuscript.

Funding: This research received no external funding.

Institutional Review Board Statement: This study was approved by the ethics committee of Milan Area 1 (protocol number: N.0000968/2023) in accordance with the Declaration of Helsinki.

Informed Consent Statement: Not applicable.

Data Availability Statement: The data that support the findings of this study are available on request from the corresponding author.

Acknowledgments: We thank Cieli Azzurri Foundation for the support given to our Fethal Therapy Unit.

Conflicts of Interest: The authors declare no conflict of interest.

References

1. Lougheed, J.; Sinclair, B.G.; Fung, K.F.K.; Bigras, J.-L.; Ryan, G.; Smallhorn, J.F.; Hornberger, L.K. Acquired right ventricular outflow tract obstruction in the recipient twin in twin-twin transfusion syndrome. *J. Am. Coll. Cardiol.* **2001**, *38*, 1533–1538. [CrossRef]
2. Karatza, A.A.; Wolfenden, J.L.; Taylor, M.J.; Wee, L.; Fisk, N.M.; Gardiner, H.M. Influence of twin-twin transfusion syndrome on fetal cardiovascular structure and function: Prospective case-control study of 136 monochorionic twin pregnancies. *Heart* **2002**, *88*, 271–277. [CrossRef]
3. Fisk, N.M.; Duncombe, G.J.; Sullivan, M.H.F. The basic and clinical science of twin–twin transfusion syndrome. *Placenta* **2009**, *30*, 379–390. [CrossRef]
4. Bajoria, R.; Ward, S.; Sooranna, S.R. Atrial natriuretic peptide mediated polyuria: Pathogenesis of polyhydramnios in the recipient twin of twin-twin transfusion syndrome. *Placenta* **2001**, *22*, 716–724. [CrossRef]
5. Senat, M.V.; Deprest, J.; Boulvain, M.; Paupe, A.; Winer, N.; Ville, Y. Endoscopic laser surgery versus serial amnioreduction for severe twin-to-twin transfusion syndrome. *N. Engl. J. Med.* **2004**, *351*, 136–144. [CrossRef]
6. Moon-Grady, A.J.; Rand, L.; Lemley, B.; Gosnell, K.; Hornberger, L.K.; Lee, H. Effect of selective fetoscopic laser photocoagulation therapy for twin-twin transfusion syndrome on pulmonary valve pathology in recipient twins. *Ultrasound Obstet. Gynecol.* **2011**, *37*, 27–33. [CrossRef]
7. Eschbach, S.J.; Ten Harkel, A.D.J.; Middeldorp, J.M.; Klumper, F.J.C.M.; Oepkes, D.; Lopriore, E.; Haak, M.C. Acquired Right Ventricular Outflow Tract Obstruction in twin-to-twin transfusion syndrome; a prospective longitudinal study. *Prenat. Diagn.* **2018**, *38*, 1013–1019. [CrossRef]
8. Quintero, R.A.; Morales, W.J.; Alien, M.H.; Bomik, P.W.; Johnson, P.K.; Kruger, M. Staging of twin-twin transfusion syndrome. *J. Perinatol.* **1999**, *19*, 550–555. [CrossRef]
9. Michelfelder, E.; Tan, X.; Cnota, J.; Divanovic, A.; Statile, C.; Lim, F.-Y.; Crombleholme, T. Prevalence, Spectrum, and Outcome of Right Ventricular Outflow Tract Abnormalities in Twin-twin Transfusion Syndrome: A Large, Single-center Experience. *Congenit. Heart Dis.* **2015**, *10*, 209–218. [CrossRef]
10. Slaghekke, F.; Lopriore, E.; Lewi, L.; Middeldorp, J.M.; van Zwet, E.W.; Weingertner, A.S.; Klumper, F.J.; DeKoninck, P.; Devlieger, R.; Kilby, M.D.; et al. Fetoscopic laser coagulation of the vascular equator versus selective coagulation for twin-to-twin transfusion syndrome: An open-label randomised controlled trial. *Lancet* **2014**, *383*, 2144–2151. [CrossRef]
11. Cantinotti, M.; Giordano, R.; Emdin, M.; Assanta, N.; Crocetti, M.; Marotta, M.; Iervasi, G.; Lopez, L.; Kutty, S. Echocardiographic assessment of pediatric semilunar valve disease. *Echocardiography* **2017**, *34*, 1360–1370. [CrossRef]
12. Baumgartner, H.; Hung, J.; Bermejo, J.; Chambers, J.B.; Evangelista, A.; Griffin, B.P.; Iung, B.; Otto, C.; Pellikka, P.A.; Quiñones, M. Echocardiographic assessment of valve stenosis: EAE/ASE recommendations for clinical practice. *Eur. J. Echocardiogr.* **2009**, *10*, 1–25. [CrossRef]

13. Van Mieghem, T.; Klaritsch, P.; Doné, E.; Gucciardo, L.; Lewi, P.; Verhaeghe, J.; Lewi, L.; Deprest, J. Assessment of fetal cardiac function before and after therapy for twin-to-twin transfusion syndrome. *Am. J. Obstet. Gynecol.* **2009**, *200*, 400.e1–400.e7. [CrossRef]
14. Chang, Y.L.; Chao, A.S.; Chang, S.D.; Cheng, P.J.; Li, W.F.; Hsu, C.C. Incidence, prognosis, and perinatal outcomes of and risk factors for severe twin-twin transfusion syndrome with right ventricular outflow tract obstruction in the recipient twin after fetoscopic laser photocoagulation. *BMC Pregnancy Childbirth* **2022**, *22*, 326. [CrossRef]
15. Faiola, S.; Casati, D.; Laoreti, A.; Amendolara, M.; Consonni, D.; Corti, C.; Mannarino, S.; Lanna, M.; Rustico, M.; Cetin, I. Right ventricular outflow tract abnormalities in monochorionic twin pregnancies without twin-to-twin transfusion syndrome: Prenatal course and postnatal long-term outcomes. *Prenat. Diagn.* **2021**, *41*, 1510–1517. [CrossRef]
16. Faiola, S.; Casati, D.; Nelva Stellio, L.; Laoreti, A.; Corti, C.; Mannarino, S.; Lanna, M.; Cetin, I. Congenital heart defects in monochorionic twin pregnancy complicated by selective fetal growth restriction. *Ultrasound Obstet. Gynecol.* **2023**, *61*, 504–510. [CrossRef]
17. Eschbach, S.J.; Boons, L.S.T.M.; Van Zwet, E.; Middeldorp, J.M.; Klumper, F.J.C.M.; Lopriore, E.; Teunissen, A.K.K.; Rijlaarsdam, M.E.; Oepkes, D.; Ten Harkel, A.D.J.; et al. Right ventricular outflow tract obstruction in complicated monochorionic twin pregnancy. *Ultrasound Obstet. Gynecol.* **2017**, *49*, 737–743. [CrossRef]
18. Faiola, S.; Casati, D.; Laoreti, A.; Corti, C.; Bianchi, S.; Nelva Stellio, L.; Cetin, I.; Lanna, M. Birth prevalence of right ventricular outflow tract abnormalities in the recipient twin of monochorionic twin pregnancies complicated by twin-to-twin transfusion syndrome: Amnioreduction versus fetoscopic laser coagulation treatment. *Ital. J. Gynæcology Obstet.* **2023**, *35*, 190–195. [CrossRef]
19. Garcia-Pavia, P.; de la Pompa, J.L. Left ventricular noncompaction: A genetic cardiomyopathy looking for diagnostic criteria. *J. Am. Coll. Cardiol.* **2014**, *64*, 1981–1983. [CrossRef]
20. Jenni, R.; Rojas, J.; Oechslin, E. Isolated noncompaction of the myocardium. *N. Engl. J. Med.* **1999**, *340*, 966–967. [CrossRef]
21. Rojanasopondist, P.; Nesheiwat, L.; Piombo, S.; Porter GAJr Ren, M.; Phoon, C.K.L. Genetic Basis of Left Ventricular Noncompaction. *Circ. Genom. Precis. Med.* **2022**, *15*, 190–200. [CrossRef] [PubMed]

Disclaimer/Publisher's Note: The statements, opinions and data contained in all publications are solely those of the individual author(s) and contributor(s) and not of MDPI and/or the editor(s). MDPI and/or the editor(s) disclaim responsibility for any injury to people or property resulting from any ideas, methods, instructions or products referred to in the content.

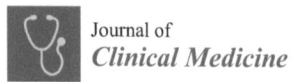

Article

Oral Glucose Tolerance Test Performed after 28 Gestational Weeks and Risk for Future Diabetes—A 5-Year Cohort Study

Esther Maor-Sagie [1,2], Mordechai Hallak [1,2], Yoel Toledano [2] and Rinat Gabbay-Benziv [1,3,*]

1. Department of Obstetrics and Gynecology, Hillel Yaffe Medical Center, Hadera 3820302, Israel; estimaorsagie@gmail.com (E.M.-S.); mottih@hymc.gov.il (M.H.)
2. Meuhedet HMO, Rehovot 7610001, Israel; yoel.t@meuhedet.co.il
3. The Ruth and Bruce Rappaport Faculty of Medicine, Technion—Israel Institute of Technology, Haifa 3200003, Israel
* Correspondence: gabbayrinat@gmail.com; Tel.: +972-4-6304313; Fax: +972-4-6314916

Abstract: Gestational diabetes mellitus (GDM) is diagnosed by an oral glucose tolerance test (oGTT), preferably performed at 24 + 0–28 + 6 gestational weeks, and is considered a risk factor for type 2 diabetes (T2DM). In this study, we aimed to evaluate the risk of T2DM associated with abnormal oGTT performed after 28 weeks. We conducted a retrospective cohort study that included parturients with available glucose levels during pregnancy and up to 5 years of follow-up after pregnancy. Data were extracted from the computerized laboratory system of Meuhedet HMO and cross-tabulated with the Israeli National Registry of Diabetes (INRD). The women were stratified into two groups: late oGTT (performed after 28 + 6 weeks) and on-time oGTT (performed at 24 + 0–28 + 6 weeks). The incidence of T2DM was evaluated and compared using univariate analysis followed by survival analysis adjusted to confounders. Overall, 78,326 parturients entered the analysis. Of them, 6195 (7.9%) performed on-time oGTT and 5288 (6.8%) performed late oGTT. The rest—66,846 (85.3%)—had normal glucose tolerance. Women who performed late oGTT had lower rates of GDM and T2DM. However, once GDM was diagnosed, regardless of oGTT timing, the risk of T2DM was increased (2.93 (1.69–5.1) vs. 3.64 (2.44–5.44), aHR (95% CI), late vs. on-time oGTT, $p < 0.001$ for both). Unlike in oGTT performed on time, one single abnormal value in late oGTT was not associated with an increased risk for T2DM.

Keywords: diabetes mellitus; gestational diabetes; prediction; pregnancy; oral glucose tolerance test

1. Introduction

Gestational diabetes (GDM) is one of the most common complications during pregnancy, with short- and long-term implications for the mother, fetus, and offspring [1]. However, despite large-scale studies, major controversies remain about its diagnosis, treatment, and future implications.

The American College of Obstetrics and Gynecology (ACOG) recommends screening all pregnant women for GDM, preferably at 24 + 0 to 28 + 6 gestational weeks [1,2]. In the United States, the preferred method for screening is the two-steps approach, which uses the glucose challenging test (GCT) followed by a diagnostic 3 h 100 g oral glucose tolerance test (oGTT) for the screen-positive women [1]. The timing of oGTT between 24 and 28 weeks of pregnancy was chosen to align with the physiological changes of pregnancy, maximizing the number of chances to detect GDM and allow for timely intervention and management.

Notably, over the last years, several publications investigated the importance of late GDM, diagnosed in the third trimester after 28 gestational weeks. In a Dutch cohort study, the authors reported GDM diagnoses in 23.5% of parturients who initially tested negative at 24–28 gestational weeks [3]. Similarly, other studies demonstrated around 25% late GDM

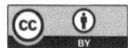

diagnoses in women who underwent late oGTT because of suspected large-for-gestational-age fetuses or polyhydramnios [4–6], with even higher rates of GDM for women with obesity [5,6].

Several studies evaluated the clinical implications of late GDM [5,7–10], emphasizing short-term maternal and neonatal outcomes with conflicting results, especially regarding the delivery of large-for-gestational-age babies and mode of delivery. To note, there was great variance among studies regarding the population, the methodology, the definition of late GDM, the GDM screening approach, and the evaluated outcomes; therefore, conclusions were hard to draw.

Regardless of that, GDM is a well-established risk factor for type 2 diabetes mellitus (T2DM). It is estimated that up to 70% of women with GDM will develop T2DM 22–28 years after pregnancy [1]. To the best of our knowledge, none of the studies that investigated late oGTT evaluated the risk of future T2DM based on the timing of GDM diagnosis during pregnancy. Thus, in this study, we aimed to investigate the risk of T2DM in women who performed abnormal late oGTT during pregnancy in a large cohort of women with 5 years of follow-up after pregnancy.

2. Materials and Methods

A retrospective cohort study aimed to evaluate the prediction performance of late 100 g oGTT during pregnancy for T2DM in a 5-year follow-up. The study included all women with documented singleton pregnancies (by pregnancy registry) without diabetes diagnosis, with last menstrual period (LMP) between 1 January 2017 and 31 December 2020. Pregnancies complicated by early GDM, defined as fasting plasma glucose at early pregnancy at or above 92 mg/dL, or women who performed oGTT at less than 24 gestational weeks were excluded. For women with more than one pregnancy during the study period, only the first pregnancy was included to ensure the longest available follow-up time. On-time oGTT was defined as oGTT performed between 24 + 0 and 28 + 6 weeks. Late oGTT was defined as oGTT performed after 28 gestational weeks. Risk for T2DM was compared between women with abnormal oGTT results—either single abnormal value (SAV) or GDM and, according to oGTT timing, on-time oGTT vs. late oGTT. Follow-up time was defined as the date of diabetes diagnosis, the date of data extraction (13 November 2022), or death—whichever came first. The study was approved by the local Institutional Review Board committee (10-18-08-21). Due to the retrospective nature of the study, informed consent was waived.

For this study, data were extracted from a dataset encompassing more than 5 years of laboratory data collected by Meuhedet HMO (health maintenance organization), cross-tabulated with a pregnancy registry, and integrated with the Israeli National Diabetes Registry (INDR). Meuhedet is one of the four Israel health insurance and medical services organizations to which Israeli residents must belong under Israel's universal healthcare framework. Maternal data included maternal age, body mass index (BMI), and diagnosis of hypertension. Delivery data included gestational age at delivery and neonatal gender. All clinical data were retrieved from the parturient electronic medical records at the time of pregnancy. Laboratory data included first-trimester fasting glucose levels, 50 g glucose challenge test (GCT), and 100 g oGTT values. T2DM diagnosis was retrieved from the INDR. As previously described [11], since 2012, all health medical organizations in Israel are required by law to report cases of diabetes to the INDR. Data in this registry were linked to the pregnancy registry and the laboratory data of Meuhedet. Diabetes diagnosis is updated daily to the registry and defined as meeting one or more of the following criteria: (1) glycated hemoglobin greater than or equal to 6.5% (47.5 mmol/mol), (2) serum glucose concentrations greater than or equal to 200 mg/dL (11.1 mmol/L) in 2 tests performed at an interval of at least 1 month, and (3) 3 or more purchases of glucose-lowering medications. The registry has a sensitivity of 95% and the positive predictive value is 93%.

By convention, and according to Israeli guidelines, all parturients are recommended to undergo fasting plasma glucose level in the first trimester to exclude overt diabetes (>125 mg/dL). Screening for GDM is recommended for all women at 24–28 gestational weeks by the two-steps approach. Late oGTT, after 28 weeks, is usually performed for latecomers or as part of large-for-gestational-age or polyhydramnios evaluation. Threshold values for GDM are consistent throughout pregnancy and defined according to the Carpenter and Coustan values [2], which require a GDM diagnosis to include at least two out of four abnormal values.

Statistical Analysis

At first, we utilized univariate analysis to evaluate differences between women who performed on-time oGTT, late oGTT, or had normal glucose tolerance. Also, we evaluated differences according to oGTT results: between women with SAV or GDM at on-time oGTT and women with SAV or GDM at late oGTT. We determined all women in the cohort without SAV or GDM diagnosis (including women with normal GCT or women with four normal values on oGTT) as women with normal glucose tolerance (control group). Maternal age and BMI were evaluated both as continuous variables and as categorical variables (with a cutoff of 35 and 40 years for age and 30 kg/m^2 for BMI). Glucose levels, gestational age at delivery, and time to follow-up were treated as continuous variables, while hypertension, GDM, neonatal gender, and T2DM were treated as categorical variables. Categorical variables were compared using χ^2 tests, and the Kruskal–Wallis test was used to test differences for continuous variables. All the tests were 2-tailed and $p < 0.05$ was considered statistically significant. Next, to account for different follow-up times, we computed Kaplan–Meier hazard curves, applied Cox regression analysis, and determined the Hazard ratio (HR) with a 95% confidence interval (CI) for the cumulative incidence of T2DM, with maternal age, BMI, and maternal hypertension as covariates, using the control group as the reference group.

Lastly, due to the large impact of obesity on future T2DM, the risk for T2DM according to oGTT results was stratified according to maternal pre-pregnancy BMI and divided into women with obesity (BMI $\geq$ 30 kg/m^2) and without obesity (BMI < 30 kg/m^2).

3. Results

3.1. Study Population

Our dataset included 88,611 women with LMP during the study period and T2DM data. After excluding all multiple pregnancies (n = 1289), women with first-trimester fasting plasma glucose levels $\geq$ 92 mg/dL (n = 8220), and women with oGTT performed prior to 24 weeks gestation (n = 776), we were left with 78,326 women who were eligible for analysis. Of them, 6195 (7.9%) women performed oGTT at 24 + 0–28 + 6 gestational weeks (on-time oGTT) and 5288 (6.8%) performed oGTT after 28 gestational weeks (late oGTT). Demographics, baseline characteristics, glucose values, and rates of T2DM according to the timing of oGTT are presented in Table 1 and Figure 1. Overall, women who performed late oGTT had lower rates of abnormal oGTT results and lower rates of T2DM during the study period. Maternal variables and risk for T2DM are further presented, stratified by oGTT results when performed on time and late in gestation (Table 2). Regardless of oGTT timing, women with GDM were older and had higher obesity levels compared to women with normal glucose tolerance. Moreover, their glucose values throughout pregnancy were higher compared to women with SAV oGTT or women with normal glucose tolerance (Table 2).

Table 1. Baseline demographic and future type 2 diabetes stratified by timing of oGTT.

	No oGTT N = 66,843	on-Time oGTT N = 6195	Late oGTT N = 5288	p Value
Maternal age, years	28.2 (24.0–33.2)	31.9 (27.4–36.1)	30.4 (25.9–35.4)	<0.001
Age ≥ 35 years	12,328 (18.4)	1943 (31.4)	1453 (27.5)	<0.001
Age ≥ 40 years	3372 (5.0)	568 (9.2)	405 (7.7)	<0.001
BMI kg/m^2	24.2 (21.5–27.8)	26.3 (23.1–30.6)	26.3 (23.1–30.6)	<0.001
BMI ≥ 30	9181 (16.8)	1667 (29.8)	1407 (29.7)	<0.001
Hypertension	478 (0.7)	101 (1.6)	54 (1)	<0.001
First-trimester fasting glucose, mg/dL	8 (76–85)	82 (78–86)	81 (76–85)	<0.001
GCT, mg/dL	97 (82–117)	151 (143–162)	133 (102–150)	<0.001
Fasting oGTT, mg/dL	--	77 (72–83)	76 (71–82)	<0.001
1 h oGTT, mg/dL	--	144 (119–170)	144 (122–166)	0.553
2 h oGTT, mg/dL	--	115 (96–138)	116 (98–137)	0.605
3 h oGTT, mg/dL	--	85 (65–104)	87 (67–105)	0.007
oGTT week	--	26.6 (25.6–27.7)	32.7 (30.4–35.6)	<0.001
oGTT results				
SAV oGTT	--	848 (13.7)	645 (12.2)	
GDM	--	654 (10.6)	446 (8.4)	<0.001
Gestational age at delivery, weeks	39.7 (38.3–40.7)	39.6 (38.6–40.6)	39.9 (38.9–40.7)	<0.001
Baby sex, male [@]	26,545 (50.7)	3147 (53.7)	2736 (54.5)	<0.001
Follow-up time	4.4 (3.4–5.2)	4.3 (3.3–5.0)	4.4 (3.4–5.1)	<0.001
Type 2 DM, cumulative				
1-Year T2DM	10 (0)	1 (0)	3 (0.1)	0.091
2-Year T2DM	77 (0.1)	12 (0.2)	9 (0.2)	0.156
3-Year T2DM	186 (0.3)	42 (0.7)	23 (0.4)	<0.001
4-Year T2DM	304 (0.5)	75 (1.2)	36 (0.7)	<0.001
5-Year T2DM	456 (0.7)	110 (1.8)	53 (1)	<0.001

Data are presented as median (IQR) for continuous variables and n (%) for categorical values. Significant differences are presented in bold ($p < 0.05$). SAV—defined as one abnormal value on oGTT (Carpenter and Coustan threshold values)[2]; GDM—defined as two abnormal values on oGTT (Carpenter and Coustan thresholds values)[2]; [@] gender results available for 63,261 deliveries. BMI—body mass index; oGTT—100 g oral glucose tolerance test; SAV—single abnormal value; GDM—gestational diabetes; T2DM—type 2 diabetes mellitus; GCT—glucose challenge test.

3.2. Incidence of Type 2 Diabetes

In the univariate analysis, for women who performed late oGTT, GDM diagnosis was associated with higher rates of T2DM compared to SAV oGTT or normal glucose tolerance. Nevertheless, unlike women with on-time oGTT, SAV results on late oGTT were not associated with an increased risk for T2DM compared to women with normal glucose tolerance.

Using the Cox-regression survival analysis, and adjusted to maternal age, BMI, and hypertension, abnormal oGTT results, either SAV or GDM, that were diagnosed from on-time oGTT (24–28 gestational weeks) indicated a higher risk for T2DM compared to SAV or GDM that was diagnosed after 28 gestational weeks (Table 3, Figure 2).

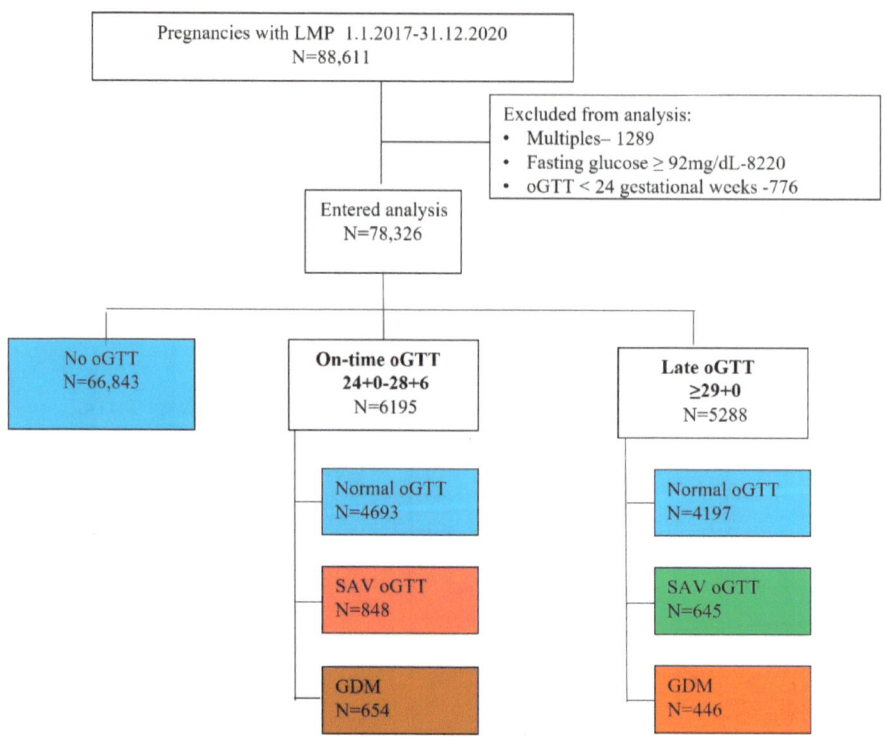

Figure 1. Study cohort. LMP—last menstrual period; oGTT—oral glucose tolerance test; GDM—gestational diabetes; SAV—single abnormal value.

Table 2. Baseline demographic and future type 2 diabetes stratified by oGTT results.

	Normal Glucose Tolerance N = 75,733	SAV Late oGTT N = 645	SAV On-Time oGTT N = 848	GDM Late oGTT N = 446	GDM On-Time oGTT N = 654	p Value
Maternal age, years	28.6 [a,b,c,d] (24.1–33.5)	31.8 [e,g] (27.1–36.1)	32.6 (28.4–37.1)	31.7 (27–37.3)	33.2 (28.7–37.1)	<0.001
Age ≥ 35 years	14,772 [a,b,c,d] (19.5)	211 [g] (32.7)	311 (36.7)	169 (37.9)	261 (39.9)	<0.001
Age ≥ 40 years	4061 (5.4) [a,b,c,d]	57 (8.8) [f]	96 (11.3)	60 (13.5)	71 (10.9)	<0.001
BMI kg/m²	24.4 [a,b,c,d] (21.7–28.1)	27.4 (23.4–32.2)	27.4 (23.8–32)	27.1 (23.8–31.4)	27.7 (32–24)	<0.001
BMI ≥ 30	11,363 [a,b,c,d] (18.1)	21 8(38)	292 (37.5)	143 (35.3)	239 (38.8)	<0.001
Hypertension	588 (0.8) [b,d]	3(0.5) [e,g]	17(2)	7(1.6)	18(2.8)	<0.001
First-trimester fasting glucose, mg/dL	80 (46–80) [a,b,c,d]	82 (78–86) [g]	83 (79–87) [i]	82 (78–86) [j]	84 (80–88)	<0.001
GCT, mg/dL	99 [a,b,c,d] (83–117)	145 [e,f,g] (129–157)	155 [h,i] (146–166)	151 [j] (136–169)	162 (150–175)	<0.001
Fasting oGTT, mg/dL	76 [a,b,c,d] (71–81)	80 [e,f,g] (74–86.5)	81 [h,i] (75–87)	83 (76–92)	83 (76–93)	<0.001
1 h oGTT, mg/dL	135 [a,b,c,d] (114–154)	181 [f,g] (161–190)	180 [h,i] (165–191)	195 (185–210)	195 (185–211)	<0.001

Table 2. Cont.

	Normal Glucose Tolerance N = 75,733	SAV Late oGTT N = 645	SAV On-Time oGTT N = 848	GDM Late oGTT N = 446	GDM On-Time oGTT N = 654	p Value
2 h oGTT, mg/dL	108 [a,b,c,d] (93–125)	144 [f,g] (125–159)	143 [h,i] (122.3–157)	171 (159.8–188)	171 (160–186)	<0.001
3 h oGTT, mg/dL	82 [a,b,c,d] (64–99)	98 [e,f,g] (72–118.5)	98 [h,i] (72–116)	113 (88.8–140)	117 (86.8–143)	<0.001
oGTT week	28.6 [a,b,c,d] (26.4–32.6)	32.1 [e,g] (30.3–34.7)	26.7 [h] (25.7–27.7)	32.1 [j] (30.1–34.5)	26.7 (25.6–27.7)	<0.001
Gestational age at delivery, weeks	39.7 [a,b,c,d] (38.4–40.7)	39.7 (38.7–40.4)	39.3 (38.4–40.3)	39.3 (38.3–40.1)	39 (38.1–39.9)	<0.001
Baby sex, male [@]	31,147(51.2)	336(55.1)	420(52.4)	225(53.1)	300(49)	0.212
Follow-up time	4.4 (3.4–5.2) [b,c,d]	4.3 (3.2–5.1) [f,g]	4.2 (3.2–5)	4.1 (2.9–5)	4 (3–4.9)	<0.001
Type 2 DM, cumulative						
1- Year T2DM	11 (0) [c]	0 (0) [f]	1 (0.1) [h]	2 (0.4) [j]	0 (0)	<0.001
2- Year T2DM	84 (0.1) [c,d]	2 (0.3) [f]	3 (0.4) [h]	5 (1.1)	4 (0.6)	<0.001
3- Year T2DM	218 (0.3) [b,c,d]	3 (0.5) [f,g]	9 (1.1) [h]	10 (2.2)	11 (1.7)	<0.001
4- Year T2DM	361 (0.5) [b,c,d]	5(0.8) [f,g]	14 (1.7) [h,i]	14 (3.1)	21 (3.2)	<0.001
5- Year T2DM	542 (0.7) [b,c,d]	10(1.6) [f,g]	22 (2.6) [i]	16 (3.6)	29 (4.4)	<0.001

Data are presented as median (IQR) for continuous variables and n (%) for categorical values. Significant differences are presented for comparison between all groups; column "p-value", significant in bold ($p < 0.05$) and for comparison between every 2 groups: a—between normal glucose tolerance and SAV on late oGTT; b—between normal glucose tolerance and SAV on on-time oGTT; c—between normal glucose tolerance and GDM on late oGTT; d—between normal glucose tolerance and GDM on on-time oGTT; e—between SAV on late oGTT and SAV on on-time oGTT; f—between SAV on late oGTT and GDM on late oGTT; g—between SAV on late oGTT and GDM on on-time oGTT; h—between SAV on on-time oGTT and GDM on late oGTT; i—between SAV on on-time oGTT and GDM on on-time oGTT; j—between GDM on late oGTT and GDM on on-time oGTT. The "normal glucose tolerance" group includes women with normal GCT or oGTT. SAV—defined as one abnormal value on oGTT (Carpenter and Coustan threshold values)[2]; GDM—defined as two abnormal values on oGTT (Carpenter and Coustan thresholds values)[2]; [@] gender results available for 63,261 deliveries. BMI—body mass index; oGTT—100 g oral glucose tolerance test; SAV—single abnormal value; GDM—gestational diabetes; T2DM—type 2 diabetes mellitus; GCT—glucose challenge test.

Table 3. Cox-regression analysis for the development of type 2 diabetes mellitus according to the study groups.

	aHR	95% CI	p Value
Maternal age, years	1.046	1.031–1.061	<0.001
BMI $\geq$ 30	8.871	7.270–10.827	<0.001
Maternal hypertension	1.843	1.099–3.091	0.021
Normal glucose tolerance	***		
SAV late oGTT	1.323	0.682–2.563	0.408
SAV on-time oGTT	2.139	1.362–3.360	<0.001
GDM late oGTT	2.933	1.685–5.105	<0.001
GDM on-time oGTT	3.642	2.441–5.436	<0.001

*** oGTT at 24 + 0–28 + 6 gestational weeks—reference group; BMI—body mass index; oGTT—100 g oral glucose tolerance test; SAV—single abnormal value; GDM—gestational diabetes.

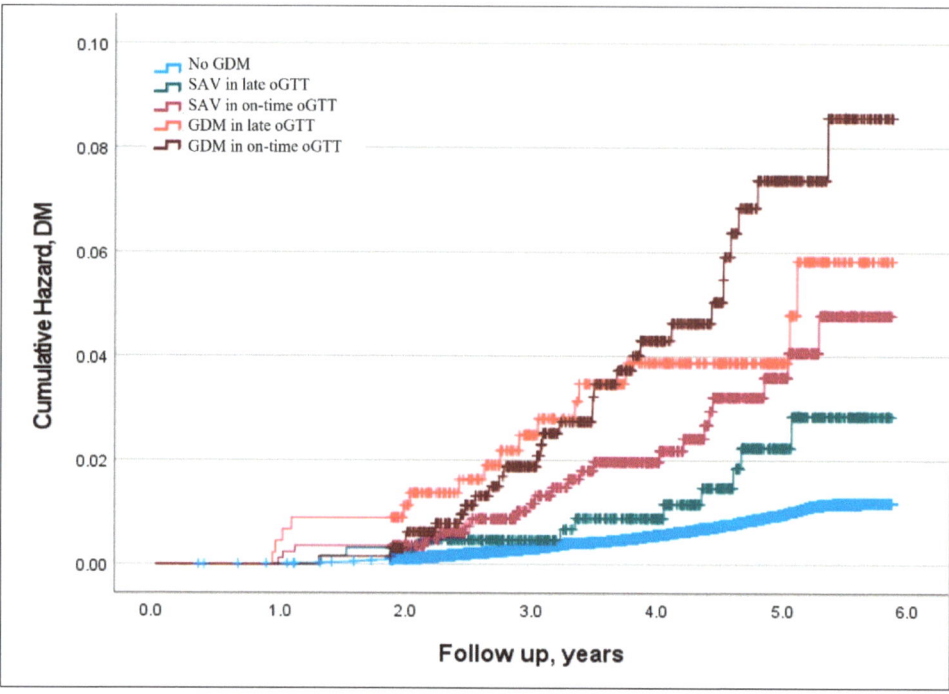

Figure 2. Abnormal oGTT and cumulative incidence of diabetes. Legend: Censored Kaplan—Meier Hazard curves for type 2 diabetes mellitus plotted for normal glucose status, single abnormal value oGTT, and GDM diagnosed at on-time oGTT (performed at 24 + 0–28 + 6 weeks) and late oGTT (performed after 28 weeks). oGTT—100 g oral glucose tolerance test; GDM—gestational diabetes; DM—diabetes mellitus; SAV—single abnormal value.

3.3. Stratification by Obesity Status

Due to the significant association between BMI and T2DM, which was also evident in our cohort, we repeated the analysis separately for women with and without obesity (Tables 4 and 5, Figure 3). The absolute incidence of T2DM was higher for women with obesity. That being said, their aHR that was solely related to abnormal oGTT results was lower compared to women without obesity.

Table 4. Cox-regression analysis for the development of type 2 diabetes mellitus according to study groups for women without obesity.

	aHR	95% CI	*p* Value
Maternal age, years	1.062	1.035–1.090	<0.001
Maternal hypertension	1.946	0.481–7.881	0.351
Normal glucose tolerance	***		
SAV late oGTT	3.300	1.048–10.398	0.041
SAV on-time oGTT	3.096	1.139–8.415	0.027
GDM late oGTT	7.708	3.140–18.920	<0.001
GDM on-time oGTT	8.939	4.503–17.743	<0.001

Results are presented as Hazard ratios (95% confidence interval), adjusted for maternal age and BMI. BMI—body mass index; oGTT—100 g oral glucose tolerance test; SAV—single abnormal value; GDM—gestational diabetes. *** The normal glucose tolerance is the reference value. The other parameters were compared to it.

Table 5. Cox-regression analysis for the development of type 2 diabetes mellitus according to study groups for women with obesity.

	aHR	95% CI	p Value
Maternal age, years	1.038	1.021–1.056	<0.001
Maternal hypertension	1.863	1.068–3.250	0.028
Normal glucose tolerance	***		
SAV late oGTT	0.999	0.445–2.244	0.999
SAV on-time oGTT	1.957	1.181–3.242	0.009
GDM late oGTT	2.091	1.035–4.226	0.040
GDM on-time oGTT	2.727	1.668–4.460	<0.001

Results are presented as Hazard ratios (95% confidence interval), adjusted to maternal age and BMI. BMI—body mass index; oGTT—100 g oral glucose tolerance test; SAV—single abnormal value; GDM—gestational diabetes. *** The normal glucose tolerance is the reference value. The other parameters were compared to it.

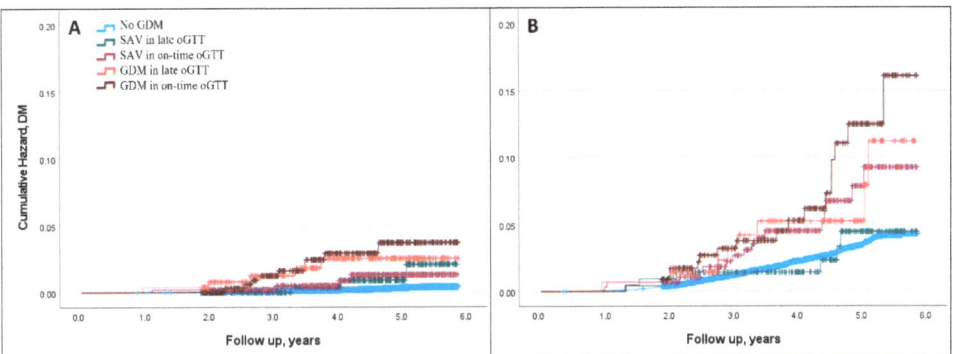

Figure 3. Abnormal oGTT and cumulative incidence of diabetes for women with and without obesity. Legend: Censored Kaplan–Meier Hazard curves for type 2 diabetes mellitus plotted for normal glucose status, SAV oGTT, and GDM diagnosed at on-time oGTT (performed at 24 + 0–28 + 6 weeks) and late oGTT (performed after 28 weeks). Curves are constructed and presented separately for women with and without obesity. (**A**) BMI < 30 kg/m^2; (**B**) BMI ≥ 30 kg/m^2; oGTT—100 g oral glucose tolerance test; GDM—gestational diabetes; DM—diabetes mellitus; SAV—single abnormal value.

4. Discussion

In this study, we aimed to investigate the risk of T2DM, over 5 years of follow-up, among women with abnormal oGTT results performed after 28 weeks of gestation (late oGTT) as compared to women who had abnormal oGTT results at 24–28 weeks of gestation (on time oGTT) and to women with normal glucose tolerance.

Our study results demonstrate the following findings: a. Women who perform late oGTT have lower rates of GDM and T2DM; b. Once GDM is diagnosed, regardless of oGTT timing, the risk of T2DM is increased even in a 5-year follow-up; c. The risk of T2DM following GDM diagnosis at late oGTT is increased for women with and without obesity; d. A SAV oGTT is associated with T2DM only if oGTT was performed prior to 28 gestational weeks.

4.1. Results in the Context of What Is Known

GDM is considered a well-established risk factor for the development of T2DM [1,2]. However, since the majority of GDM cases are diagnosed between 24 + 0 and 28 + 6 weeks, none of the studies evaluated the risk of T2DM specifically when GDM was diagnosed later in gestation.

Prior studies that evaluated the clinical implication of late oGTT investigated the maternal and neonatal short-term outcomes with conflicting results [5,7,10]. Thus, there is no consensus on yield and indications for performing oGTT in late pregnancy. Our results demonstrated that women who performed late oGTT had a lower prevalence of abnormal oGTT results, both SAV and GDM. This result is probably related to the different maternal characteristics and the indications for performing oGTT. Women who performed late oGTT were younger, with lower rates of hypertension and lower glucose levels in the first trimester and at GCT compared to women who performed on-time oGTT. Moreover, although indications for late oGTT were unavailable for this dataset, we assume that indications included latecomers or women with large-for-gestational-age fetuses or polyhydramnios with a previous normal GCT screening. Accordingly, this group represents women with lower pre-pregnancy metabolic risk and, therefore, lower abnormal oGTT risk and lower risk for T2DM.

According to our results, once GDM was diagnosed, regardless of the timing of the oGTT, the risk for T2DM was about three folds higher compared to women with normal glucose tolerance during gestation. Nevertheless, women with only a SAV oGTT had a statistically significant increased risk for T2DM only if oGTT was performed between 24 + 0 and 28 + 6 gestational weeks. Several possibilities can explain this difference. First, insulin resistance during pregnancy is mainly increased from 16 to 26 weeks of gestation, with a mild increase thereafter [12]. It is possible that late GDM, diagnosed to a large extent after normal GCT screening, represents milder insulin insensitivity when compared to on-time oGTT; therefore, when using the same thresholds for diagnosis, abnormal oGTT results will be associated with lower rates of T2DM compared to on-time oGTT. This is supported by the fact that SAV in late oGTT, unlike in on-time oGTT, was not statistically associated with an increased risk of T2DM in our cohort. These women may be prone to T2DM later in life, and our limited 5-year follow-up was too short to detect the risk. A second possible explanation considers the need for different thresholds for GDM diagnosis at a more advanced stage of pregnancy. O'Sullivan, who set the first thresholds for GDM, tested women in their second and third trimesters [13]. Further studies have tried to determine the correct thresholds during the third trimester regarding fetal outcomes [14]. The authors compared the glucose levels by home glucose monitoring between 2 groups of women who conducted oGTT after 33 weeks due to risk factors. One group was diagnosed with GDM and the other was negative. They found that the distribution of glucose values between the groups was significantly different nevertheless, with overlapping. Women who were diagnosed and treated reached lower glucose values in the third trimester and had lower rates of macrosomia and cesarean deliveries. These results were explained by the continuity effect of hyperglycemia. The authors concluded that high-risk women who do not fulfill the criteria for GDM diagnosis should be treated with the same attention as GDM parturients due to their risk factors and that no different thresholds should be set. Lastly, it is possible that the reproducibility of the oGTT decreases with advanced gestational age; therefore, there are more false positive and negative results for late oGTT [15].

4.2. Obesity and Type 2 Diabetes Incident

The underlying mechanism for T2DM is thought to be different among women with and without obesity [16]. A common underlying mechanism for GDM development is relative pancreatic insufficiency or β-cell dysfunction, which is possibly the predominant mechanism in women with normal BMI. Advanced gestation insulin resistance increases in order to preserve fetal demands, leading to accelerating ongoing pancreatic β-cell exhaustion and an increased risk of postpartum T2DM. Alternatively, in women with obesity, excessive adiposity may promote a proinflammatory state and insulin resistance, which contribute to both GDM development and later T2DM [17].

Prior studies that evaluated combinations of risk factors and postpartum dysglycemia [16] demonstrated that GDM alone had a comparable risk for T2DM, such as having two risk factors—obesity or post-delivery weight retention, for example. Having GDM on top of these risk factors exacerbates the effect of GDM on T2DM development. Concordant with that observation, our results showed that women with obesity had a significantly higher risk of developing T2DM compared to women without obesity. That being said, GDM diagnosis increased the risk of T2DM in women with and without obesity.

4.3. Research Implications

Our results emphasize the need to set universal standards for late oGTT, regarding indications, thresholds of diagnosis, and treatment advantage. Further studies should focus on both short-term and long-term outcomes for the mother and offspring and the extent of improvement in outcomes.

Since hyperglycemia is a continuum throughout pregnancy, and several studies have demonstrated increased fetal and maternal risk with increasing glucose levels even within the normal range [18,19], we need models with a longer follow-up time to determine the actual risk of late GDM and SAV diagnosis. Understanding the long-term implications of the late GDM diagnosis might clarify the underlying mechanism and contribute to the follow-up and therapeutic approach to these patients.

4.4. Clinical Implications

Our results imply that GDM diagnosed in late gestation represents a true metabolic disturbance and is not just a matter of threshold. This may imply its significance when managing GDM diagnosed in late gestation. Moreover, our results suggest that women with late GDM diagnoses should be further evaluated for risk factors and be tested for diabetes postpartum according to the ADA guidelines [2] in a similar way to women diagnosed with GDM at 24 + 0 and 28 + 6 gestational weeks. Regarding SAV, our findings do not support the need for GDM follow-up postpartum for women with late SAV solely based on this diagnosis. However, as long as we continue to diagnose late GDM with the same thresholds, we should treat these women with caution and recruit them to follow up according to their risk factors, regardless of their GDM status.

4.5. Strength and Limitations

The strengths of this study include the large cohort and the linkage of two detailed databases with systematic data collection measured rather than reported. Our results were based directly on the laboratory glucose values and INDR solid criteria and not on reported GDM or T2DM diagnosis. To avoid prediabetes patients, we only included women with fasting glucose less than 92 mg/dL and women with oGTT performed after 20 weeks. Nevertheless, our study was not free of limitations, mainly due to its retrospective nature. First, the Meuhedet HMO pregnancy registry has been limited to the last five years. Second, we lacked data on other covariates, such as a family history of T2DM or possible after-pregnancy interventions such as weight reduction or lifestyle modifications that might have interfered with the risk for T2DM. Third, we did not have the indication for late oGTT performance or if an oGTT was performed for the second time during pregnancy. Lastly, the INRD does not include prediabetic state and T2DM diagnosis by 75GR oGTT; however, only a few participants went through this test, and we assume all of them were captured by the INRD diagnostic criteria postpartum.

5. Conclusions

When diagnosed after 28 weeks, GDM, but not SAV, is associated with an increased risk of T2DM over 5 years of follow-up. Further studies are needed to standardize late oGTT regarding indications, thresholds for diagnosis, short- and long-term implications, and yield for treatment.

Author Contributions: Conceptualization, E.M.-S. and R.G.-B.; Data curation, R.G.-B.; Formal analysis, R.G.-B. and E.M.-S.; Investigation, M.H. and E.M.-S.; Methodology, Y.T. and R.G.-B.; Supervision, R.G.-B. and M.H.; Writing—original draft, E.M.-S.; Writing—review & editing, Y.T., M.H. and R.G.-B. All authors have read and agreed to the published version of the manuscript.

Funding: This research received no external funding.

Institutional Review Board Statement: This study was approved by the institutional review board in accordance with the Helsinki Declaration. IRB 10-18-08-21 was given at 18 August 2021.

Informed Consent Statement: Patient consent was waived since the research subjects' identities were not known to the researchers.

Data Availability Statement: Data may by available upon request.

Conflicts of Interest: The authors declare no conflict of interest.

References

1. Bulletins-Obstetrics, C. ACOG Practice Bulletin No. 190: Gestational Diabetes Mellitus. *Obstet. Gynecol.* **2018**, *131*, e49–e64.
2. American Diabetes Association. Classification and Diagnosis of Diabetes: Standards of Medical Care in Diabetes—2021. *Diabetes Care* **2021**, *44* (Suppl. S1), S15–S33, Erratum in *Diabetes Care* **2021**, *44*, 2182.
3. de Wit, L.; Bos, D.M.; van Rossum, A.P.; van Rijn, B.B.; Boers, K.E. Repeated oral glucose tolerance tests in women at risk for gestational diabetes mellitus. *Eur. J. Obstet. Gynecol. Reprod. Biol.* **2019**, *242*, 79–85. [CrossRef] [PubMed]
4. Sasson, A.M.; Shats, M.; Goichberg, Z.; Mazaki-Tovi, S.; Morag, I.; Hendler, I. Oral glucose tolerance test for suspected late onset gestational diabetes. *J. Matern. Neonatal Med.* **2021**, *34*, 3928–3932. [CrossRef] [PubMed]
5. Abu Shqara, R.; Or, S.; Wiener, Y.; Lowenstein, L.; Wolf, M.F. Clinical implications of the 100-g oral glucose tolerance test in the third trimester. *Arch. Gynecol. Obstet.* **2023**, *307*, 421–429. [CrossRef] [PubMed]
6. Abu Shqara, R.; Or, S.; Nakhleh Francis, Y.; Wiener, Y.; Lowenstein, L.; Wolf, M.F. Third trimester re-screening for gestational diabetes in morbidly obese women despite earlier negative test can reveal risks for obstetrical complications. *J. Obstet. Gynaecol. Res.* **2023**, *49*, 852–862. [CrossRef] [PubMed]
7. Chionuma, J.; Akinola, I.; Dada, A.; Ubuane, P.; Kuku-Kuye, T.; Olalere, F. Profile of insulin resistance of pregnant women at late third trimester in Nigeria: A descriptive cross-sectional report. *Niger. J. Clin. Pract.* **2022**, *25*, 1736–1744. [CrossRef] [PubMed]
8. Wolf, M.F.; Peleg, D.; Stahl-Rosenzweig, T.; Kurzweil, Y.; Yogev, Y. Isolated polyhydramnios in the third trimester: Is a gestational diabetes evaluation of value? *Gynecol. Endocrinol.* **2017**, *33*, 849–852. [CrossRef] [PubMed]
9. Arbib, N.; Gabbay-Benziv, R.; Aviram, A.; Sneh-Arbib, O.; Wiznitzer, A.; Hod, M.; Chen, R.; Hadar, E. Third trimester abnormal oral glucose tolerance test and adverse perinatal outcome. *J. Matern.-Fetal Neonatal Med.* **2017**, *30*, 917–921. [CrossRef] [PubMed]
10. Shindo, R.; Aoki, S.; Nakanishi, S.; Misumi, T.; Miyagi, E. Impact of gestational diabetes mellitus diagnosed during the third trimester on pregnancy outcomes: A case-control study. *BMC Pregnancy Childbirth* **2021**, *21*, 246. [CrossRef] [PubMed]
11. Twig, G.; Zucker, I.; Afek, A.; Cukierman-Yaffe, T.; Bendor, C.D.; Derazne, E.; Lutski, M.; Shohat, T.; Mosenzon, O.; Tzur, D.; et al. Adolescent Obesity and Early-Onset Type 2 Diabetes. *Diabetes Care* **2020**, *43*, 1487–1495. [CrossRef] [PubMed]
12. Stanley, K.; Fraser, R.; Bruce, C. Physiological changes in insulin resistance in human pregnancy: Longitudinal study with the hyperinsulinaemic euglycaemic clamp technique. *BJOG Int. J. Obstet. Gynaecol.* **1998**, *105*, 756–759. [CrossRef] [PubMed]
13. O'sullivan, J.B.; Mahan, C.M. Criteria for the oral glucose tolerance test in pregnancy. *Diabetes* **1964**, *13*, 278–285. [PubMed]
14. Cauldwell, M.; Chmielewska, B.; Kaur, K.; Van-De-L'Isle, Y.; Sherry, A.; Coote, I.W.; Steer, P.J. Screening for late-onset gestational diabetes: Are there any clinical benefits? *BJOG Int. J. Obstet. Gynaecol.* **2022**, *129*, 2176–2183. [CrossRef] [PubMed]
15. Libman, I.M.; Barinas-Mitchell, E.; Bartucci, A.; Robertson, R.; Arslanian, S. Reproducibility of the oral glucose tolerance test in overweight children. *J. Clin. Endocrinol. Metab.* **2008**, *93*, 4231–4237. [CrossRef] [PubMed]
16. Chen, L.-W.; Soh, S.E.; Tint, M.-T.; Loy, S.L.; Yap, F.; Tan, K.H.; Lee, Y.S.; Shek, L.P.-C.; Godfrey, K.M.; Gluckman, P.D.; et al. Combined analysis of gestational diabetes and maternal weight status from pre-pregnancy through post-delivery in future development of type 2 diabetes. *Sci. Rep.* **2021**, *11*, 5021. [CrossRef] [PubMed]
17. Šimják, P.; Cinkajzlová, A.; Anderlová, K.; Pařízek, A.; Mráz, M.; Kršek, M.; Haluzík, M. The role of obesity and adipose tissue dysfunction in gestational diabetes mellitus. *J. Endocrinol.* **2018**, *238*, R63–R77. [CrossRef] [PubMed]
18. Bo, S.; Monge, L.; Macchetta, C.; Menato, G.; Pinach, S.; Uberti, B.; Pagano, G. Prior gestational hyperglycemia: A long-term predictor of the metabolic syndrome. *J. Endocrinol. Investig.* **2004**, *27*, 629–635. [CrossRef] [PubMed]
19. Riskin-Mashiah, S.; Younes, G.; Damti, A.; Auslender, R. First-trimester fasting hyperglycemia and adverse pregnancy outcomes. *Diabetes Care* **2009**, *32*, 1639–1643. [CrossRef] [PubMed]

Disclaimer/Publisher's Note: The statements, opinions and data contained in all publications are solely those of the individual author(s) and contributor(s) and not of MDPI and/or the editor(s). MDPI and/or the editor(s) disclaim responsibility for any injury to people or property resulting from any ideas, methods, instructions or products referred to in the content.

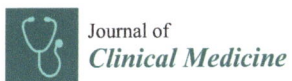

Article

Placenta Accreta Spectrum Prophylactic Therapy for Hyperfibrinolysis with Tranexamic Acid

Tiyasha Hosne Ayub [1,*], Brigitte Strizek [1], Bernd Poetzsch [2], Philipp Kosian [1], Ulrich Gembruch [1] and Waltraut M. Merz [1]

1. Department of Obstetrics and Prenatal Medicine, University Hospital Bonn, Venusberg Campus 1, 53127 Bonn, Germany
2. Institute for Experimental Hematology and Transfusion Medicine, University Hospital Bonn, Venusberg Campus 1, 53127 Bonn, Germany
* Correspondence: tiyasha_hosne.ayub@ukbonn.de

Abstract: Background: To report on prophylactic therapy for hyperfibrinolysis with tranexamic acid (TXA) during expectant management (EM) in the placenta accreta spectrum (PAS). Methods: This is a monocentric retrospective study of women with PAS presenting at our hospital between 2005 and 2021. All data were retrospectively collected through the departmental database. Results: 35 patients with PAS were included. EM was planned in 25 patients prior to delivery. Complete absorption of the retained placenta was seen in two patients (8%). Curettage was performed in 14 patients (56%). A hysterectomy (HE) was needed in seven (28%) patients; 18 patients (72%) underwent uterus-preserving treatment without severe complications. The mean duration of EM was 107 days. The mean day of onset of hyperfibrinolysis and beginning of TXA treatment was day 45. The mean nadir of fibrinogen level before TXA was 242.4 mg/dL, with a mean drop of 29.7% in fibrinogen level. Conclusions: Our data support EM as a safe treatment option in PAS. Hyperfibrinolysis can be a cause of hemorrhage during EM and can be treated with TXA. To our knowledge, this is the first cohort of patients with EM of PAS in whom coagulation monitoring and use of TXA have been shown to successfully treat hyperfibrinolysis.

Keywords: placenta accreta spectrum; expectant management; hyperfibrinolysis; disseminated intravascular coagulopathy; tranexamic acid; fibrinogen; D-dimer

1. Introduction

Placenta accreta spectrum (PAS) is associated with high maternal morbidity [1–4]. The rising incidence is mainly attributed to increasing cesarean section (CS) rates [5–10]. Retained placenta after vaginal delivery and placenta previa are other risk factors [11–14]. Forcibly removing an invasive placenta may lead to massive obstetric hemorrhage and a life-threatening coagulopathy. Therefore, cesarean hysterectomy (CS-HE) is considered the gold standard of treatment [15–19]. However, surgical complications should not be disregarded, especially in placenta percreta, when adjacent organs like the bladder are infiltrated and bladder or ureter injuries with associated long-term complications like vesicouterine fistula can be caused [2]. Furthermore, hypervascularization via additional blood supply, mainly from the external iliac arteries, increases the risks of major blood loss even in experienced hands [16–18]. Partial excision of invasive placental areas, another treatment option, is also associated with high blood loss. Additional procedures like embolization, vessel ligation, or temporal internal iliac balloon occlusion can reduce blood loss, but there are no randomized controlled trials comparing these procedures [2,19].

Expectant management (EM), leaving the placenta in situ after the delivery of the fetus without any manipulation of the placenta, is associated with a more than 50% reduction in blood loss and need for transfusions [2,20]. A favorable outcome has been reported in up to 85% of cases, avoiding hysterectomy in 19 to 60% of cases [21–30]. Delayed secondary hysterectomy may be required in 58% within 9 months after delivery [2,25]. Indications include infections and hemorrhage, which may trigger disseminated intravascular coagulopathy (DIC) [23,31,32]. In contrast, hyperfibrinolysis is induced by a massive release of plasminogen activators resulting in increased plasmin concentration and proteolysis of fibrinogen/fibrin. Tranexamic acid (TXA), a synthetic antifibrinolytic agent, inhibits the conversion of plasminogen into plasmin, thus inhibiting hyperfibrinolysis, and is approved for the treatment of hyperfibrinolytic bleeding complications [33]. The uterus and placenta are both rich in plasminogen activators promoting hyperfibrinolysis [31]. Therefore, hemorrhage in PAS may be the result of primary hyperfibrinolysis and may occur without inflammation.

We aimed to report on the prevention and management of hyperfibrinolysis with TXA during EM of PAS.

2. Materials and Methods

All patients with PAS presenting at our center between 2005 and 2021 were included. The outcome of 19 patients has already been published, focusing on physical, mental, and reproductive sequelae after the treatment of PAS [31,34]. Antenatal diagnosis of PAS was made using 2D ultrasound, color Doppler, and transvaginal ultrasound [35,36]. Ultrasound criteria included loss of the clear zone or decidua, partial or complete absence of the myometrium layer, sub-placental lacunae, a sudden break-off in the outline of the calcifications characteristic for third-trimester placental basal plates, increased vascular perfusion between the uteroplacental interface reaching the uterine serosa, bladder wall interruption, placental bulge, and exophytic mass hypervascularity (Figure 1) [8,35–38].

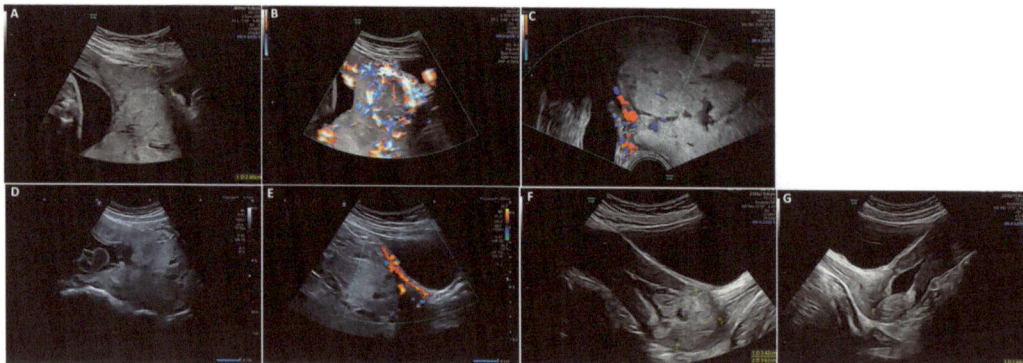

Figure 1. (A–C) PAS in 34 + 0 weeks of gestation with loss of decidua, bladder wall interruption, placental bulge, and exophytic mass hypervascularity. (D,E) Placenta in situ on day 13 after CS with persistent bladder wall interruption. (F) Placenta in situ on day 63 after CS with a diameter of about 3.5 cm, well separated from the uterine wall, without perfusion. (G) Day 122 after CS; fluid-filled uterine cavity surrounded by a hyperechogenic rim.

Treatment options (leaving the placenta in situ, partial excision of invasive placental areas, and CS-HE) were discussed in detail with the patients before making an informed decision about further management. Surgery was performed by a team of senior obstetricians and anesthetists with neonatologic stand-by, mainly under general anesthesia. The placenta was avoided by a uterine fundal transverse or longitudinal incision after abdominal access by supraumbilical or lower midline incision (Figure 2) [39]. An intraoperative ultrasound was performed at the surgeon's discretion to locate the placenta. Uterotonic agents were not administered [40].

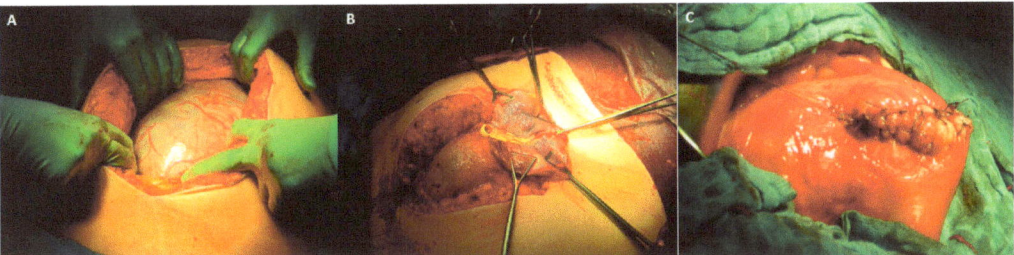

Figure 2. (**A**): A large area of PAS is seen on the front wall of the uterus after abdominal access by a supraumbilical midline incision. (**B**) Uterine fundal longitudinal incision on the back wall of the uterus avoiding the placenta. (**C**) Closed uterotomy after leaving the placenta in situ.

Once we observed a decrease in the fibrinogen level and a corresponding increase in the D-dimer level, we started with TXA therapy with an initial dose of 1 g t.i.d. The changes in the concentrations of fibrinogen and the D-dimer were calculated in percent. Completion of EM was defined by the absence of any remaining placental tissue, either by complete absorption, curettage, or HE. Additionally, successful EM was defined as uterus preservation. On the other hand, a failed EM was defined as loss of the uterus. The outcome of hyperfibrinolysis management with TXA therapy was defined as normalization of coagulation screening and prevention or cessation of vaginal bleeding.

Maternal and fetal outcomes, laboratory and ultrasound reports, and follow-ups were retrospectively collected. The Institutional Review Board of the University of Bonn Medical Faculty does not require formal approval for retrospective observational studies. Only basic statistical tests were performed. This included the calculation of the mean value and plotting the values in a figure using Microsoft Office Professional Plus 2016 (Microsoft Corp., Redmond, WA, USA).

3. Results

During the study period, thirty-five patients with PAS were included. The diagnosis was established antenatally in 32 (91.4%) patients. A large area of PAS was detected during delivery in three patients. There was no maternal death. Details of the study population are listed in Table 1 and Figure 3. The mean week of gestation at first diagnosis was 28 + 4 weeks, and at delivery, it was 35 + 0 weeks. Thirty (85.7%) patients had at least one previous CS, and eleven (31.4%) patients had at least one curettage. Seven (20%) patients had a history of both CS and curettage. Placenta previa totalis was diagnosed in 24 (68.6%) patients. Two (5.7%) patients reported a history of PAS. Five (14.3%) patients had no prior CS, and one of these suffered PAS in her first pregnancy with smoking as a sole risk factor. Uterine malformations such as uterus bicornis were seen in three (8.6%) patients. Placenta membranacea was present in four (11.4%) patients, of whom two had large parts of scattered ingrown placenta on the front and back walls of the uterus. Scheduled elective CS-HE was performed in seven (20%) patients, with the latest in 2017. Two (5.7%) patients were delivered by emergency CS in the 28th week of gestation due to vaginal hemorrhage. An elective CS-HE due to completed family planning was chosen by five (14.3%) patients.

Table 1. Patient characteristics.

Total number of patients	35
Maternal age, mean (range)	32.8 (21–41)
Gravidity, mean (range)	3.6 (1–13)
Parity, mean (range)	2.2 (0–11)
Timing of diagnosis, n (%)	
antepartum	32/35 (91.4%)
Intrapartum	3/35 (8.6%)

Table 1. *Cont.*

Type of PAS	
increta	17/35 (48.6%)
percreta	14/35 (40%)
increta/percreta and membranacea	4/35 (11.4%)
Placenta previa in current pregnancy	26/35 (74.3%)
total	24/35 (68.6%)
Partial	2/35 (5.7%)
GA at diagnosis (weeks), mean (range)	28 + 4 (9 + 2–36 + 3)
GA at delivery (weeks), mean (range)	35 + 0 (27 + 2–37 + 1)
Risk factors, n (%) (multiple risk factors possible)	
Previous CS	30/35 (85.7%)
1 CS	18/30 (60%)
2 CS	5/30 (16.7%)
3 CS	3/30 (10%)
>3 CS	4/30 (13.3%)
Number of patients without previous CS	5/35 (14.3%)
Curettages	2/5 (40%)
Placenta previa in current pregnancy	1/5 (20%)
History of placenta increta	1/5 (20%)
Smoking	1/5 (20%)
Curettages (number of curettages)	11(1–5)/35 (31.4%)
Uterus bicornis/arcuatus	3/35 (8.6%)
History of endomyometritis	1/35 (2.9%)
Asherman syndrome	1/35 (2.9%)
History of intrauterine device	1/35 (2.9%)
History of placenta increta	2/35 (5.7%)
Assisted reproduction by IVF/ICSI	2/35 (5.7%)
Smoking	4/35 (11.4%)
EM	28/35 (80%)
Planned EM	25/28 (89%)
Intrapartum diagnosis (unplanned), managed with EM	3/28 (11%)
Successful uterus-preserving management	21/35 (60%)
Successful uterus-preserving management in planned EM	18/25 (72%)
Antenataelly intended CS-HE	7/35 (20%)
Unplanned CS-HE/HE	7/25 (28%)

PAS—placenta accreta spectrum; GA—gestational age; CS—cesarean section; IVF—in vitro fertilization; ICSI—intracytoplasmic sperm injection; HE—hysterectomy; EM—expectant management.

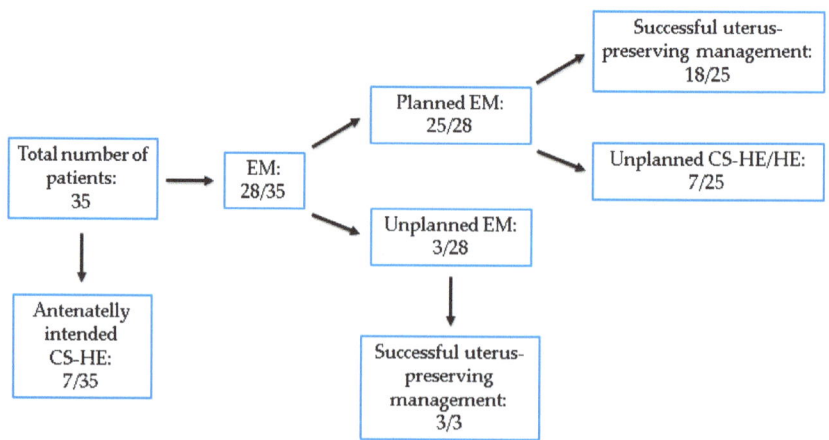

Figure 3. Placenta accreta spectrum: management and outcome. EM—expectant management; CS—cesarean section; HE—hysterectomy.

3.1. Planned EM, Failed

EM was the intended approach for the treatment of PAS in 25 (89.3%) patients after 2007 (Tables 1 and 2). In two (8%) patients, partial placental detachment occurred during CS. Complete removal of the placenta was achieved in both cases. In the first patient, hemostatic treatment consisted of the insertion of a chitosan-coated gauze (Celox®, Crewe, UK) and a Bakri balloon. The estimated blood loss (EBL) was 4.000 mL. The patient received an intravenous bolus injection of 1 g TXA, five units of packed red cells (PRC), and four units of fresh frozen plasma (FFP). The second patient, who presented with placenta increta and membranacea required compression sutures of the placental bed, insertion of tabotamp, and chitosan-coated gauze (Celox®) for control of hemorrhage. EBL was 3.000 mL, with a transfusion of three units of PRC and four units of FFP.

Table 2. Outcome of cases with EM (n = 28).

EM n (%)	28
Mean duration of EM (days)	107 (8–589)
Planned EM	25/28 (89.3%)
Complete placental absorption	2/25 (8%)
Planned curettage	14/25 (56%)
Emergency curettage due to bleeding	1/25 (4%)
Intraoperative placental detachment, complete removal during CS	2/25 (8%)
HE	7/25 (28%)
HE during CS	1/25 (4%)
Unplanned HE	4/25 (16%)
Planned HE	2/25 (8%)
Unplanned EM (one vaginal delivery, one operative vaginal delivery, one CS)	3/28 (10.7%)
Complete placental absorption	3/3 (100%)
Complications following planned EM, n (%) (multiple possible)	25
Abnormal coagulation screening	11/25 (44%)
Infection	11/25 (44%)
Abdominal pain	6/25 (24%)
Nausea	1/25 (4%)
Gingival bleeding	1/25 (4%)
Dysuria	1/25 (4%)
Blood transfusions (2–26 units)	11/25 (44%)
During HE (8–26 units)	5/7 (71.4%)
During curettage (2–11 units)	4/14 (28.6%)
During CS (4 units)	2/2 (100%)

CS—cesarean section; HE—hysterectomy; EM—expectant management.

3.2. Planned EM, Successful

In total, two (8%) of the twenty-five patients with intended EM showed complete absorption of the retained placenta (Figures 1 and 4). Fourteen patients (56%) underwent secondary curettage with complete removal of the placenta. Four (28.5%) patients received units of PRC during curettage (two, four, and eleven units). One patient presented with fever and vaginal bleeding and needed an early discontinuation of therapy due to bleeding on day 18 after CS (Table 2). An emergency curettage was performed with the insertion of a chitosan-coated gauze (Celox®). The following day, a second curettage was performed due to bleeding. This time, a Bakri balloon was inserted into the uterus. The patient received nine units of PRC and six FFP in total. Secondary HE was needed in seven patients (28%): one during CS due to severe bleeding, one due to massive intravesical bleeding because of suspected invasion of the bladder wall on day 8 after CS, one after failed placental removal during curettage on day 52 after CS, and two due to infection and perforation during curettage on days 56 and 86 after CS, respectively. Planned secondary HEs were performed in two (8%) patients, one due to a residual large area of placenta previa et increta near the cervix on day 121 after CS, and the other due to completed family planning on day 59 after CS (Tables 2 and 3). Thus, 18 patients (72%) were successfully treated with uterus-preserving methods; in 15 (93.7%) patients, this was without severe complications (Table 1).

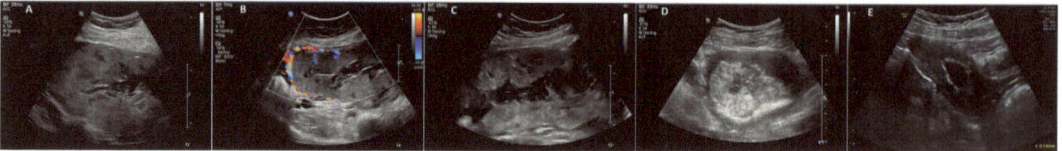

Figure 4. (**A**) Placenta in situ on day 9 after CS. (**B**) Placenta in situ on day 15 after CS. (**C**) Regressively altered placenta in situ on day 64 after CS. (**D**) Placenta in situ well separated from the uterine wall without perfusion on day 106 after CS. (**E**) Day 194 after CS with a hyperechogenic rim around a fluid-filled uterine cavity.

Table 3. Characteristics of patients with treatment of hyperfibrinolysis with tranexamic acid.

Pat.	Start of TXA (Day)	Fibrinogen (mg/dL) at Start of TXA (Previous Value), Normal Range 180–355 mg/dL	D-Dimer (mg/L) at Start of TXA (Previous Value), Normal Range: 0–0.5 mg/L	Therapy Outcome	Duration of EM (Days)
1	71	64 (ND)	ND	Curettage	119
2	56	159 (437)	21.75 (3.9)	Curettage	109
3	52	216 (360)	ND	HE due to infection and perforation with injury of bladder during curettage (24 PRC transfusion)	86
4	34	431 (503)	11.02 (3.6)	Complete absorption (Figure 1)	152
5	58	229 (326)	ND	Curettage	82
6	38	243 (339)	ND	Curettage, laparotomy due to perforation and injury of bladder without HE	71
7	28	325 (362)	5.66 (3.86)	Curettage (two PRC transfusion)	102
8	45	315 (401)	10.83 (5.77)	Curettage	91
9	28	198 (240)	17.41 (13.89)	Curettage, but residual placenta	116
10	35	218 (318)	ND	Elective HE due to large area of placenta previa et percreta near the cervix	121
11	45	268 (454)	14.45 (4.46)	Elective HE due to completed family planning	59
Mean	45 (28–71)	242.4 (64–431) mean % drop: 29.7%	13.5 (5.7–21.7) mean % rise: 273.7%		101 (59–152)

TXA—tranexamic acid; Pat.—patient; ND—not determined; PRC—packed red cells; HE—hysterectomy.

3.3. Uplanned EM, Successful

In three (10.7%) patients, the diagnosis was established during delivery, and parts of abnormally invasive tissue were left in utero (Table 2). Of these, two patients delivered vaginally and one via CS. All three were successfully treated with complete absorption of the residual placenta. The first patient had a curettage for incomplete placenta after operative vaginal term delivery. An abnormally invasive placental area of approximately

7 × 6 cm on the uterine fundus was detected, and it was left in situ due to stable bleeding and proper uterus contraction. EM was followed, with spontaneous tissue loss on day 70 after delivery. The second patient had a curettage for retention of the placenta after full-term vaginal delivery. An abnormally invasive placental area in the uterine fundus was found. This patient was additionally treated with methotrexate. The increased part of the placenta was completely absorbed after 153 days, and she became pregnant again one year later. The outcome of the following pregnancy was a secondary CS in the 30 + 2 weeks of gestation due to contractions after a preterm premature rupture of membranes in the 22 + 6 weeks of gestation. The placenta was adherent but could be removed completely. The EBL was 700 mL. The third patient had an elective CS at term for breech presentation. During surgery, the abnormally invasive placental area was left in situ. Fifteen u-shape and three B-Lynch sutures were placed for hemostatic control. EBL was 1.800 mL, and she did not require units of PRC. The follow-up of the patient was conducted at 589 days. The patient had a very thin myometrium on the back wall of the uterus. Curettage was assessed to be high risk and was, therefore, not performed. The placenta was eventually completely absorbed.

3.4. Follow-Up during EM (n = 25)

The mean duration of EM was 107 days (range 8–589 days, Table 2). All patients were monitored weekly for six to eight weeks after delivery. Thereafter, monitoring was extended to monthly check-ups. Each visit included a clinical examination, ultrasound, and laboratory investigations (ß-hCG, PAPP-A, CRP, full blood count, fibrinogen, D-dimer, prothrombin time, activated partial thromboplastin time, and antithrombin). ß-hCG decreased steadily and became negative before cessation of blood flow in the retained placenta [2]. Prothrombin time, activated partial thromboplastin time, and antithrombin concentration remained within normal ranges. In case of abnormal findings, surveillance was intensified. Eleven patients (44%) required readmission for febrile complications, including one case of coxitis, which occurred two weeks after unplanned HE 86 days after CS (Table 2). Coxitis was assumed to be a complication of bacteremia and was treated by arthrotomy and lavage; for details see Table 2.

3.5. Hyperfibrinolysis Management

Hyperfibrinolysis, which is defined as a combination of decreased fibrinogen and elevated D-dimer levels, was detected in 11 out of 25 (44%) patients. The platelet count was normal in all these patients. The outcome of these patients is summarized in Table 3.

The mean day of onset of hyperfibrinolysis and initiation of treatment with TXA was post-operative day 45 (range 28–71). The mean duration of EM in this subgroup was 101 days (range 59–152) under continued TXA medication. The mean fibrinogen nadir before TXA was 242.4 mg/dL (range 64–431 mg/dL, normal range 180–355 mg/dL), with a mean drop of 29.7% in fibrinogen levels (Figure 5). D-dimer levels were available for six patients, as shown in Figure 6. The mean D-dimer concentration before initiation of TXA treatment was 13.5 mg/L (range 5.7–21.7 mg/L; normal range: 0–0.5 mg/L), with a mean increase of 273.7%. Our starting dose of TXA was 1 g t.i.d. during TXA therapy, close monitoring was continued to adjust the dose, if necessary. The maximum dose of TXA was 1.5 g t.i.d. Curettage was performed in seven (63.6%) patients (Table 3). One patient required a laparotomy due to a bladder injury. Another patient presented with complete absorption of the placenta. A planned HE was performed on two patients. Emergency HE for intractable bleeding after uterine perforation with a bladder injury during curettage was required in one patient at day 86 post-partum. The patient received 26 units of PRC and 20 units of FFP. Therefore, in this subgroup, eight patients (72.7%) could be treated by uterus-preserving methods. Eight weeks after CS, one patient presented with massive bleeding and not detectable fibrinogen levels. The patient had received TXA therapy but, due to normalized fibrinogen levels, TXA had been stopped one week prior to the bleeding. Curettage could be performed on this patient. The patient needed a transfusion of eleven units of PRC, six units of FFP, two units of platelet concentrates, and a Bakri catheter. However, this patient could not be included in Table 3 and Figure 5 due to a lack of regular measurements of her coagulation profile before curettage. There were no thromboembolic complications (deep venous thrombosis or pulmonary embolism) in any of the patients.

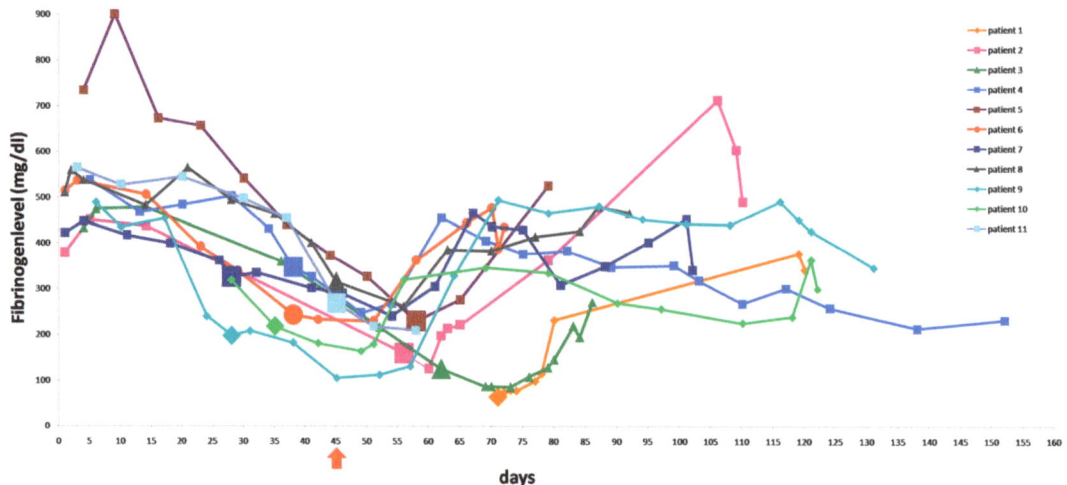

Figure 5. Fibrinogen during EM and treatment with TXA in 11 patients. The days when TXA therapy was started are highlighted in bold. The mean day of initiating TXA therapy after CS was day 45 (arrow).

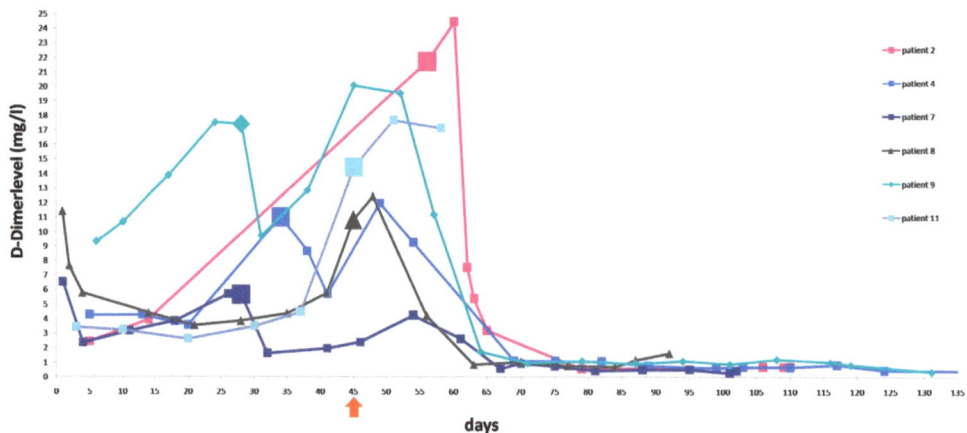

Figure 6. D-dimer during EM and treatment with TXA in six patients. The days when TXA therapy was started are highlighted in bold. The mean day of initiating TXA acid therapy after CS was day 45 (arrow).

A further follow-up showed that three of our patients conceived again after PAS; one patient among them conceived three times. One patient developed Asherman syndrome, and one suffered from short-term depression. The mean duration of inpatient stay was eight days (range 2–34). One infant died two months after delivery at 27 + 2 weeks of gestation because of vaginal hemorrhage, corresponding to a 2.8% infant mortality rate, and most of the newborns were discharged with their mothers within the first week after delivery.

4. Discussion

PAS is a challenging problem worldwide, with a high maternal morbidity [1,2,7]. Although conservative management for PAS is associated with lower surgical morbidity at

CS, CS-HE is still the gold standard of treatment [41]. Antenatal diagnosis and centralized management are associated with lower maternal and fetal morbidity [20,42]. Exact placenta localization is mandatory for the determination of the uterine incision.

Advantages of EM include fertility preservation and reduction of surgical complications such as severe hemorrhage [2,20]. Differentiating DIC from hyperfibrinolysis is essential for the correct management [30,31]. Infection is the most likely cause of DIC, and removing the focus of infection surgically is essential to reduce further complications [30]. If secondary hyperfibrinolysis occurs in the context of DIC, TXA treatment will fail to control bleeding. TXA treatment should be considered only in isolated hyperfibrinolysis. Thus, regular evaluation of coagulation and inflammation parameters is recommended in patients with EM. The coagulation screening in our center included weekly measurements of fibrinogen and D-dimer levels. Any changes should be considered an indication for initiation of 1 g TXA t.i.d. In our study, we detected a mean decrease in fibrinogen levels of 29.7% and a concomitant D-dimer increase of 273.7% before the start of TXA. We initiated TXA in patients with a relevant mean drop of 128.7 mg/dL (range 37–278 mg/dL) in fibrinogen even if it was still above the normal range (355 mg/dL) for non-pregnant patients. Close monitoring should be continued under TXA treatment to adjust the dose. In case of insufficient increase of the fibrinogen level, continuous decrease in the level, or vaginal bleeding under TXA therapy, the dose of TXA was increased up to 1.5 g t.i.d. Prothrombin time, activated partial thromboplastin time, and antithrombin were not relevant parameters for monitoring in our cohort [31]. Coagulation screening should include platelet count to exclude DIC. All our patients treated with TXA had normal platelet counts.

Close monitoring during EM is recommended, with weekly follow-ups in the first eight weeks after delivery, with special attention to coagulation parameters in the second month after delivery (Table 4) [43]. If the patient is stable, monitoring intervals can be extended to monthly from the third month. Every check-up should include a clinical examination for bleeding, abdominal pain, and temperature, as well as an ultrasound with measurement of the size and perfusion of the residual placenta and assessment of fluid retention as a sign of partial detachment of the retained placenta. Furthermore, laboratory tests should include infection parameters, blood count, and ß-hCG in addition to coagulation screening [2].

Table 4. Our monitoring protocol of expectant management of placenta accreta spectrum.

Suggested Follow Up
Weekly follow-up in the first two month, thereafter every two-four weeks
Clinical examination
Ultrasound
Laboratory tests
(for detailed algorithm for coagulation screening we refer to Schröder et al., 2015 [31])

Hyperfibrinolysis did not occur in the first four weeks after CS in our study. The mean beginning of TXA therapy was on day 45 after CS. Fibrinogen levels can normalize under TXA therapy, but treatment should be continued in our opinion. Severe bleeding in one of our patients eight weeks after CS might have been prevented if TXA had been continued.

Patient management may be difficult due to the long duration and frequent check-ups required with EM (up to six months) [2]. This information needs to be included in the initial counseling. The patient should be briefed about symptoms like abdominal pain, bad smell of vaginal discharge, risk of infection, bleeding, and dysuria. Any decision about further treatment should be made jointly. In one of our previous publications, we discovered that 50% of women after HE reported difficulties in accepting the loss of fertility. All women with prenatally diagnosed high-grade invasive disease were satisfied with their choice of treatment [34].

5. Conclusions

In conclusion, although CS-HE is still the gold standard for treatment of PAS, EM of PAS is a safe treatment option with the intention of reduced blood loss at the time of delivery and reduced perioperative complications if delayed hysterectomy is performed [2,20,25]. Close clinical and laboratory follow-up is mandatory, with special attention to early signs of hyperfibrinolysis, which usually appear four to six weeks after CS. TXA can safely be used to treat hyperfibrinolysis and prevent severe bleeding complications and should be continued even after normalized coagulation screening.

In our retrospective cohort, we hypothesize that the use of TXA contributed to successful EM of PAS and reduced complications during follow-up. Two-thirds of our patients with planned EM successfully underwent uterus-preserving treatment; in the subgroup of patients treated with TXA, the rate increased to nearly three-quarters. Hyperfibrinolysis occurred in 11 (44%) patients during EM. To our knowledge, this is the first case series of patients with prospective management of PAS in whom coagulation monitoring combined with TXA treatment successfully reverted hyperfibrinolysis. Further details remain to be investigated in prospective studies. This refers, e.g., to fibrinogen cut-off values for evaluating initiation and discontinuation of TXA therapy and dose-finding.

Author Contributions: Conceptualization: W.M.M. and U.G.; methodology: T.H.A., W.M.M. and U.G.; formal analysis: T.H.A. and B.S.; investigation: T.H.A., B.S. and B.P.; data curation: T.H.A.; writing—original draft preparation: T.H.A.; writing—review and editing: B.S., P.K., U.G., W.M.M. and B.P.; supervision: W.M.M. and U.G. All authors have read and agreed to the published version of the manuscript.

Funding: This research received no external funding.

Institutional Review Board Statement: This study was conducted in accordance with the Declaration of Helsinki. Ethical review and approval were waived in view of the retrospective nature of the study by the Ethics Committee of the Medical Faculty of the University of Bonn.

Informed Consent Statement: Patient consent was waived due to retrospective analysis. Patients were not contacted, and data collection was within the scope of routine patient care.

Data Availability Statement: The datasets used and/or analyzed during the current study are available from the corresponding author upon reasonable request.

Conflicts of Interest: The authors declare no conflicts of interest.

References

1. Poder, L.; Weinstein, S.; Maturen, K.E.; Feldstein, V.A.; Mackenzie, D.C.; Oliver, E.R.; Shipp, T.D.; Strachowski, L.M.; Sussman, B.L.; Wang, E.Y.; et al. ACR Appropriateness Criteria® Placenta Accreta Spectrum Disorder. *J. Am. Coll. Radiol.* **2020**, *17*, S207–S214. [CrossRef] [PubMed]
2. Sentilhes, L.; Kayem, G.; Chandraharan, E.; Palacios-Jaraquemada, J.; Jauniaux, E. FIGO Placenta Accreta Diagnosis and Management Expert Consensus Panel FIGO Consensus Guidelines on Placenta Accreta Spectrum Disorders: Conservative Management. *Int. J. Gynecol. Obstet.* **2018**, *140*, 291–298. [CrossRef] [PubMed]
3. Silver, R.M.; Barbour, K.D. Placenta Accreta Spectrum. *Obstet. Gynecol. Clin. N. Am.* **2015**, *42*, 381–402. [CrossRef] [PubMed]
4. Jauniaux, E.; Chantraine, F.; Silver, R.M.; Langhoff-Roos, J. FIGO Placenta Accreta Diagnosis and Management Expert Consensus Panel FIGO Consensus Guidelines on Placenta Accreta Spectrum Disorders: Epidemiology. *Int. J. Gynecol. Obstet.* **2018**, *140*, 265–273. [CrossRef] [PubMed]
5. Jauniaux, E.; Collins, S.; Burton, G.J. Placenta Accreta Spectrum: Pathophysiology and Evidence-Based Anatomy for Prenatal Ultrasound Imaging. *Am. J. Obstet. Gynecol.* **2018**, *218*, 75–87. [CrossRef] [PubMed]
6. Jauniaux, E.; Jurkovic, D. Placenta Accreta: Pathogenesis of a 20th Century Iatrogenic Uterine Disease. *Placenta* **2012**, *33*, 244–251. [CrossRef]
7. Parra-Herran, C.; Djordjevic, B. Histopathology of Placenta Creta: Chorionic Villi Intrusion into Myometrial Vascular Spaces and Extravillous Trophoblast Proliferation Are Frequent and Specific Findings with Implications for Diagnosis and Pathogenesis. *Int. J. Gynecol. Pathol.* **2016**, *35*, 497–508. [CrossRef]
8. Jauniaux, E.; Alfirevic, Z.; Bhide, A.; Belfort, M.; Burton, G.; Collins, S.; Dornan, S.; Jurkovic, D.; Kayem, G.; Kingdom, J.; et al. Placenta Praevia and Placenta Accreta: Diagnosis and Management: Green-top Guideline No. 27a. *BJOG* **2019**, *126*, E1–E48. [CrossRef]

9. Eshkoli, T.; Weintraub, A.Y.; Sergienko, R.; Sheiner, E. Placenta Accreta: Risk Factors, Perinatal Outcomes, and Consequences for Subsequent Births. *Am. J. Obstet. Gynecol.* **2013**, *208*, 219.e1–219.e7. [CrossRef]
10. Solheim, K.N.; Esakoff, T.F.; Little, S.E.; Cheng, Y.W.; Sparks, T.N.; Caughey, A.B. The Effect of Cesarean Delivery Rates on the Future Incidence of Placenta Previa, Placenta Accreta, and Maternal Mortality. *J. Matern.-Fetal Neonatal Med.* **2011**, *24*, 1341–1346. [CrossRef]
11. Nikolajsen, S.; Løkkegaard, E.C.L.; Bergholt, T. Reoccurrence of Retained Placenta at Vaginal Delivery: An Observational Study. *Acta Obstet. Gynecol. Scand.* **2013**, *92*, 421–425. [CrossRef] [PubMed]
12. Cahill, A.G.; Beigi, R.; Heine, R.P.; Silver, R.M.; Wax, J.R. Placenta Accreta Spectrum. *Am. J. Obstet. Gynecol.* **2018**, *219*, B2–B16. [CrossRef] [PubMed]
13. Sandall, J.; Tribe, R.M.; Avery, L.; Mola, G.; Visser, G.H.; Homer, C.S.; Gibbons, D.; Kelly, N.M.; Kennedy, H.P.; Kidanto, H.; et al. Short-Term and Long-Term Effects of Caesarean Section on the Health of Women and Children. *Lancet* **2018**, *392*, 1349–1357. [CrossRef] [PubMed]
14. Silver, R.M.; Landon, M.B.; Rouse, D.J.; Leveno, K.J.; Spong, C.Y.; Thom, E.A.; Moawad, A.H.; Caritis, S.N.; Harper, M.; Wapner, R.J.; et al. Maternal Morbidity Associated With Multiple Repeat Cesarean Deliveries. *Obstet. Gynecol.* **2006**, *107*, 1226–1232. [CrossRef] [PubMed]
15. Fox, K.A.; Shamshirsaz, A.A.; Carusi, D.; Secord, A.A.; Lee, P.; Turan, O.M.; Huls, C.; Abuhamad, A.; Simhan, H.; Barton, J.; et al. Conservative Management of Morbidly Adherent Placenta: Expert Review. *Am. J. Obstet. Gynecol.* **2015**, *213*, 755–760. [CrossRef]
16. Kingdom, J.C.; Hobson, S.R.; Murji, A.; Allen, L.; Windrim, R.C.; Lockhart, E.; Collins, S.L.; Soleymani Majd, H.; Alazzam, M.; Naaisa, F.; et al. Minimizing Surgical Blood Loss at Cesarean Hysterectomy for Placenta Previa with Evidence of Placenta Increta or Placenta Percreta: The State of Play in 2020. *Am. J. Obstet. Gynecol.* **2020**, *223*, 322–329. [CrossRef]
17. Allen, L.; Jauniaux, E.; Hobson, S.; Papillon-Smith, J.; Belfort, M.A.; Tikkanen, M. FIGO Placenta Accreta Diagnosis and Management Expert Consensus Panel FIGO Consensus Guidelines on Placenta Accreta Spectrum Disorders: Nonconservative Surgical Management. *Int. J. Gynecol. Obstet.* **2018**, *140*, 281–290. [CrossRef]
18. Tan, S.G.; Jobling, T.W.; Wallace, E.M.; Mcneilage, L.J.; Manolitsas, T.; Hodges, R.J. Surgical Management of Placenta Accreta: A 10-year Experience. *Acta Obstet. Gynecol. Scand.* **2013**, *92*, 445–450. [CrossRef]
19. Sentilhes, L.; Goffinet, F.; Kayem, G. Management of Placenta Accreta. *Acta Obstet. Gynecol. Scand.* **2013**, *92*, 1125–1134. [CrossRef]
20. Fitzpatrick, K.; Sellers, S.; Spark, P.; Kurinczuk, J.; Brocklehurst, P.; Knight, M. The Management and Outcomes of Placenta Accreta, Increta, and Percreta in the UK : A Population-based Descriptive Study. *BJOG* **2014**, *121*, 62–71. [CrossRef]
21. Kayem, G.; Davy, C.; Goffinet, F.; Thomas, C.; Clément, D.; Cabrol, D. Conservative Versus Extirpative Management in Cases of Placenta Accreta. *Obstet. Gynecol.* **2004**, *104*, 531–536. [CrossRef] [PubMed]
22. Timmermans, S.; Van Hof, A.C.; Duvekot, J.J. Conservative Management of Abnormally Invasive Placentation. *Obstet. Gynecol. Surv.* **2007**, *62*, 529–539. [CrossRef] [PubMed]
23. Sentilhes, L.; Ambroselli, C.; Kayem, G.; Provansal, M.; Fernandez, H.; Perrotin, F.; Winer, N.; Pierre, F.; Benachi, A.; Dreyfus, M.; et al. Maternal Outcome After Conservative Treatment of Placenta Accreta. *Obstet. Gynecol.* **2010**, *115*, 526–534. [CrossRef] [PubMed]
24. Sentilhes, L.; Kayem, G.; Ambroselli, C.; Provansal, M.; Fernandez, H.; Perrotin, F.; Winer, N.; Pierre, F.; Benachi, A.; Dreyfus, M.; et al. Fertility and Pregnancy Outcomes Following Conservative Treatment for Placenta Accreta. *Hum. Reprod.* **2010**, *25*, 2803–2810. [CrossRef] [PubMed]
25. Clausen, C.; Lönn, L.; Langhoff-Roos, J. Management of Placenta Percreta: A Review of Published Cases. *Acta Obstet. Gynecol. Scand.* **2014**, *93*, 138–143. [CrossRef] [PubMed]
26. Pather, S.; Strockyj, S.; Richards, A.; Campbell, N.; De Vries, B.; Ogle, R. Maternal Outcome after Conservative Management of Placenta Percreta at Caesarean Section. A Report of Three Cases and a Review of the Literature. *Aust. N. Z. J. Obstet. Gynaecol.* **2014**, *54*, 84–87. [CrossRef] [PubMed]
27. Kayem, G.; Deneux-Tharaux, C.; Sentilhes, L. The PACCRETA group PACCRETA: Clinical Situations at High Risk of Placenta ACCRETA/Percreta: Impact of Diagnostic Methods and Management on Maternal Morbidity. *Acta Obstet. Gynecol. Scand.* **2013**, *92*, 476–482. [CrossRef]
28. Bretelle, F.; Courbière, B.; Mazouni, C.; Agostini, A.; Cravello, L.; Boubli, L.; Gamerre, M.; D'Ercole, C. Management of Placenta Accreta: Morbidity and Outcome. *Eur. J. Obstet. Gynecol. Reprod. Biol.* **2007**, *133*, 34–39. [CrossRef]
29. Matsuzaki, S.; Yoshino, K.; Endo, M.; Tomimatsu, T.; Takiuchi, T.; Mimura, K.; Kumasawa, K.; Ueda, Y.; Kimura, T. Successful Anticoagulant Therapy for Disseminated Intravascular Coagulation during Conservative Management of Placenta Percreta: A Case Report and Literature Review. *BMC Pregnancy Childbirth* **2017**, *17*, 443. [CrossRef]
30. Biele, C.; Kaufner, L.; Schwickert, A.; Nonnenmacher, A.; Von Weizsäcker, K.; Muallem, M.Z.; Henrich, W.; Braun, T. Conservative Management of Abnormally Invasive Placenta Complicated by Local Hyperfibrinolysis and Beginning Disseminated Intravascular Coagulation. *Arch. Gynecol. Obstet.* **2021**, *303*, 61–68. [CrossRef]
31. Schröder, L.; Pötzsch, B.; Rühl, H.; Gembruch, U.; Merz, W.M. Tranexamic Acid for Hyperfibrinolytic Hemorrhage During Conservative Management of Placenta Percreta. *Obstet. Gynecol.* **2015**, *126*, 1012–1015. [CrossRef] [PubMed]
32. Levi, M.; Ten Cate, H. Disseminated Intravascular Coagulation. *N. Engl. J. Med.* **1999**, *341*, 586–592. [CrossRef] [PubMed]
33. McCormack, P.L. Tranexamic Acid: A Review of Its Use in the Treatment of Hyperfibrinolysis. *Drugs* **2012**, *72*, 585–617. [CrossRef] [PubMed]

34. Welz, J.; Keyver-Paik, M.-D.; Gembruch, U.; Merz, W.M. Self-Reported Physical, Mental, and Reproductive Sequelae after Treatment of Abnormally Invasive Placenta: A Single-Center Observational Study. *Arch. Gynecol. Obstet.* **2019**, *300*, 95–101. [CrossRef] [PubMed]
35. Merz, W.; Van De Vondel, P.; Strunk, H.; Geipel, A.; Gembruch, U. Diagnosis, Treatment and Application of Color Doppler in Conservative Management of Abnormally Adherent Placenta. *Ultraschall Med.* **2008**, *30*, 571–576. [CrossRef] [PubMed]
36. Jauniaux, E.; D'Antonio, F.; Bhide, A.; Prefumo, F.; Silver, R.M.; Hussein, A.M.; Shainker, S.A.; Chantraine, F.; Alfirevic, Z. Delphi consensus expert panel Modified Delphi Study of Ultrasound Signs Associated with Placenta Accreta Spectrum. *Ultrasound Obstet. Gynecol.* **2023**, *61*, 518–525. [CrossRef] [PubMed]
37. Comstock, C.H. Antenatal Diagnosis of Placenta Accreta: A Review: Antenatal Diagnosis of Placenta Accreta. *Ultrasound Obstet. Gynecol.* **2005**, *26*, 89–96. [CrossRef] [PubMed]
38. Collins, S.L.; Ashcroft, A.; Braun, T.; Calda, P.; Langhoff-Roos, J.; Morel, O.; Stefanovic, V.; Tutschek, B.; Chantraine, F.; on behalf of the European Working Group on Abnormally Invasive Placenta (EW-AIP). Proposal for Standardized Ultrasound Descriptors of Abnormally Invasive Placenta (AIP). *Ultrasound Obstet. Gynecol.* **2016**, *47*, 271–275. [CrossRef]
39. Shukunami, K.; Hattori, K.; Nishijima, K.; Kotsuji, F. Transverse Fundal Uterine Incision in a Patient with Placenta Increta. *J. Matern.-Fetal Neonatal Med.* **2004**, *16*, 355–356. [CrossRef]
40. Matsubara, S. Measures for Peripartum Hysterectomy for Placenta Previa Accreta: Avoiding Uterotonic Agents and "Double Distal Edge Pickup" Mass Ligation. *Arch. Gynecol. Obstet.* **2012**, *285*, 1765–1767. [CrossRef]
41. Youssefzadeh, A.C.; Matsuzaki, S.; Mandelbaum, R.S.; Sangara, R.N.; Bainvoll, L.; Matsushima, K.; Ouzounian, J.G.; Matsuo, K. Trends, Characteristics, and Outcomes of Conservative Management for Placenta Percreta. *Arch. Gynecol. Obstet.* **2022**, *306*, 913–920. [CrossRef] [PubMed]
42. Van Beekhuizen, H.J.; Stefanovic, V.; Schwickert, A.; Henrich, W.; Fox, K.A.; MHallem Gziri, M.; Sentilhes, L.; Gronbeck, L.; Chantraine, F.; Morel, O.; et al. A Multicenter Observational Survey of Management Strategies in 442 Pregnancies with Suspected Placenta Accreta Spectrum. *Acta Obstet. Gynecol. Scand.* **2021**, *100*, 12–20. [CrossRef] [PubMed]
43. Judy, A.E.; Lyell, D.J.; Druzin, M.L.; Dorigo, O. Disseminated Intravascular Coagulation Complicating the Conservative Management of Placenta Percreta. *Obstet. Gynecol.* **2015**, *126*, 1016–1018. [CrossRef] [PubMed]

Disclaimer/Publisher's Note: The statements, opinions and data contained in all publications are solely those of the individual author(s) and contributor(s) and not of MDPI and/or the editor(s). MDPI and/or the editor(s) disclaim responsibility for any injury to people or property resulting from any ideas, methods, instructions or products referred to in the content.

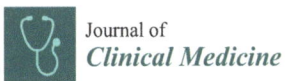

Article

Neonatal Outcomes of Infants Diagnosed with Fetal Growth Restriction during Late Pregnancy versus after Birth

Ohad Houri [1,2,*], Meytal Schwartz Yoskovitz [1,2], Asnat Walfisch [1,2], Anat Pardo [1,2], Yossi Geron [1,2], Eran Hadar [1,2] and Ron Bardin [1,2]

[1] Helen Schneider Hospital for Women, Rabin Medical Center, Petach Tikva 4941492, Israel; meytalsch7@gmail.com (M.S.Y.); asnatwa@clalit.org.il (A.W.); pardoanat@gmail.com (A.P.); yosgeron@gmail.com (Y.G.); eranh42@gmail.com (E.H.); ronbardin@gmail.com (R.B.)
[2] Faculty of Medicine and Health Science, Tel Aviv University, Tel Aviv 6997801, Israel
* Correspondence: ohadhouri@gmail.com; Tel.: +972-50-6954123

Abstract: Objective: The aim of this study was to investigate the potential differences in the outcomes of neonates in whom FGR was diagnosed late in pregnancy as compared to those in whom growth restriction was diagnosed after birth. **Methods:** A retrospective study was conducted in a tertiary medical center between 2017 and 2019. The study included women carrying a single infant with an estimated fetal weight below the tenth percentile in whom FGR was diagnosed during late pregnancy, after 32 gestational weeks (known late-onset FGR; study group) or only after birth (unknown FGR; control group). Data were collected by review of the electronic health records. The primary outcome measure was the rate of composite adverse neonatal outcome. **Results:** A total of 328 women were included, 77 (23.47%) in the known-FGR group and 251 (75.53%) in the unknown-FGR group. In the known-FGR group, an etiology for the FGR was identified in 28.57% cases, most commonly placental insufficiency (21.74%). Compared to the unknown-FGR group, the known-FGR group was characterized by significantly higher rates of elective cesarean delivery (15.58% vs. 9.96%, $p < 0.001$), preterm birth (18.18% vs. 3.98%, $p < 0.01$), and labor induction (67.53% vs. 21.51%, $p < 0.01$). A significantly higher proportion of neonates in the known-FGR group had a positive composite adverse outcome (38.96% vs. 15.53%, $p < 0.01$). For multivariate regression analysis adjusted for maternal age, gestational age at delivery, and mode of delivery, there was no difference between groups in the primary outcome (aOR 1.73, CI 0.89–3.35, $p = 0.1$). Every additional gestational week at delivery was a protective factor (aOR = 0.7, 95% CI 0.56–0.86, $p < 0.01$). **Conclusions:** A prenatal diagnosis of late-onset FGR is associated with higher intervention and preterm birth rates as compared to a diagnosis made after birth. Fetuses diagnosed with late-onset FGR during pregnancy should undergo specific and personalized assessment to determine the cause and severity of the growth delay and the best management strategy. This study highlights the importance of careful decision-making regarding the induction of labor in late-onset FGR.

Keywords: fetal growth restriction; adverse neonatal outcomes

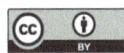

1. Background

Fetal growth restriction (FGR) is a condition in which the fetus has not reached its full growth potential. It is defined as an estimated fetal weight (EFW) below the 10th percentile for gestational age [1,2]. FGR is divided into early and late onset based on the time of diagnosis: before (20–30%) and after (70–80%) 32 gestational weeks (GW). There are differences in pathogenesis, severity, course, and outcomes between the two types [3–5].

In cases of FGR, delivery is timed to achieve maximum fetal growth and maturity while minimizing short- and long-term morbidity and mortality [6]. There is currently no consensus on the optimal timing of delivery [2,7].

Numerous studies have investigated the timing and effectiveness of prenatal diagnosis, monitoring, and treatment of FGR to improve maternal and neonatal outcomes [7–13], but the findings are unclear [2,7]. Some showed that diagnosing FGR during pregnancy improved immediate neonatal outcomes and reduced intrauterine mortality [8–10], whereas others suggested that diagnosing FGR prenatally increases maternal and neonatal complications [11–13], while no significant positive impact on overall mortality is apparent [14]. The aim of this study was to investigate differences in neonatal outcomes between late-FGR neonates who were diagnosed during pregnancy or only after delivery.

2. Methods

2.1. Design and Setting

A retrospective study was conducted between January 2017 and September 2019 at a single tertiary medical center.

2.2. Study Population

The study included women with singleton gestations and a normal pregnancy course (including nuchal translucency, routine fetal anomaly scans at 18–22 weeks gestation, and a glucose challenge test) who gave birth to infants with a birthweight below the 10th percentile for gestational age according to the national growth charts [15]. Participants were classified into two groups: late-onset FGR diagnosed during pregnancy based on sonographic EFW after 32 gestational weeks (known FGR; study group), and FGR first diagnosed at birth according to the actual birthweight (Unknown FGR; comparison group).

In this study, we included only women who had completed recommended fetal investigations before 32 GW with normal results in all antenatal follow up tests. The tests included nuchal translucency, first- and second-trimester biochemical markers, routine anatomical scans, and EFW prior to 32 gestational weeks.

In the known-FGR group, we included only women who have been followed at our high-risk clinic and ultrasound unit.

Exclusion criteria were any anatomical or genetic fetal malformations known before 32 GW, chronic maternal disease (pre-pregnancy diabetes, chronic hypertension, hypo/hyperthyroidism, asthma, epilepsy, lupus, APLA syndrome), known early-onset FGR (before 32 GWs), multiple gestation, missing information on pregnancy follow-up or outcome.

The known-FGR group was further subdivided by etiology of FGR (identified av not identified) during pregnancy.

2.3. Definitions and Practice Guidelines

Late-onset FGR was defined as a sonographic EFW below the 10th percentile for gestational age (SMFM, 2020) according to the nationally accepted growth curves representing the norm in the Israeli population, that was diagnosed for the first time after 32 gestational weeks [1,2,7,15].

Uteroplacental insufficiency was defined as a pulsatility index (PI) above the 95th percentile for gestational age in the umbilical artery (UA) or a PI below the fifth percentile for gestational age in the middle cerebral artery (MCA) [2].

Gestational age was calculated according to the date of the last menstrual period and was confirmed by a first-trimester measurement of the crown-rump length. Gestational age was changed if the gap was more than 4 days before 10 gestational weeks [1].

In our health system, an EFW scan is routinely done at 32 GWs. The scan is fully covered by public health insurance. When the EFW is at or below the 10th percentile, Doppler indices are sought as part of the immediate evaluation. This is followed by a comprehensive maternal-fetal evaluation of the medical and maternal history and a thorough physical examination, including weight, height, and weight gain during pregnancy as well as blood pressure measurement to rule out pregnancy-related hypertensive morbidity. According to the Israeli guidelines, when fetal causes are suspected (an EFW less than the third percentile, polyhydramnios, an abnormal anatomical scan, personal family history of genetic disease), a more detailed investigation is offered which is also fully covered by public health insurance [1]. It consists of genetic counseling, late amniocentesis for evaluation of chromosome microarray analysis (CMA), with optional further genetic investigation by whole-exome sequencing (WES), late repeated anatomical scan, fetal echocardiogram, and laboratory tests for viral infections (CMV, toxoplasma). These tests are usually offered and are fully covered even in the absence of additional risk factors for fetal abnormalities except for the EFW.

When late FGR is diagnosed, women are followed at designated maternal–fetal medicine clinics. The EFW is assessed every 2 weeks, and a non-stress test (NST) and biophysical profile (BPP) along with a UA and MCA Doppler assessment are performed weekly. The timing and mode of delivery are based on these findings as well as on gestational age and pattern of fetal growth. Cesarean delivery (CD) is performed for standard obstetric indications. In cases of absent or reverse UA diastolic flow, delivery is recommended at 34 or 32 gestational weeks, respectively. At 37 gestational weeks, if the EFW is lower than the third percentile or Doppler indices are abnormal, oligohydramnios or lack of growth is detected, or there are other physician/maternal concerns, induction of labor is recommended. At the time of this study, the common practice at our center was to deliver any fetus with an EFW or AC below the 10th percentile at 37 GWs, even if there were no other risk factors.

2.4. Data Collection

Data were collected by review of the computerized medical records. The hospital's healthcare databases are valid and highly reliable, including diagnoses based on codes and fixed texts as well as fields for categorical and continuous variables. In cases of uncertainty and/or missing data, a manual reading/scan of the patient's file was performed.

Maternal, fetal, obstetric, and neonatal parameters were collected. Maternal parameters included age, height, and weight (pre-pregnancy and at delivery) and medical and obstetric history. Fetal parameters included gestational week (GW), EFW, and fetal biometry at the time of the FGR diagnosis. pregnancy follow-up data of up to 32 gestational weeks, including nuchal translucency, first- and second-trimester biochemical markers, anatomical scans, glucose challenge test, and the EFW before 32 gestational weeks. Also recorded were results of the definitive tests performed from week 32 onwards: advanced anatomical ultrasound scan, Doppler flow in various vessels (from diagnosis until delivery), amniotic fluid index, fetal echocardiography, genetic analyses (CMA, WES), infections and serology status (CMV, Toxoplasma), and coagulopathies (APLA, any other). Obstetric variables included the induction of labor, mode of delivery, GW at delivery, and birth weight/percentile. Neonatal parameters included gender, Apgar scores at 1 and 5 min, fetal arterial pH, admission to the neonatal intensive care unit (NICU) and neonatal morbidity, namely jaundice, transient tachypnea of the newborn (TTN), respiratory distress syndrome (RDS), sepsis, seizures, asphyxia, mechanical ventilation, necrotizing enterocolitis (NEC), intraventricular hemorrhage (IVH), hypoxic-ischemic encephalopathy (HIE), acidosis, meconium aspiration syndrome (MSA), and neonatal death.

2.5. Outcome Measures

The primary outcome was defined as a composite of neonatal outcomes. This was defined as at least one of the following: an Apgar score of less than 7 at 1 or 5 min, a fetal arterial pH of less than 7.1, admission to the NICU, jaundice, TTN, RDS, sepsis, seizures, asphyxia, mechanical ventilation, NEC, IVH, HIE, and death. Severe composite neonatal outcomes include asphyxia, HIE, IVH, meconium aspiration syndrome, seizures, intrauterine fetal death, and neonatal death.

2.6. Statistical Analysis

Statistical analysis was performed using SAS software, version 34.0 (SAS Corp. Cary, NC, USA). Descriptive statistics are presented by number and percentage for categorical variables and mean and standard deviation for continuous variables. Variables were compared between groups using chi-square test or one-way analysis of variance, as appropriate. Multivariate analysis was performed for the primary outcome, adjusting for maternal age, gestational week at delivery, and mode of delivery. The data are presented as an adjusted odds ratio (aOR) with 95% confidence interval (CI). A p-value below 0.05 was considered statistically significant.

2.7. Ethical Approval

The study was approved by the Institutional Review Board of Rabin Medical Center (approval no. 0727-17-RMC). Informed consent was waived by the Institutional Review Board due to the study's retrospective design.

3. Results

Of the 791 women who gave birth to a newborn weighing below the 10th percentile (by gender and gestational age) during the study period, 79 were excluded because of maternal chronic diseases, 30 due to multifetal pregnancies, and 354 cases had missing data or were not followed in our clinic. This left 328 pregnancies for analysis. Of them, 77 (23.47%) with known late-onset FGR were diagnosed prenatally (known FGR, study group) and 251 (75.53%) were first diagnosed after birth (unknown FGR; control group). Their background and obstetric characteristics are shown in Tables 1 and 2, respectively. The mean maternal age in the study group was 30.6 ± 5.2 years (range 19–46 years). There were no differences between the groups in rates of gestational diabetes (6.49% vs. 4.78%, p = 0.56) and hypertensive disorders of pregnancy (5.19% vs. 2.79%, p = 0.29). The unknown-FGR group had a significantly higher rate of previous CD (14.74% vs. 5.19%, p = 0.02) and Caucasians (100% vs. 92%, p = 0.04). The known-FGR group had higher rates of current CD (no trial of labor, 15.58% vs. 9.96%, p < 0.01) and labor induction (67.53% vs. 21.51%, p < 0.01). The other differences between the groups were not statistically significant.

Table 1. Clinical characteristics of women with FGR pregnancies diagnosed prenatally (known FGR) or postnatally (unknown FGR).

Characteristics	Control Group Unknown FGR (n = 251)	Study Group Known FGR (n = 77)	p-Value
Age, years	30.55 ± 5.56	30.69 ± 5.26	0.74
Pre-pregnancy weight, Kg	56.96 ± 11.11	57.17 ± 12.07	0.92
Weight at birth, Kg	67.92 ± 10.98	67.57 ± 12.67	0.87
Gestational weight gain, Kg	10.79 ± 4.31	9.52 ± 3.68	0.13
Height, cm	160.01 ± 5.84	161.34 ± 6.99	0.25
Body mass index, Kg/m^2	19.56 ± 8.06	21.04 ± 7.10	0.32
Gravidity	2 (1–3)	2 (1–3)	0.43
Parity	1 (0–2)	1 (0–2)	0.4
Previous cesarean delivery	37 (14.74)	4 (5.19)	0.02
Ethnicity			0.04
Caucasian	231 (92.03)	77 (100)	
Non-Caucasian	13 (5.18)	0 (0)	
Smoking during pregnancy	0 (0)	0 (0)	-
Alcohol consumption during pregnancy	0 (0)	0 (0)	-
Illicit drug use during pregnancy	0 (0)	0 (0)	-
Spontaneous conception	193 (76.89)	67 (87.01)	0.30

Data are presented as mean ± standard deviation for continuous variables or n (%) or median (range) for categorical variables.

Table 2. Obstetric characteristics of FGR pregnancies diagnosed prenatally (known FGR) or postnatally (unknown FGR).

Characteristics	Control Group Unknown FGR (n = 251)	Study Group Known FGR (n = 77)	p-Value
Cholestasis of pregnancy	0 (0)	0 (0)	
Gestational diabetes	12 (4.78)	5 (6.49)	0.56
Hypertensive disorders during pregnancy	7 (2.79)	4 (5.19)	0.29
Onset of labor			
Planned Cesarean delivery, no trial of labor	25 (9.96)	12 (15.58)	<0.01
Induction of labor	54 (21.51)	52 (67.53)	
Spontaneous	172 (68.53)	13 (16.88)	
Mode of delivery			
Vaginal	192 (76.49)	56 (72.73)	0.11
Vacuum-assisted	28 (11.16)	5 (6.49)	
Cesarean	31 (12.35)	16 (20.78)	
Type of cesarean			
Elective	21 (8.37)	11 (14.29)	1.0
Intrapartum	10 (3.98)	5 (6.49)	

Data are presented as n (%) for categorical variables.

The neonatal outcomes are shown in Table 3. The known-FGR group had a lower mean GW at delivery (37.6 ± 1 vs. 39.3 ± 1, $p < 0.01$), a higher rate of preterm deliveries prior to 37 gestational weeks (18.18% vs. 3.98%, $p < 0.01$), and a lower mean birthweight (2232 ± 292 vs. 2500 ± 200 g, $p < 0.01$).

Table 3. Neonatal outcomes of FGR pregnancies diagnosed prenatally (known FGR) or postnatally (unknown FGR).

Neonatal Outcomes	Control Group Unknown FGR (n = 251)	Study Group Known FGR (n = 77)	p-Value
Gestational age at birth, week	39.3 ± 1	37.6 ± 1	<0.01
Preterm birth (<37 + 0 weeks)	10 (3.98)	14 (18.18)	0.01
Birthweight, grams	2500.34 ± 200.87	2232.83 ± 292.05	<0.01
Head circumference, cm	34.63 ± 23.81	32.08 ± 1.07	0.19
Neonatal gender, male	121 (48.21)	41 (53.25)	0.51
Umbilical cord pH	7.32 ± 0.07	7.33 ± 0.05	0.39
Umbilical cord pH < 7.1	11 (4.38)	1 (1.30)	0.3
1 min Apgar score ≤ 7	8 (3.19)	0 (0)	0.2
5 min Apgar score ≤ 7	3 (1.20)	0 (0)	1.0
Asphyxia	3 (1.20)	0 (0)	1.0
Seizure	0 (0)	2 (2.60)	0.05
Hypoxic-ischemic encephalopathy	0 (0)	0 (0)	-
Intraventricular hemorrhage	0 (0)	2 (2.60)	0.05
Jaundice	21 (8.37)	17 (22.08)	0.02

Table 3. *Cont.*

Neonatal Outcomes	Control Group Unknown FGR (n = 251)	Study Group Known FGR (n = 77)	p-Value
Transient tachypnea of the newborn	1 (0.40)	2 (2.60)	0.13
Sepsis	8 (3.19)	8 (10.39)	0.02
Mechanical ventilation	2 (0.80)	0 (0)	1.0
NICU admission	5 (1.99)	6 (7.79)	0.02
Meconium aspiration syndrome	3 (1.20)	0 (0)	1.0
Respiratory distress syndrome	0 (0)	0 (0)	-
Necrotizing enterocolitis	0 (0)	0 (0)	-
Intrauterine fetal death	1 (0.40)	0 (0)	1.0
Neonatal death	0 (0)	0 (0)	-
Composite neonatal outcome *	39 (15.53)	30 (38.96)	0.01
Severe composite neonatal outcome **	7 (2.78)	5 (6.49)	0.04

Data are presented as mean ± standard deviation for continuous variable or n (%) for categorical variables. * Composite neonatal outcome includes all the above. ** Severe composite neonatal outcome includes asphyxia, hypoxic–ischemic encephalopathy, intraventricular hemorrhage, meconium aspiration syndrome, intrauterine fetal death and neonatal death.

The composite neonatal outcome was positive in 69 of the 328 neonates (21.03%). The rate was significantly higher in the known-FGR group than in the unknown-FGR group (38.96% vs. 15.53%, respectively; $p = 0.01$). The rate of severe composite neonatal outcome was also significantly higher in the known-FGR group (6.49% vs. 2.78%, respectively; $p = 0.04$). Isolated neonatal complications were also more frequent in the known-FGR group, but the differences did not reach statistical significance: sepsis (10.39% vs. 3.19%), TTN (2.60% vs. 0.4%), IVH (2.60% vs. 0), and NICU admission (7.79% vs. 1.99%). In the unknown-FGR group, there were cases of neonatal asphyxia (1.2%), need for mechanical ventilation (0.8%), meconium aspiration (1.2%), and an Apgar score less than or equal to 7 at 5 min (1.2%); none of these complications were found in the known-FGR group.

There was a single case of intrauterine fetal death in the unknown-FGR group, at 38 gestational weeks, following an uneventful pregnancy course. Two weeks earlier, a normal BPP had been recorded. The EFW at 32 gestational weeks was normal (25th percentile), with an actual birthweight below the third percentile. There were no cases of intrauterine death in the known-FGR group.

Within the known-FGR group, there was an etiological explanation for the FGR in only 22 cases (28.47%, Table 4). In the remainder (71.43%), the cause of the FGR was not determined. The most common etiology was placental insufficiency, in 15 cases (21.74%). Four women (5.19%) had, for the first time, an abnormal anatomical scan in late pregnancy, showing a small kidney, cardiomegaly, a dilated third ventricle, and a dilated renal pelvis. Three women (3.89%) tested positive for APLA, and one was diagnosed with fetal toxoplasmosis infection. The positive composite neonatal outcome rate was 45.45% in the FGR subgroup with an identified etiology and 36.6% in the FGR subgroup in which no etiology was identified ($p = 0.6$). The difference between each subgroup in the known-FGR group versus the entire unknown-FGR group was statistically significant ($p = 0.01$ and $p = 0.01$, respectively, Table 4).

Multivariate analysis, adjusted for maternal age, gestational age at delivery, and mode of delivery, yielded no differences between the known- and unknown-FGR groups for the composite neonatal outcome (aOR 1.73, CI 0.89–3.35, $p = 0.1$). Each additional week of gestational age at delivery was found to be protective (aOR = 0.7, 95% CI 0.56–0.86, $p < 0.01$).

Table 4. Obstetric and neonatal outcomes in pregnancies with known and unknown FGR, stratified by FGR etiology (identified, not identified).

Neonatal Outcomes	Control Group Unknown FGR (N = 251)	Known FGR Etiology Identified (N = 55)	Known FGR Etiology Not Identified (N = 22)	p-Value
Birthweight, grams	2500 ± 200	2249 ± 290	2192 ± 297	0.29 [b]
Umbilical cord pH < 7.1	11 (4.38)	1 (1.82)	0 (0)	0.7 [a] 0.6 [b] 1.0 [c]
1 min Apgar score ≤ 7	8 (3.19)	0 (0)	0 (0)	0.35 [a] 1.0 [b] 1.0 [c]
5 min Apgar score ≤ 7	3 (1.20%)	0 (0)	0 (0)	1.0 [a,b]
Asphyxia	3 (1.20)	0 (0)	0 (0)	1.0 [a,b]
Seizure	0 (0)	2 (3.64)	0 (0)	0.03 [a] 1.0 [c]
Hypoxic ischemic encephalopathy	0 (0)	0 (0)	0 (0)	-
Intraventricular hemorrhage	0 (0)	1 (1.82)	1 (4.55)	0.18 [a] 0.08 [b] 0.49 [c]
Jaundice	21 (8.37)	11 (20)	6 (27.27)	0.02 [a] 0.01 [b] 0.54 [c]
Transient tachypnea of the newborn	1 (0.40)	1 (1.82)	1 (4.55)	0.32 [a] 0.15 [b] 0.49 [c]
Sepsis	8 (3.19)	7 (12.73)	1 (4.55)	0.08 [a] 0.53 [b] 0.42 [c]
Mechanical ventilation	2 (0.80)	0 (0)	0 (0)	1.0 [a b]
NICU admission	5 (1.99)	3 (5.45)	3 (13.64)	0.16 [a] 0.02 [b] 0.34 [c]
Meconium aspiration syndrome	3 (1.20)	0 (0)	0 (0)	1.0 [a]
Respiratory distress syndrome	0 (0)	0 (0)	0 (0)	-
Necrotizing enterocolitis	0 (0)	0 (0)	0 (0)	-
Intrauterine fetal death	1 (0.4)	0 (0)	0 (0)	-
Neonatal death	0 (0)	0 (0)	0 (0)	-
Composite outcome *	39 (15.53)	20 (36.36)	10 (45.45)	0.01 [a] 0.01 [b] 0.6 [c]

Data are presented as mean ± standard deviation for continuous variables or n (%) for categorical variables. [a] Comparison of unknown-FGR group with subgroup of known FGR of unidentified etiology; [b] comparison of unknown-FGR group with subgroup of known FGR with an identified etiology; [c] comparison of unknown-FGR group with the entire known-FGR group. * Composite neonatal outcome includes all the above.

4. Discussion

In this study, we sought to determine if the diagnosis of late-onset FGR and its corresponding workup and management during pregnancy affects neonatal outcomes. Our primary findings in a cohort of 328 neonates showed that the immediate outcomes were less favorable in those diagnosed with late-onset FGR during pregnancy as compared to those first diagnosed at birth. These included a lower gestational age of approximately 1.5 weeks at delivery, resulting in a 4.5-fold preterm birth rate. The intervention rate was significantly higher in this group as well. Most of the FGRs diagnosed during pregnancy were probably constitutional. When the cause was identified, it was most commonly uteroplacental insufficiency. On a multivariate regression analysis adjusted for maternal age, gestational age at delivery, and mode of delivery, there was no difference in the primary outcome between the groups.

Our findings are supported by several studies linking higher rates of obstetric complications in FGR pregnancies to the higher rate of interventions taken, such as induction of labor and elective cesarean delivery, resulting in an earlier gestational age at delivery and a higher likelihood of preterm birth and lower birthweight, both absolute and relative to gestational age [11–13]. Ohel et al. [12] found that the mean gestational age at delivery in patients diagnosed with FGR during pregnancy was 38.8 weeks versus 39.4 weeks in patients diagnosed only at birth. Corresponding values in the study of Nohuz et al. [16] were 37.7 and 39.4 weeks. Similarly, in our study, the gestational age at delivery of fetuses diagnosed with late-onset FGR during pregnancy was 1.5 weeks lower than that of fetuses diagnosed at birth, corresponding to a 4.5-fold preterm delivery rate. A more advanced gestational age at birth was found on multivariate analysis to be an independent protective factor for adverse neonatal outcomes. The neonatal composite outcome was statistically higher in the known-FGR group, regardless of whether the etiology was identified or not (Table 4). The main difference between the groups was the gestational week at delivery. However, due to the small size of the groups, the multivariate analysis was conducted between the two groups rather than three.

There is no consensus on the timing of delivery in late-onset FGR because of the lack of randomized trials based on Doppler indices. Guidelines for the management of FGR are highly variable [17], as the timing and route of delivery of FGR pregnancies are based on a combination of factors, including findings on Doppler, BPP, and NST coupled with the gestational age and EFW. The ISOUG [2] and ACOG [7] guidelines recommend that in FGR pregnancies with a normal Doppler study and a reassuring NST, delivery after 38 + 0 gestational weeks may be considered, but should not be delayed beyond 39 + 0 weeks to reduce the risk of severe growth restriction or stillbirth. In the only randomized control trial (DIGITAT), which included 650 patients with FGR, the randomly assigned cutoff for induction of labor or expectant monitoring was 36 gestational weeks [18]. The induction group gave birth 10 days earlier and had a neonatal birthweight of 130 g less than the expectantly managed group, but contrary to our results, the composite neonatal outcome rates were similar (6.1 and 5.3%) as were the cesarean delivery rates (approximately 14%). However, similar to our results, the study found that NICU admission was less likely when FGR fetuses were delivered after 38 GWs [19], suggesting a benefit of deferring delivery as long as the fetus is closely monitored and there are no other indications for early delivery. The authors of the DIGITAT study concluded that in cases of late-onset FGR, patients who are keen on non-intervention can safely choose expectant management and that it is reasonable to opt for labor induction to prevent possible neonatal morbidity and stillbirth.

In our study, among all the fetuses diagnosed with late-onset FGR during pregnancy, 38.96% had a positive composite neonatal outcome compared to 15.53% of the fetuses diagnosed with growth restriction at birth. Some previous studies support our findings whereas others contradict them [9–11,19,20]. The variations among the studies, including the DIGITAT trial [18,19], can be explained by different definitions and inconsistent neonatal outcome measures, as well as the lack of distinction between late- and early-onset FGR. According to some reports, neonates diagnosed with FGR during pregnancy had a significantly better immediate outcome, which they attributed to better management of pregnancy and delivery than cases of FGR diagnosed at birth [9–11]. However, not only did these studies fail to differentiate between late- and early-onset FGR, but their neonatal outcome measures were also different from those examined here. For instance,

Verlijsdonk et al. [9] evaluated the primary outcomes of intrauterine death: a 5 min Apgar score less than 7, an umbilical artery pH less than 7.05, and a secondary outcome of NICU admission. Fratelli et al. [11] evaluated clinical and perinatal characteristics and found that identifying fetuses with growth delay during pregnancy could improve perinatal outcomes. Yet, they also found NICU admission to be more common in the group diagnosed with FGR during pregnancy, which was likely due to more frequent monitoring and higher rates of interventions in these cases, as well as more severe growth restriction. In our research, as in the DIGITAT trial, NICU admission was considered part of the composite outcome, and the rate was significantly higher in the known-FGR as compared to the unknown-FGR group. We have also distinguished between severe composite neonatal outcome and total adverse neonatal outcomes, with both being more prevalent in the study group.

A comparison of the mode of delivery between the groups revealed that most deliveries in the known-FGR group were initiated by induction and most in the unknown-FGR group were spontaneous. Additionally, the rate of cesarean delivery was lower in the unknown-FGR group, although the difference was not significant. Thus, when FGR is unknown, there seems to be a lower likelihood of any intervention, especially cesarean delivery. Despite the lack of statistical significance, these findings support previous studies showing higher rates of induction of labor and cesarean delivery in pregnancies with known FGR [9–11]. In the DIGITAT trial [19], the rate of cesarean delivery was similar in the two groups.

The prenatally diagnosed group in our study was further divided by etiology (identified or not identified), and each subgroup was compared with the unknown-FGR group for neonatal outcomes. The subgroup in which the etiology was identified had the highest composite neonatal morbidity rate, followed, in order, by the subgroup with unknown etiology and the control group. These findings are consistent with previous reports suggesting that fetuses with growth restriction due to a pathological cause have a higher rate of morbidity and mortality than constitutionally small fetuses [14,15,19,20], possibly because of the high incidence of early delivery and its consequences. They highlight the importance of accurate diagnosis, identification of the etiology, and categorization of fetuses into early- and late-onset groups as a primary measure to avoid unnecessary interventions and early delivery.

When growth restriction is diagnosed during pregnancy, especially if it is placenta-related, more frequent fetal monitoring is mandated. This is a double-edged sword. On one hand, it might lead to early intervention to prevent stillbirth, and on the other hand, it may be associated with a higher rate of preterm birth and adverse neonatal outcomes mainly due to complications of early-term delivery.

The strengths of our study include the specific definition of FGR, the relatively large number of women and infants, careful patient selection to avoid biases of background diseases and/or other complications prior to the time of diagnosis, and uniform follow-up and management policies under the same protocols of a single tertiary center.

The main limitation of our study is the retrospective design. Additionally, not all women in the study group underwent all possible diagnostic options (Doppler examination was performed on 86.61%, CMV serology test on 68.83%, toxoplasma serology test on 61.0%, fetal echo on 16.88%, and amniocentesis for genetic testing on 18.18%). This could have confounded the results, as women in whom there was a higher chance of finding a specific cause for FGR were referred for relevant diagnostic tests for that specific cause while other diagnostic tests were not performed, even though a complete workup was offered and is free. Moreover, due to the small size of the groups, the multivariate analysis was conducted between the known- and unknown-FGR groups, rather than between all three groups. In addition, long-term neonatal outcomes following hospital discharge were beyond the scope of the study. In addition, pregnancies that were not followed up in our clinics were excluded in order to use only valid in-house data.

5. Conclusions

A prenatal diagnosis of late FGR is associated with higher intervention and preterm birth rates compared to a diagnosis made after birth. This study emphasizes the importance of identifying fetuses with late-onset FGR during pregnancy and performing a specific and personalized assessment for each, to determine the cause and severity of the growth delay. Utilizing a combination of third-trimester anatomical surveys, genetic investigations, and Doppler criteria correlates with the likelihood of adverse perinatal outcomes in cases of late-onset FGR. In addition, it highlights the importance of caution when deciding to induce labor in cases of late-onset FGR in an attempt to avoid preterm delivery while maintaining close fetal monitoring.

Author Contributions: All authors contributed to the study's conception and design. O.H. wrote the manuscript. A.P. and Y.G. prepared the material and collected the data. M.S.Y. analyzed the data. A.W. prepared the tables. E.H. and R.B. interpreted the data. The first draft of the manuscript was written by O.H., and all authors commented on previous versions of the manuscript. All authors have read and agreed to the published version of the manuscript.

Funding: This research received no external funding.

Institutional Review Board Statement: All methods were carried out in accordance with relevant guidelines and regulations. This study was performed in line with the principles of the Declaration of Helsinki. Approval was granted by the Rabin Medical Center Institutional Review Board (approval no. 0727-17-RMC). Informed consent was waived by The Rabin Medical Center Institutional Review Board because of the retrospective study design. The data were anonymized before use.

Informed Consent Statement: Informed consent was waived by the Institutional Review Board due to the study's retrospective design.

Data Availability Statement: The datasets generated and analyzed during the current study are not publicly available due to ethical committee regulations but are available from the corresponding author on reasonable request.

Conflicts of Interest: The authors have no relevant financial or non-financial interests to disclose. No competing financial interests exist. The authors declare no conflict of interest.

Abbreviations

BPP, biophysical profile; CMA, chromosome microarray analysis; CMV, cytomegalovirus; EFW, estimated fetal weight; FGR, fetal growth restriction; HIE, hypoxic–ischemic encephalopathy; IVH, intraventricular hemorrhage; MCA, middle cerebral artery; MSA, meconium aspiration syndrome; NEC, necrotizing enterocolitis; NICU, neonatal intensive care unit; NST, non-stress test; RDS, respiratory distress syndrome; TTN, transient tachypnea of the newborn; UA, uterine artery; WES, whole exome sequencing.

References

1. Israel Association of Obstetrics and Gynecology. Position Paper Number 10. Pregnancy Management of a Suspected IUGR Fetus. November 2019. (In Hebrew). Available online: https://cdn.mednet.co.il/2015/04/%D7%A4%D7%92-%D7%AA%D7%95%D7%A7%D7%A3-13.pdf (accessed on 1 November 2020).
2. Lees, C.C.; Stampalija, T.; Baschat, A.; da Silva Costa, F.; Ferrazzi, E.; Figueras, F.; Hecher, K.; Kingdom, J.; Poon, L.C.; Salomon, L.J.; et al. ISUOG Practice Guidelines: Diagnosis and management of small-for-gestational-age fetus and fetal growth restriction. *Ultrasound Obstet. Gynecol.* **2020**, *56*, 298–312. [CrossRef] [PubMed]
3. Figueras, F.; Gratacos, E. An integrated approach to fetal growth restriction. *Best. Pract. Res. Clin. Obstet. Gynaecol.* **2017**, *38*, 48–58. [CrossRef] [PubMed]
4. Savchev, S.; Figueras, F.; Sanz-Cortes, M.; Cruz-Lemini, M.; Triunfo, S.; Botet, F.; Gratacos, E. Evaluation of an optimal gestational age cut-off for the definition of early- and late-onset fetal growth restriction. *Fetal Diagn. Ther.* **2014**, *36*, 99–105. [CrossRef] [PubMed]
5. Nawathe, A.; Lees, C. Early onset fetal growth restriction. *Best. Pract. Res. Clin. Obstet. Gynaecol.* **2017**, *38*, 24–37. [CrossRef] [PubMed]

6. Israel Association of Obstetrics and Gynecology. Position Paper Number 8. Guidelines for Ultrasound in Pregnancy. 1 December 2012. (In Hebrew). Available online: https://cdn.mednet.co.il/2017/01/%D7%A0%D7%99%D7%99%D7%A8-%D7%A2%D7%9E%D7%93%D7%94-%D7%9E%D7%A2%D7%95%D7%93%D7%9B%D7%9F-8.pdf (accessed on 1 December 2012).
7. Fetal Growth Restriction: ACOG Practice Bulletin, Number 227. *Obstet Gynecol.* **2021**, *137*, e16–e28. [CrossRef] [PubMed]
8. Gardosi, J.; Francis, A.; Turner, S.; Williams, M. Customized growth charts: Rationale, validation and clinical benefits. *Am. J. Obstet. Gynecol.* **2018**, *218*, S609–S618. [CrossRef] [PubMed]
9. Verlijsdonk, J.W.; Winkens, B.; Boers, K.; Scherjon, S.; Roumen, F. Suspected versus non-suspected small-for-gestational-age fetuses at term: Perinatal outcomes. *J. Matern. Fetal Neonatal Med.* **2012**, *25*, 938–943. [CrossRef]
10. Lindqvist, P.G.; Molin, J. Does antenatal identification of small-for-gestational age fetuses significantly improve their outcome? *Ultrasound Obstet. Gynecol.* **2005**, *25*, 258–264. [CrossRef]
11. Fratelli, N.; Valcamonico, A.; Prefumo, F.; Pagani, G.; Guarneri, T.; Frusca, T. Effects of antenatal recognition and follow-up on perinatal outcomes in small-for-gestational age infants delivered after 36 weeks. *Acta Obstet. Gynecol. Scand.* **2013**, *92*, 223–229. [CrossRef]
12. Ohel, G.; Ruach, M. Perinatal outcome of idiopathic small for gestational age pregnancies at term: The effect of antenatal diagnosis. *Int. J. Gynaecol. Obstet.* **1996**, *55*, 29–32. [CrossRef] [PubMed]
13. Aviram, A.; Yogev, Y.; Bardin, R.; Meizner, I.; Wiznitzer, A.; Hadar, E. Small for gestational age newborns—Does pre-recognition make a difference in pregnancy outcome? *J. Matern. Fetal Neonatal Med.* **2015**, *28*, 1520–1524. [CrossRef] [PubMed]
14. Walker, D.M.; Marlow, N.; Upstone, L.; Gross, H.; Hornbuckle, J.; Vail, A.; Wolke, D.; Thornton, J.G. The Growth Restriction Intervention Trial: Long-term outcomes in a randomized trial of timing of delivery in fetal growth restriction. *Am. J. Obstet. Gynecol.* **2011**, *204*, 34.e1–34.e9. [CrossRef] [PubMed]
15. Dollberg, S.; Haklai, Z.; Mimouni, F.B.; Gorfein, I.; Gordon, E.S. Birth weight standards in the live-born population in Israel. *Isr. Med. Assoc. J.* **2005**, *7*, 311–314. [PubMed]
16. Nohuz, E.; Rivière, O.; Coste, K.; Vendittelli, F. Prenatal identification of small-for-gestational age and risk of neonatal morbidity and stillbirth. *Ultrasound Obstet. Gynecol.* **2020**, *55*, 621–628. [CrossRef] [PubMed]
17. McCowan, L.M.; Figueras, F.; Anderson, N.H. Evidence-based national guidelines for the management of suspected fetal growth restriction: Comparison, consensus, and controversy. *Am. J. Obstet. Gynecol.* **2018**, *218*, S855–S868. [CrossRef] [PubMed]
18. Boers, K.E.; Vijgen, S.M.; Bijlenga, D.; van der Post, J.A.; Bekedam, D.J.; Kwee, A.; van der Salm, P.C.M.; van Pampus, M.G.; Spaanderman, M.E.A.; de Boer, K.; et al. DIGITAT study group. Induction versus expectant monitoring for intrauterine growth restriction at term: Randomized equivalence trial (DIGITAT). *BMJ* **2010**, *341*, c7087. [CrossRef] [PubMed]
19. Boers, K.E.; van Wyk, L.; van der Post, J.A.; Kwee, A.; van Pampus, M.G.; Spaanderam, M.E.; Duvekot, J.J.; Bremer, H.A.; Delemarre, F.M.C.; Bloemenkamp, K.W.M.; et al. Neonatal morbidity after induction vs. expectant monitoring in intrauterine growth restriction at term: A subanalysis of the DIGITAT RCT. *Am. J. Obstet. Gynecol.* **2012**, *206*, 344.e1–344.e7. [CrossRef] [PubMed]
20. Ananth, C.V.; Vintzileos, A.M. Distinguishing pathological from constitutional small for gestational age births in population-based studies. *Early Hum. Dev.* **2009**, *85*, 653–658. [CrossRef] [PubMed]

Disclaimer/Publisher's Note: The statements, opinions and data contained in all publications are solely those of the individual author(s) and contributor(s) and not of MDPI and/or the editor(s). MDPI and/or the editor(s) disclaim responsibility for any injury to people or property resulting from any ideas, methods, instructions or products referred to in the content.

MDPI AG
Grosspeteranlage 5
4052 Basel
Switzerland
Tel.: +41 61 683 77 34

Journal of Clinical Medicine Editorial Office
E-mail: jcm@mdpi.com
www.mdpi.com/journal/jcm

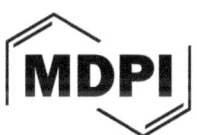

Disclaimer/Publisher's Note: The statements, opinions and data contained in all publications are solely those of the individual author(s) and contributor(s) and not of MDPI and/or the editor(s). MDPI and/or the editor(s) disclaim responsibility for any injury to people or property resulting from any ideas, methods, instructions or products referred to in the content.

www.ingramcontent.com/pod-product-compliance
Lightning Source LLC
LaVergne TN
LVHW072326090526
838202LV00019B/2359